Ann Green
2280 Ardmore Cove
Memphis, TN. 38127

Medicare Made Easy

A PEOPLE'S MEDICAL SOCIETY BOOK

MEDICARE · MADE · EASY

Charles B. Inlander
President, People's Medical Society

Charles K. MacKay

Addison-Wesley Publishing Company, Inc.
Reading, Massachusetts ▪ Menlo Park, California ▪ New York
Don Mills, Ontario ▪ Wokingham, England ▪ Amsterdam
Bonn ▪ Sydney ▪ Singapore ▪ Tokyo ▪ Madrid ▪ San Juan

Bausell/Rooney/Inlander, *How to Evaluate and Select a Nursing Home,* © 1988 by People's Medical Society. Pages 14 and 49–61. Reprinted with permission of Addison-Wesley Publishing Co., Inc., Reading, Massachusetts.

Library of Congress Cataloging-in-Publication Data

Inlander, Charles B.
  Medicare made easy.

  "A People's Medical Society book."
  Includes index.
  1. Medicare.   2. Medicare — Claims administration.
  I. MacKay, Charles K.   II. Title.
  HD7102.U4156   1989   343.73′0226   88-7536
  ISBN 0-201-17269-0   347.303226

Cover design by Hannus Design Associates
Text design by Joyce C. Weston
Set in 12-point Sabon by Compset, Inc., Beverly, MA

  CDEFGHIJ-AL-89
Third printing, August 1989

To Amy, Dale and Ginny

Acknowledgments

No book can be written by the authors alone. In this case, many hard working and dedicated people assisted. We would like to thank the dedicated employees of the Health Care Financing Administration (HCFA), the people who administer the Medicare program. Especially we thank Rodger Goodacre, Director, Division of Beneficiary Services; Carole Weinberg, Administrative Assistant; Jane Shipley, Dick Getrost, Steve Pusateri and Carol Sampson, all HCFA public affairs specialists; and many other fine people at the Baltimore headquarters.

Also, special thanks to the staff of the Senate Special Committee on Aging for their assistance in helping us to better understand the Catastrophic coverage that goes into effect in 1989 and beyond.

In addition, Jean Perih, Legislative Assistant to U.S. Congressman Don Ritter, was instrumental in our receiving the forms used under the Medicare program.

Most importantly three persons deserve our sincere thanks and eternal gratefulness. They are our Addison-Wesley editor Jane Isay who wanted this book even before we wrote the basic proposal; Gail Ross, our agent, who has been our greatest fan and supporter since we began working together three years ago; and, Michael Rooney, director of Special Projects for the People's Medical Society. Michael Rooney is in fact the third author of this book. He is responsible for the overall coordination of the book, the gathering of the forms, creation of the charts and general supervision of the two people whose names appear on the cover.

Finally, our thanks to the members and staff of the People's Medical Society. With people like them life is made so much easier.

Contents

Introduction

Since 1983, when we created the People's Medical Society, I have traveled over one million miles listening and talking to people about medicine and health care. I have heard tales of horror and stories of inspiration. I have met victims of the medical system and persons alive today because of it.

And we get mail as well. In fact, on average, the People's Medical Society receives several thousand pieces a week. And just as I find when on the road, the stories and questions cover the entire medical/health care gamut.

By meeting and corresponding with hundreds of thousands of people, I have reached the following conclusions:

- Medical consumers want to be more involved in and in charge of their health care.
- The majority want reliable information about the quality of the services available so they can make informed medical decisions.
- Nobody can figure out Medicare!

Medicare has been around for almost twenty-five years, and more than thirty-two million Americans are covered by the program. Over $100 billion is paid out each year by Medicare to doctors and hospitals for services to elderly and to certain disabled citizens. That's almost 3 percent of the gross national product.

But that's not all. Over $100 billion more is paid out each year from either the pockets of Medicare beneficiaries or their private supplemental insurers to pay for services Medicare did not cover entirely or at all.

Yet, despite the enormity of the program — Medicare is the costliest government entitlement program in the world — virtually no Medicare recipient really understands how it works or how it can work for him or her. In fact, many people deny themselves medical care, pay out-of-pocket for services Medicare will cover, refuse to appeal a denial of coverage, or allow themselves to be bullied or buffaloed by a doctor's receptionist, hospital accounting clerk, or insurance carrier's telephone representative simply because they do not understand Medicare.

People who are under the age of 65, are not disabled, or have not directly assisted a senior or disabled citizen in traversing the Medicare maze find it hard to believe that Medicare is such a complicated program. What could be so hard, they ask? You hit 65 or have a disability, you head down to the Social Security office and sign up for the program, and the rest is a smooth sail down an idyllic, albeit costly, medical stream.

Little do they know. In fact, a very alert 92-year-old woman once confided in me that she could not wait until the next year when her 64-year-old son would become eligible for Medicare. Her reason — now he would not think she was suffering from senile dementia every time she complained about her problems with Medicare.

Why is Medicare so complicated? Why can't reasonably intelligent people — the majority of whom are able to wend their way through the Internal Revenue Service's long income tax form without getting audited and incarcerated — make heads or tails out of Medicare?

The answer is simple. There has not been a single publication printed by the government (or anyone else, for that matter) that explains fully and clearly how to use the program, what it does and does not cover, how to appeal individual rulings and decisions, and most important, how to make Medicare work for the consumer.

Wait a minute. Doesn't Medicare itself publish a variety of publications that explains it all? The answer is both yes and no.

Yes, it does publish many publications. All are useful to one extent or another. In fact, the primary publication, *Your Medicare Handbook* — the one everyone gets after signing up — is a straightforward booklet that gives the basic information one needs. *But,* and this is a big, qualified but, it does nothing more than give a basic description of services.

The other Medicare publications are also helpful — most are single-topic brochures covering a specific issue or situation. Most people do not even know these publications exist, however.

The major gap in Medicare's own publications is what they do not, and in some instances cannot, say.

Because Medicare is a government program, initiated by Congress, administered by a governmental bureaucracy, and partially operated by contracted insurance companies and paying private doctors, hospitals, and health maintenance organizations, the publications it produces must go through layer upon layer of review not only to ensure accuracy but also to avoid opening any of the parties involved to problems.

For example, the Medicare laws and regulations do not require doctors to accept "assignment." Assignment is government talk for accepting what Medicare pays as full payment for services rendered.

Medicare's publications explain that. But what they do not tell you is the following:

- Most doctors do not accept assignment 100 percent of the time.
- You can negotiate with any doctor who does not accept assignment and possibly, in your case, get him or her to do so.

These are two glaring omissions. They are also extremely important bits of information for you, the beneficiary.

In other words, Medicare's publications are like the instructions you get with your federal income tax forms each year — they give you basic information, tell you what form you need, when and where to file, and so on. But they do not tell you how to get the maximum benefits, tactics and techniques you can use to save money, or how to make the most of the program.

That is why we have written *Medicare Made Easy*. It is time for the

Medicare beneficiary to have not only the basic information but all of the information needed to use and get the maximum benefit from the program.

We also wrote this book to help the reader cut through the bureaucratic red tape that envelops Medicare.

Medicare Made Easy goes way beyond what Medicare tells its beneficiaries. We show readers what they need to know to get their benefits on the very first day eligible. We describe how one consumer can pay less for doctor and hospital services than a friend or neighbor who has the exact same coverage. We help beneficiaries in their selection of a Medicare supplemental insurance program (something Medicare itself cannot even talk about).

As the nation's largest consumer health advocacy organization, the People's Medical Society has no ax to grind, no insurance to sell, and no conflicts of interest. We exist for one purpose: to help medical consumers get the most from the health care system.

This book is designed to fulfill that goal. Everything in it is meant to help you.

Medicare is a very complicated and confusing program. In 1989, it will become more so with the catastrophic provisions and other expansions Congress adopted in 1988. The cost to Medicare beneficiaries is going up dramatically and will continue to do so over the coming years. It is essential that every Medicare beneficiary know and understand how to get the maximum benefit from a program that is probably the most important government service any American citizen ever receives.

Medicare is not a charity program. All beneficiaries have paid a premium, before being eligible, through Social Security taxes withheld while employed. As a Medicare recipient one continues to pay through monthly premiums, copayments and deductibles, and, beginning in 1989 for many beneficiaries, a new levy on one's annual federal income tax.

Use this book as a reference, a tool, a guide. It is designed to cut through the jargon, explain by example, and direct beneficiaries to additional resources. You should not be intimidated by a program your government established for you.

Remember, Medicare is your health insurance plan. You pay for it; you elect the people who have the oversight responsibility for it. In our democracy, you are the chairperson of the board. And just like any chief executive, make sure you are treated with the respect, dignity, and service you deserve.

CHARLES B. INLANDER
PRESIDENT, PEOPLE'S MEDICAL SOCIETY
ALLENTOWN, PENNSYLVANIA

In this chapter you will learn: How Medicare began ▪ The role of the Social Security Administration ▪ The role of the Health Care Financing Administration ▪ The role of Medicare Carriers and Intermediaries ▪ The role of the Peer Review Organizations

---

1. Understanding Medicare

Medicare is probably the largest and the most expensive single program that the federal government runs. It is also one of the most complex, because passage of the Medicare law in 1965 required a good deal of horse-trading, especially with the American Medical Association (AMA) and various health insurers. If at times Medicare seems not to make sense to you, keep in mind that it was never supposed to. The current law is the result of a long series of political deals that had to satisfy diverse interests in order for there to be any law at all.

You won't think too much about Medicare until you have occasion to file a claim. Assume that your health problems are simple and uncomplicated. Assume that all the care you need is within the bounds of what the program pays for. Assume that you have enough income to pay the Medicare Part B (doctor insurance) premium, the catastrophic insurance premium, and the premium for a good supplemental policy easily. Assume that you have selected a good Medicare supplemental insurance policy. Assume that everything each of your doctors does is clearly medically necessary. Assume that you get well or die quickly. If all of these assumptions are met, Medicare will appear benign and friendly. You will wonder why anyone ever has problems with it.

If Medicare is your only source of payment for health care, you can't afford supplemental insurance or pick a poor policy, and you require care in a nursing home, you are likely to have a nightmare. You will wonder how anyone could have designed a monstrosity that does to people what Medicare may well do to you. What you know can determine what kind of experience you will have with Medicare.

We have tried to keep this book short, simple, and to the point. Our goal is to put *you* in the driver's seat when you, as a Medicare beneficiary, deal with doctors, hospitals, the assorted Medicare carriers and intermediaries, and the needlessly large amount of paperwork involved. When we depart from the goal of KISS — Keep It Short and Simple — it is to provide you with background that you need to deal effectively with Medicare.

Medicare has been reformed almost continuously since it began, but it has been reformed piecemeal, with layers of controls being added atop one another. To avoid cluttering up the text with definitions and footnotes that the subject almost seems to demand, and to help you break the code language of Medicare and medicine, we've chosen to print special words in **boldface** the first few times they occur in the book (or in a chapter) as a clue that they are defined in the glossary at the back of the book. Points that we want to emphasize are in *italics*.

The American health care system embodies even more deals between the various parties involved than Medicare itself. They aren't public deals. Those who pay for health care in both the private and the public sectors still don't feel as involved as they would like to be. Patients, consumers of medical services — you — have been involved in an effective way only in the last decade or so. Only in the last five years have really effective health care consumer organizations emerged.

The impetus for Medicare arose in the early 1960s as part of the wave of New Frontier and Great Society programs started by President John F. Kennedy and continued by President Lyndon Johnson. A repeatedly quoted figure was that the elderly, at the time the law was passed, spent about 15 percent of their incomes on health care — a figure that was thought to be intolerable, as Senator Hubert Humphrey proclaimed with tears streaming down his face, arguing for passage of the law on the floor of the Senate. That was in 1965.

Yet today the elderly again spend more than 15 percent of their income on health care, even with Medicare. Does this mean that Medicare is a failure? Not really, if we measure it by other standards. Without it, the elderly and the disabled would spend far more than 15 percent of their incomes on health care, many would have to do without it, and the American people would have even less control over doctors and hospitals than they do today. And Medicare has helped to establish the idea that those who pay the bills in health care should make at least some of the rules.

Medicare has established, through the **Peer Review Organization** programs and their predecessors, that the medical profession and the hospital industry cannot really be trusted to guarantee quality care on their own. The Peer Review Organizations are groups of doctors who make judgments about the medical necessity of what Medicare pays for. But they do it under contract with Medicare and aim at targets set by Medicare. They are constantly producing evidence that doctors need professional checkups as much as their patients need medical ones. (A list of the Peer Review Organizations is provided in appendix J.)

The recently enacted **Diagnosis-Related Groups (DRG) system,** which we explain later, has shown that hospitals can give adequate care even if they are not rewarded with an endless shower of money. But Medicare has *not* relieved the elderly of the burden of paying for health care. It has only lightened it — and the elderly are paying more now, as a percentage of income, than when the law was passed.

Medicare does not pay for some of the services you may need the most. A common misimpression, for example, is that Medicare pays for nursing home care. This misimpression may have tragic consequences. Medicare will pay if you need short-term care in a **Skilled Nursing Facility** to recover further after a hospital stay. But no other nursing home care is paid for. "Custodial" care — care that you need because you can no longer function with complete independence — is *not* covered.

Medicare requires cost-sharing for most services. The average annual income from Social Security for a retired individual is $5,856; the average income for a retired couple is $9,996. This does not leave much room to pay more than 15 percent for health care, a burden that this program was supposed to alleviate.

Medicare imposes this burden on you because it is committed to the principle of cost-sharing. This is, in theory, a good idea. In practice, it has meant the loss of the original goals — somewhat equal access to health care and elimination of the threat of impoverishment because of illness — for many Americans. The amounts that you must pay for the Part B premiums (the part of Medicare that pays for doctor bills), for hospital care, and for doctors' services are raised automatically as the result of a formula, without regard for your ability to pay.

Medicare has never been able to establish national standards for payments to doctors, even though it has succeeded in doing so for hospitals. This means that Medicare itself pays varying amounts in the same locality for services provided by doctors with exactly the same skills and training. Worse yet, because doctors are not required to accept **assignment** — to agree to take what Medicare decides is a fair payment for their services — Medicare beneficiaries can have doctor bills, after Medicare has paid, that are two to three times what Medicare regards as fair payment *in full*. Only in Massachusetts are doctors required to accept what Medicare pays.

A national pay scale has been nearly unthinkable in part because doctors are not required to treat Medicare beneficiaries. Ensuring access to health care for older Americans without such a requirement is a chicken-and-egg problem. Older Americans need money to pay for health care. They also need doctors who will see them for the amounts that they can afford. Contrary to the image of the sainted doctor tending all the sick, the American Medical Association has maintained in its recent codes of ethics that a doctor has no obligation to treat any individual. (Stopping treatment against a patient's wishes is different, and it's considered unethical. It's called "abandonment" — but watch how fast you get abandoned if you can't pay your bill.) The AMA lobbied hard to ensure that no provision requiring doctors to treat beneficiaries went into the Medicare bill.

Medicare has never been able to pay enough to get a majority of doctors to accept Medicare patients and take what it pays as payment in full, but it pays enough that virtually all doctors will take the check and bill the Medicare patient for more. Not requiring that doctors treat Medicare patients for what Medicare will pay has been a losing strategy. It created a black hole that has sucked up tax dollars without really reducing the proportionate cost of health care to the elderly.

There are, of course, Medicare supplemental insurance plans that claim to cover the costs that Medicare doesn't cover. Some of them do a decent job, but others don't; nearly all of them fail to provide coverage for long-term care, which imposes the greatest risk of financial ruin on the elderly. (Relatively few of the elderly run up hospital bills that are enormous compared to others, and Medicare still picks up most of the tab for the usual length of hospital stay. It is long-term care, which about 5 percent of the over-65 population are using at any one time, that poses the real financial threat.) Some of the plans, frankly, are pure rip-offs. In this book, we show how to go about picking an affordable Medicare supplemental plan that fits your needs.

Medicare — and medicine — involve many special terms. Some have the purpose of efficiently substituting one special word for several plain English ones. (Example: "assignment" instead of "the doctor's agreeing to take what Medicare determines is the fair price, handling the paperwork with Medicare for the patient, getting a check for 80 percent of the price directly from Medicare, and charging the patient or the patient's insurer only 20 percent," which could get cumbersome.) Others are just medical or bureaucratic jargon, having the effect of giving the laity less control over the process by introducing what can amount to the secret language of a club.

Who Dealt This Mess, Anyway?

Who really runs Medicare? The answers may surprise you.

The Law

Medicare, as it currently exists, is a compromise between politicians' desire to provide what they thought was good-quality medical care to the elderly and their fear of what it would cost. It's between doctors and hospitals who fear loss of control over patients and medicine in general and their desire for federal dollars. It's between the public's notion that health care is a right and the reality that even the federal government cannot enforce such rights throughout fifty states and four territories. Add the desire of large health insurers, such as Blue Cross and Blue Shield, not to be locked out of the picture. Like the camel, it is a horse put together by a committee. And Medicaid — another federal health insurance program primarily for the nonelderly poor, which even the most starry-eyed legislators had not expected to see passed — was tacked on at the last second.

Like other benefits provided by the federal government to the middle class, the current form of Medicare has become something of a sacred cow. Legislators and the public fear changing it, because they fear losing what has been gained.

This means that, in contrast to some other federal programs, much of the driving force for change comes from the small professional bureaucracy that runs it and from the small segments of the other parts of government and the public that have learned to deal with them. Some of them toil on the staffs of congressional committees. Some work in the domestic policy section of the **Office of Management and Budget (OMB)**. Others work in the **Congressional Budget Office**. Some are in universities. The inner workings of the Medicare program are almost as far removed from public scrutiny as those of the Department of Defense.

Congress could never adjourn if all the details of federal program management were worked out on the floor of the House and Senate. Laws passed by Congress broadly authorize the programs; appropriations passed as part of the federal budget each year provide money for them. Everything else is left to the various **executive departments**, which write regulations for them that "have the force of law." This means that they are just like laws passed by Congress, but Congress never passed them, and most congresspersons never see them. Except in very special situations, all of them are published in the *Federal Register* before they take effect. Try finding the *Federal Register* at your local newsstand someday.

There's nothing sinister about this. It's a necessary compromise needed to make democracy work in a complicated society with thousands of government programs, a $1,000,000,000,000 (one trillion dollar) budget, and only 535 congresspersons and senators to look over the whole thing. But it does mean that Medicare beneficiaries have to enter the fray along with the doctors, the hospitals, the insurers, and all the other interest groups if they want their wishes to be heard, let alone heeded.

So here's who runs the parts of the show:

The Social Security Administration

The **Social Security Administration** is charged with administering determinations of eligibility for Medicare. If you are applying on the basis of reaching age 65 and not on the basis of disability or end stage renal disease, this almost always amounts to proving that you are who you say you are and that you were born when you say you were. If you are applying on the basis of disability, things usually get sticky (see chapter 8). The moment you are found eligible, your concerns with the Social Security Administration end. It passes on information to beneficiaries, and local offices act as a contact point for Medicare, but once the Social Security Administration has determined that you're eligible, you immediately become the responsibility of

The Health Care Financing Administration (HCFA)

The **Health Care Financing Administration (HCFA)** was set up in the early days of the Carter administration to bring control of all federally funded health programs under one roof. (When we say "Medicare" in this book, we mean HCFA and the Medicare program as run by it.) The idea was that health financing issues should be dealt with as such, not as issues peculiar to the funding program, such as Medicare, Medicaid, the Indian Health Service, and so on. What happened in practice is that a lot of public servants who had been under different roofs were lodged under one roof. Medicare and Medicaid have shared good ideas, and come to resemble each other a lot more than they once did, but nothing miraculous has happened, except for the **diagnosis-related groups (DRG) system.** This represents a major loss of power by the medical profession and hospitals, and a major gain for the government. It is a model for moving the health care system away from professional interests and toward public interests. It may or may not be repeated while HCFA is around. (Incoming presidents and cabinet secretaries love to reorganize things. It gives the appearance of action while they try to figure out what is going on and tears the reins of power out of the hands of the civil service, which gives the political appointees a chance to grab them, but only a chance. The civil service usually catches them again in the end.)

Medicare controls every aspect of what happens to you as a Medicare recipient from the moment you are determined eligible. You are not handed back to the Social Security Administration until you die, when the Social Security Administration makes the determination on survivor's benefits.

In the last eight years, HCFA has been charged with controlling the cost of medical care. In the course of trying to do that, it realized that Medicare and Medicaid laws only looked like they left a lot of decisions in the hands of the **carriers** and the medical profession. Medicare has begun to assert control in almost every area, including many that doctors and hospitals, or even the **Food and Drug Administration (FDA)**, another part of the federal government, consider their own. Medicare has decided to release figures on the death rates and readmission rates for patients in hospitals around the nation. It is safe to say that as pressure to reduce the federal deficit mounts, Medicare will discover more things in the law that it has the power to do. Again, there's nothing sinister about this. Medicare always had the power to do much of what has been done by regulation. It has always had the power to find the prices charged by some doctors "inherently unreasonable" and refuse to pay them. Only recently has it found the will to do so.

HCFA can usually be counted on to try to do the right thing. But the medical profession and health care providers still retain enormous power in political circles, even if that power has diminished in recent years. The mood in Congress, the pressure to control health care costs, and the activism of groups such as the People's Medical Society and the American Association of Retired Persons have created a climate in which HCFA can be used as a lever to expand the power of consumers in the health care system. This situation is not guaranteed to last, and Medicare has to be watched. You can deal with it in two ways: first, as a member of an association that asserts the rights of Medicare beneficiaries, and second, as an individual beneficiary.

What HCFA cannot do on its own, Congress has often been willing to do. Congressional committee staffers and the civil servants in HCFA talk to each other, and ideas are passed around. The regulations that Medicare lawyers discovered that Medicare did not have the power to issue have shown a tendency to become laws in the very next Congress.

It is not editorializing, but just pointing to a fact, to say that this situation has come about because the hospitals and organized medicine have deeply offended some powerful congresspersons and senators in the last few years. Health care is so complicated that congresspersons who take the time to educate themselves about it are routinely deferred to by their colleagues. The current discord between Congress and organized medicine creates a great opportunity for ordinary people to have a very loud voice in the way Medicare operates.

The Carriers and Intermediaries

When the Medicare law was passed, health insurers demanded a role. Basically, they argued that Medicare was socialized medicine, and therefore unacceptable, if the federal government ran it itself, but was a boon to the public if the federal government gave them contracts to run it. They won, sort of.

Medicare contracts with health insurance organizations, called **carriers** or **intermediaries**, to process Medicare claims. A list of carriers for the various parts of the United States can be found in appendix A.

Medicare periodically holds competitions for the contract to be a Medicare carrier for a particular area. Those who want the contract write large, detailed proposals and submit them to Medicare. Medicare selects the one that looks like it can do the job at the lowest overall cost. Medicare then monitors the carrier's performance. A look at the list of intermediaries shows that the Blue Cross and Blue Shield plans were certainly not locked out, as they feared.

The carriers and intermediaries try to implement the results of changes in the law and regulations according to manuals issued by Medicare. Sometimes they fail. The key to dealing with them is accurate paperwork and meticulous record-keeping. We've provided a Medicare Claims Log in appendix B to simplify the job.

The Peer Review Organizations

The peer review organizations are groups of doctors who make decisions on the medical necessity of health care under contract with Medicare. We explain how to deal with them in chapter 6, which deals with hospitals, and in chapter 8. They are becoming an increasingly greater force within Medicare as the Health Care Financing Administration relies on them for cost control.

How to Deal with All of the Above

In this section we discuss some points to remember in dealing with all of the above. We hope that things will go smoothly for you and that you will never have occasion to use them.

The most fundamental point is that *Medicare is not a gift. You paid for it while you were working.* Medicare owes you services in just the same way that a health insurer to whom you have paid premiums owes them to you. You still pay a premium for Part B (doctor insurance). There is a contractual obligation to provide you with the services you've paid for, even if the federal government is the one with whom you have the contract.

Second, *being a Medicare beneficiary does not deprive you of any right you would have as a holder of private health insurance.* In fact, as you'll see in chapter 8, you have *more* rights than holders of private health insurance in all but a few states. Third, the price of health care has reached a level that very few individuals can afford. Everyone is dependent on someone else — an employer, a parent, or the government — for health care. It has priced itself out of the private market. As far as health care is concerned, everyone is poor. Everyone needs help.

The Rest of the Book

This book has seven more chapters. Chapter 2 gives you an essential overview. Chapter 3 tells you exactly what Medicare does and doesn't cover. Chapter 4 describes supplemental insurance. Chapter 5 tells you how to negotiate with your doctor about fees and treatment. Chapter 6 explains how to deal with hospitals and the peer review organizations. Chapter 7 covers Medicare and nursing homes. Chapter 8 covers the problems that can arise and what you can do to solve them yourself or how to get help when you need it. We've also provided fourteen appendices that contain other sources of help.

A final note: We believe that health care in one's later years should be a source of security and not one of endless worry. We hope that this book helps make it so.

As this book was going to press, Congress passed the Medicare catastrophic coverage law that substantially revised the way many matters in Medicare are handled and increased benefits in some areas. We revised the book to reflect the language of the law. Actual implementation of these changes will require the writing of regulations, a process that had barely begun when this book was finished. The regulations, when written, may alter some of the material herein in minor ways. Your Social Security office can provide information about changes; beneficiaries will also receive general explanations by mail.

In this chapter you will learn: How Social Security and Medicare are linked ▪ When you're eligible and how to apply ▪ How to overcome barriers and claim the benefits you earned ▪ The correct forms to use to speed your application on its way ▪ What Medicare covers and what it doesn't ▪ How to file a claim

2. The Basics

Many are unaware of how relatively little of a person's necessary medical care Medicare covers. It's around 50 percent now, and that number is falling, for many reasons. Medical care has become more expensive than Congress anticipated, and legislation would be required to close the gap. At a time when federal deficits and the stability of the Medicare Trust Fund are major concerns, Congress is reluctant to increase benefits as long as beneficiaries will tolerate the situation. Doctors' fees have risen dramatically. The majority of the nation's doctors do not accept Medicare **assignment** for all patients, and Medicare has only recently begun to use its power to limit what it pays doctors. The combination of these factors drives up the doctor bill for both beneficiaries and the Medicare program. The situation is unlikely to get much better. A rare exception is the catastrophic care law, which went into effect on January 1, 1989. This will help, but most Medicare patients do not face catastrophes of the sort the new law is designed to cover. Instead their resources are drained nickel by nickel, dime by dime.

This chapter deals, of necessity, with Social Security. Social Security and the Medicare program are entangled in the area of Medicare eligibility. Since we'll be talking about Social Security, it's worth noting that many people are unaware of how little of preretirement income Social Security is intended to replace — about 42 percent, on average.

(The proportion falls as preretirement earnings rise. Lower-paid workers have a much higher replacement ratio than more highly paid ones.)

For both these reasons, it is important to know your Medicare and Social Security status *before* you retire. It is equally important to know what Medicare covers before retiring — possibly losing any coverage you might have through your employer — or dropping any personal medical insurance coverage you might have.

Who May Apply for Medicare and Who Is Eligible

Anyone who thinks he or she is in one of the groups that Medicare covers can apply for it. In fact, if there is any doubt at all — in your mind or in the mind of the representative of Social Security at the Social Security office where you apply for Medicare — about whether you are eligible, you should apply.

The Basic Coverage Groups

Medicare was originally intended for "the elderly" — people 65 or older. It now covers the following:

- *The elderly* — those who are 65 or older
- Those who are **permanently and totally disabled**
- Those who have **end stage renal disease,** the medical term for kidney disease that is severe enough to require dialysis or a transplant

Of course, things are not really this simple. Most, but not all, of the elderly are covered. The permanently and totally disabled are covered, but only if they meet the Social Security Administration's current definition of "permanently and totally disabled" and have received Social Security disability payments for at least two years. Those with end stage renal (kidney) disease are covered, but only if they meet the current definition of end stage renal disease. For most people, becoming eligible is just a matter of turning 65 and applying. For a few, it can be a frustrating process involving lawyers, appeals, and a lot of expense and anguish. What we will try to do in this chapter is make the process as easy as possible for everyone involved.

Eligibility Requirements for Medicare Coverage

To be eligible for Medicare, in any of the coverage groups, *one has to be a citizen of the United States, either by birth or naturalization, or an alien admitted for permanent residence who has resided in the United States for at least five years.*

Eligible people must also have reached age 65. If they are not yet 65, they must be disabled or suffering from end stage renal disease. A common misconception is that you will be covered if you are receiving Social Security. *This is not true unless you meet the requirements above.* The requirements for Social Security and Medicare are different. For example, it is possible to start receiving Social Security payments at age 62, but you will not be covered by Medicare until you reach 65.

In addition, to be eligible for Medicare you must be *entitled to payments under the Social Security Act or the Railroad Retirement Act.* This means, in general, that you must have worked for at least ten years (or, alternatively, six quarters out of the last thirteen) in a job that was covered under the Social Security Act, or be covered *based on the earnings record of someone who is covered.*

The language Americans use daily makes almost no distinction between "eligible" (for something) and "entitled" (to something.) The Social Security and Medicare laws use the words differently. You are "eligible" for Medicare as soon as, and whenever, you meet the eligibility requirements that apply to you. You are "entitled" to Medicare only after you have *applied and are officially determined (sometimes after a session in court, pitting you against the federal government) to be eligible.*

We've tried to keep the language of this book simple. We tried substituting "receiving Social Security payments" for "entitled," but that doesn't work because you can be entitled and not receiving payments (for example, if you keep on working after age 62 and make enough to reduce your Social Security payments to zero). Our following translation of the legalese is the best we can do; the important thing to keep in mind is that in order to receive Medicare, *you must apply.* There's only one exception to this: if you are already entitled to Social Security payments and turn age 65, you are enrolled in (and entitled to) both parts of Medicare unless you advise the Social Security Administration that you do not want Part B. There are two exceptions to the exception. You're not automatically enrolled, even if you're receiving checks, if you are entitled to Medicare on the basis of government employment or you are residing outside the United States. Otherwise, you *must apply*. The upshot is, *if you want it, apply for it.*

The Work Requirement

A quarter is one-fourth of a year, or three months. While you can be covered with as little as six quarters, the majority of Social Security recipients have worked for the ten-year (forty-quarter) period the Social Security Act specifies. There is an alternative requirement for persons who have died or attained age 62 without having forty quarters. (Death prior to age 62 is relevant because it is possible to be entitled to Medicare on the earnings record of someone who has died.) Finally, it is also possible to be covered if one has worked for six out of the last thirteen quarters, ending with the one in which one becomes entitled to Social Security benefits. The eligibility conferred under the last option, however, can be lost. Eligibility under the first two is permanent.

The alternative requirement is this: To be eligible, one must have one quarter of coverage for each year elapsing after 1950 or the year they reached age 21, whichever is later, and the year before the year in which they attained age 62 or died, whichever is earlier. Alternatively, they can have six quarters in the thirteen-quarter period (three years and three months) in which they become entitled to Social Security payments. A minimum of six quarters is always required.

This last option can be thought of as a window of eligibility that is linked to the month you apply for, and are found eligible for, Social Security. Obviously, if you wait to apply until you have no longer worked for six out of the last thirteen quarters, counting backward from the quarter in which the application occurs, you can lose your eligibility under this option. The two tables on page 20 may help make this a bit clearer.

For a quarter in which you worked to count for Medicare (and Social Security) purposes, you must have earned a certain amount during the quarter. You must also have earned it from an employer covered under Social Security. The amount you had to earn each quarter was $250 for years before 1979, and

- $260 in 1979
- $290 in 1980
- $310 in 1981
- $340 in 1982
- $370 in 1983
- $390 in 1984
- $410 in 1985
- $440 in 1986
- $460 in 1987

Social Security (and Medicare) Eligibility Alternatives:
Quarters of Coverage Required

OPTION 1	OPTION 2	OPTION 3
40 quarters, regardless of when earned.	One quarter for each calendar year after age 21, not to exceed 40 quarters. or One quarter for each calendar year after 1950, until age 62, not to exceed 40 quarters.	Six out of the last thirteen quarters.

Social Security (and Medicare) Eligibility Alternatives:
Quarters of Coverage Required

YEAR OF BIRTH	YEAR AGE 21 REACHED (OR 1950)	YEAR AGE 62 REACHED	QUARTERS REQUIRED
1920	1950	1982	31
1925	1950	1987	36
1930	1951	1992	40
1935	1956	1997	40
1940	1961	2002	40
1945	1966	2007	40
1950	1971	2015	40

The exception that allows less than forty quarters of coverage applies primarily to individuals who returned to, or entered, the work force late in life and became disabled or died before age 62 and aliens who have entered the United States and have resided here for at least five years. (Aliens must be *legal residents* for five years to receive Medicare, but their work counts toward coverage as soon as they start working.) Let's look at some examples:

Marge Smith, who had never worked before, started working in the first quarter of 1985, because her husband was disabled, and worked continuously. She was born in 1926, turned 21 in 1947, and turned 62 in 1988. She needs thirty-seven quarters of coverage, (because the number of years after 1950 and before 1988 is thirty-seven), or six out of the thirteen-quarter period before her entitlement to Social Security payments. Although she is 62 in 1988, she does not yet have thirteen quarters. She first becomes eligible for Social Security payments after the first quarter of 1989 (in April 1989). She is covered at this point, and will be eligible for Medicare when she becomes 65, but she should apply for Social Security now to be entitled to Medicare. *(If her husband is covered, she can be entitled based on his earnings record.)*

Why should Marge apply now? Because if she stops work and more than seven quarters go by before she applies, *she will no longer meet the alternative six-out-of-the-last-thirteen quarters requirement* for getting Medicare. The connection with entitlement to Social Security is what makes the magic work, because it sets the point from which one starts counting backward.

John Smith, Marge's son, attained age 21 in 1986. He became disabled in 1991. He started working in 1987, right after he graduated from college, and worked until he was disabled. He needs six quarters. (He has, of course, four for each of the years 1987, 1988, 1989, and 1990, a total of sixteen; he needs four to be covered by the formula above [one each for 1987–1990], but the minimum is six.) He is covered, because he has at least six quarters. He will be eligible for Medicare when he has been entitled to Social Security disability payments for two years.

John meets the minimum-of-six-quarters requirement *and* the six-out-of-the-last-thirteen requirement. He has to meet *both* to be entitled to Social Security. He is *not* eligible for Medicare until he has been entitled to Social Security for two years.

Victoria Smith-Jones, Marge Smith's English cousin, enters the country as a lawfully admitted alien in the first quarter of 1988, because Marge's situation is difficult and the two want to be together. She was born in 1926 and becomes age 62 in 1988. She has a job waiting for her, and works continuously. She needs thirty-seven quarters of coverage (because the number of years after 1950 and before 1988 is thirty-seven), or six out of the thirteen-quarter period before her entitlement to Social Security payments. She becomes eligible for Social Security payments at age 62, as does Marge, and is wise enough to apply to protect her eligibility for Medicare, but she is not actually eligible for Medicare until she has resided in the United States for five years. She meets this requirement in the first quarter of 1993. She is eligible *for Social Security (and entitled to) in the second quarter of 1992, but is not eligible for Medicare until the first quarter of 1993, after she has lived in the United States for five years. The fact that she hits 65 in 1991 is not relevant here, because Victoria is an alien.*

For reasons known only to Congress, the five-year residency requirement applies to Part B of Medicare, not Part A. An alien can qualify for Part A as soon as he or she is entitled to Social Security, but must wait five years for Part B, regardless of entitlement.

For a long time, federal and state workers and some workers in organizations run by religions that objected to Social Security were not covered; most of them are now covered. Congress has changed the laws from time to time to include more groups. Often this was done to ensure that more taxes were collected to keep the Social Security and Medicare trust funds from running out. Other groups were given the option of being covered.

The requirement of forty quarters of covered work has been scaled back, as we've shown in the examples above, for people who Congress knew could not have worked so long. These include most of the disabled and most of those with end stage renal disease. (From now on we'll use the word "disabled" to mean those who meet the current legal definition of "permanently and totally disabled." We understand that this definition excludes many people who cannot, in fact, obtain work.)

Do not assume that you do not meet this requirement. Many people do not know about the alternative ways of becoming eligible and erroneously think that they have to have worked for forty continuous quarters. This is not always true, as we've seen.

Another reason not to assume that you are not eligible is that you may be eligible based on the earnings record of someone who is covered. For example, widows and widowers are covered if they were married to their spouses at least one year before the death of the spouse. Divorced persons are eligible if they were married to the covered person for at least ten years.

Also:

- *Wives* are eligible if they have attained age 65 and if their husbands are covered.
- *Divorced wives* are eligible if they were married to the person on whose earnings record they are covered, have attained age 65, and have not remarried.

- *Husbands* are eligible under the same conditions as wives.
- *Divorced husbands* are eligible under the same conditions as divorced wives.
- *Widows and widowers* are eligible if they are over 65.
- *Mothers and fathers* of covered children are eligible if they have attained the age of 65.
- *Surviving parents* of children eligible for Social Security who were receiving at least one-half of their support from their child at the time of the child's death or disability are eligible when they reach age 65.

You now have to deal with a division of labor in the federal government. Until you have been determined to be eligible for Medicare, you are the responsibility of the Social Security Administration, which makes eligibility determinations for both Medicare and Social Security benefits. Once you are eligible for Medicare, you will deal with the **Health Care Financing Administration (HCFA)**, which runs Medicare and Medicaid. (For the sake of brevity and avoidance of alphabet soup, we'll use "Medicare" to refer to the HCFA from now on, unless there's a clear need to distinguish the program from those who run it.) We talk about the application process later in the chapter. For the moment, please believe that we are not trying to confuse Social Security issues with Medicare issues. Until you are found eligible for Medicare, the two are tied together in a Gordian knot. Most of the advice we give on Medicare will also help you preserve or increase your benefits under Social Security. Right now, we want to give you some information (and encouragement) about

What to Do if You Are Not Eligible Now

Remember, you cannot get Medicare unless you are eligible for Social Security. (There is an option to purchase Medicare as insurance if you're not eligible. We'll discuss that later.) In order to make sure you are eligible for Medicare, qualify for Social Security (and, if you're a resident alien, make sure you meet the five-year requirement).

You are likely to be found ineligible only if you don't meet the age, alien residency, or work requirement. Only time will cure the first two.

If you are found not to be eligible because you do not have enough covered work, there's only one answer: more work, earning at least $540 (for 1988) in each quarter, until you meet either the standard test or the alternative. The standard test, as we discussed above, is one quarter of work for each of the years after the year you turned 21 and

---

FOLD HERE

REQUEST FOR STATEMENT OF EARNINGS
(PLEASE PRINT IN INK OR USE TYPEWRITER)

	FOR SSA USE ONLY	
AX		●
SP		●

I REQUEST A SUMMARY STATEMENT OF EARNINGS FROM MY SOCIAL SECURITY RECORD

NH — Full name you use in work or business

First	Middle Initial	Last
		,

●

SN — Social Security number shown on your card

	DB	Your date of birth			**A**
		Month	Day	Year	

●

MA — Other Social Security number(s) you have used

● **SX** — Your Sex — ☐ Male   ☐ Female

AK — Other name(s) you have used (Include your maiden name)

FOLD HERE

PRIVACY STATEMENT

The Social Security Administration (SSA) is authorized to collect information asked on this form under section 205 of the Social Security Act. It is needed so SSA can quickly identify your record and prepare the earnings statement you requested. While you are not required to furnish the information, failure to do so may prevent your request from being processed. The information will be used primarily for issuing your earnings statement.

I am the individual to whom the record pertains. I understand that if I knowingly and willingly request or receive a record about an individual under false pretenses I would be guilty of a Federal crime and could be fined up to $5000.

▶ Sign your name here: (Do not print)	TELEPHONE NO. (Area Code)	DATE

SEND THE STATEMENT TO: (to be completed in ALL cases.)

PN — Name

●

AD — Address (Number and Street, Apt. No., P.O. Box, or Rural Route)

●

City and state	**ZP**	Zip Code	
●		●	

Form **SSA-7004-PC-OP1** (9/85)
Destroy prior editions

---

before the year you turned 62 or became disabled (in the eyes of Social Security). (The standard is forty for most of us.) The alternative is six out of the last thirteen quarters before you apply for Social Security. But you should eliminate the possibility that you've been found ineligible due to an error:

Make Sure Your Earnings Record Is Accurate

You can obtain a statement of your earnings record every three years by obtaining a Form 7004PC (see form and instructions, page 24) from your local Social Security office and sending it to the Social Security Administration. You can also send a letter. The letter below is a suggested format for this.

Your name
Your street address
Your city, state, and ZIP code

Date

Social Security Administration
P.O. Box 57
Baltimore, MD 21203

Dear Madam or Sir:

Please send me a copy of my earnings record. My Social Security number is [*fill in your number*]. My date of birth is [*fill in date*]. [*If you have used any other names:*] I am also known as [*fill in the other names*].

Thank you for your attention to this request.

Sincerely yours,
Your signature

If your earnings record does not show that you have enough covered quarters to be covered now, the first thing to do is make sure that the record is accurate. It can be in error regarding *whether or not* there were any earnings in a quarter. This can affect your eligibility for Social Security and Medicare. It can also be in error about the *amount* you earned. This can affect your eligibility for both programs and the amount of your Social Security benefits.

Errors in earnings records happen for a number of reasons. Failure of employers to report earnings to the **Social Security Administration (SSA)** is probably the most common reason now. In the past, there were many problems with making sure that each person working under Social Security had a unique number. In one case, a wallet manufacturer included a dummy Social Security card in its wallets. The number used was not obviously a fake one, such as 000-00-000, and the card looked just like the real thing. Many people who bought the wallets used the card and the number it carried as their **Social Security**

number (SSN). In other cases, all members of a family used the same Social Security number.

To straighten out an earnings record that has errors in it, Social Security has to check it against other records that are correct. This is where the hard part begins. Ideally, you will have all the paycheck stubs or pay envelopes that were ever issued to you, and you will have all of your federal, state, and local tax returns for your entire working life. You will have the name and address of all your former employers. None of them will have shut down, moved, or changed its name. If all this is true, straightening out your earnings record will be snap.

The foregoing is almost never true. Fortunately, all you usually have to provide is information on the last five years of earnings, which are typically the highest-earning years (your SSA payment is based on the "high five"). Those five years contain twenty of the forty quarters you need to show that you worked, so all that is necessary is proving that you worked some in twenty other quarters.

Personnel at your local SSA district office can help you straighten out your earnings record. The SSA has specialists in this at regional offices if the local office can't help you, and your case can be sent to them as a last resort. The problem is that all of this will take time. For this reason, it is important to start early — before you need Medicare.

You may think you can see that your earnings record is right, but it's still a good idea to check it against your tax returns for the last five years. The figure recorded should equal the total of the Social Security Wages boxes on your W-2 forms. If you earned more than the maximum amount taxed for the year, only the maximum earnings for the year will be shown. If more is shown, you can apply to the IRS, via an amended tax return for the years in which too much was collected, to get a refund of the excess. See the example on page 27.

Work,
More Work

This is yet another reason to check your earnings record. Don't retire from your job, assuming that the SSA will provide more than enough to live on and Medicare will take care of all your bills, until you know you are eligible and what your benefits will be. Social Security has a form (see illustration on pages 42–43) that allows you to estimate your benefit. Find out if you need more quarters of work to be covered.

This advice is obviously of no benefit if you have already quit and can't get your job back (or any job) or if you are permanently and totally disabled. We advise you to seek almost any sort of work you can do in order to obtain coverage. The benefits, although not as great as perhaps they should be, are well worth it.

Excess Social Security Taxes: Getting a Refund

In 1987, the maximum amount taxable for Social Security was $43,800 and the Social Security tax rate for employees was 7.15 percent.

By working two jobs, you earned $47,800. One paid $35,000 and the other $12,800. Neither employer reached $43,800 in wages for you for the year, so neither stopped collecting Social Security taxes from your paycheck.

You paid: $35,000 × 7.15% = $2,502.50
         $12,800 × 7.15% = $ 915.20
         Total: $3,417.70

You should have paid: $43,800 × 7.15% = $3,131.70

Refund due: $3,417.70 − $3,115.00 = $ 302.70

Applying for a refund of this amount will *not* reduce your Social Security benefits, because no more than $43,800 can be counted toward them for 1987.

If you feel that you are disabled, you should apply for disability benefits. The necessary quarters of coverage are reduced, based on the year you became disabled.

Proving that You Really Are Disabled

You may be denied coverage if you do not qualify for Social Security benefits as a permanently and totally disabled person. Congress, in adding disabled person coverage, was acutely aware of the problems that had arisen in state Workers' Compensation programs, and structured the law so that only unquestionably disabled persons would qualify. The definition used to accomplish this seems absurdly strict:

*The term "disability" means (A) inability to engage in any substantial gainful activity by reason of any medically determined physical or mental impairment which can be expected to result in death or has lasted or can be expected to last for a continuous period of not less than 12 months, or (B) blindness; and the term "blindness" means central visual acuity of 20/200 or less in the better eye with the use of a correcting lens. (**Social Security Act, Sec. 216(i)(1)**)*

The application for disability insurance benefits is shown on pages 28–33.

APPLICATION FOR DISABILITY INSURANCE BENEFITS

I apply for a period of disability and/or all insurance benefits for which I am eligible under title II and title XVIII of the Social Security Act, as presently amended.

PART I—INFORMATION ABOUT THE DISABLED WORKER

1. (a) PRINT your name ⟶ FIRST NAME, MIDDLE INITIAL, LAST NAME

   (b) Enter your name at birth if different from item (a) ⟶

   (c) Check (√) whether you are ⟶   ☐ Male   ☐ Female

2. Enter your Social Security Number ⟶ __ __ __ / __ __ / __ __ __ __

3. (a) Enter your date of birth ⟶ MONTH, DAY, YEAR

   (b) Enter name of State or foreign country where you were born. ⟶

   If you have already presented, or if you are now presenting, a public or religious record of your birth established before you were age 5, go on to item 4.

   (c) Was a public record of your birth made before you were age 5?   ☐ Yes   ☐ No   ☐ Unknown

   (d) Was a religious record of your birth made before you were age 5?   ☐ Yes   ☐ No   ☐ Unknown

4. (a) What is your disabling condition? (Briefly describe the injury or illness that prevents, or has prevented, you from working.)

   (b) Is your injury or illness related to your work in any way? ⟶   ☐ Yes   ☐ No

5. (a) When did you become unable to work because of your disabling condition? ⟶ MONTH, DAY, YEAR

   (b) Are you still disabled? (If "Yes," go on to item 6.)
   (If "No," answer (c).) ⟶   ☐ Yes   ☐ No

   (c) If you are no longer disabled, enter the date your disability ended. ⟶ MONTH, DAY, YEAR

6. (a) Have you (or has someone on your behalf) ever filed an application for Social Security benefits, a period of disability under Social Security, supplemental security income, or hospital or medical insurance under Medicare? ⟶   ☐ Yes (If "Yes," answer (b) and (c).)   ☐ No (If "No," or "Unknown" go on to item 7.)   ☐ Unknown

   (b) Enter name of person on whose Social Security record you filed other application. ⟶

   (c) Enter Social Security Number of person named in (b). (If unknown, so indicate) ⟶ __ __ __ __ / __ __ / __ __ __ __

7. (a) Were you in the active military or naval service (including Reserve or National Guard active duty or active duty for training) after September 7, 1939 and before 1968? ⟶   ☐ Yes (If "Yes," answer (b) and (c).)   ☐ No (If "No," go on to item 8)

   (b) Enter dates of service ⟶ FROM: (month, year)   TO: (month, year)

   (c) Have you ever been (or will you be) eligible for a monthly benefit from a military or civilian Federal agency? (include Veterans Administration benefits only if you waived military retirement pay) ⟶   ☐ Yes   ☐ No

FORM **SSA-16-F6** (1-85)   Page 1 (Previous editions are obsolete)

8.	Have you or your spouse worked in the railroad industry for 7 years or more?	☐ Yes	☐ No

9.

(a) Have you filed (or do you intend to file) for any other public disability benefits? (Include workers' compensation and Black Lung benefits)

☐ Yes (If "Yes," answer (b).)   ☐ No (If "No," go on to item 10.)

(b) The other public disability benefit(s) you have filed (or intend to file) for is (Check as many as apply):

☐ Veterans Administration Benefits   ☐ Welfare

☐ Supplemental Security Income   ☐ Other (If "Other," complete a Workers' Compensation/Public Disability Benefit Questionnaire)

10.

(a) Have you ever engaged in work that was covered under the social security system of a country other than the United States? (If "Yes," answer (b).) (If "No," go on to item 11.)

☐ Yes   ☐ No

(b) List the country(ies):

11. Enter below the names and addresses of all the persons, companies, or Government agencies for whom you have worked this year, last year, and the year before last.
If the above does not apply, write "NONE" below and go on to item 13.

NAME AND ADDRESS OF EMPLOYER (If you had more than one employer, please list them in order beginning with your last (most recent) employer)	Work Began		Work Ended (If still working show "Not ended")	
	MONTH	YEAR	MONTH	YEAR
(If you need more space, use "Remarks" space on page 3.)				

12.	May the Social Security Administration or the State agency reviewing your case ask your employers for information needed to process your claim?	☐ Yes	☐ No

13. THIS ITEM MUST BE COMPLETED, EVEN IF YOU WERE AN EMPLOYEE.

(a) Were you self-employed this year, last year, or the year before? (If "Yes," answer (b).) (If "No," go on to item 14.)

☐ Yes   ☐ No

(b) Check the year or years in which you were self-employed	In what kind of trade or business were you self-employed? (For example, storekeeper, farmer, physician)	Were your net earnings from your trade or business $400 or more? (Check "Yes" or "No")	
☐ This Year			
☐ Last Year		☐ Yes	☐ No
☐ Year before last		☐ Yes	☐ No

14.

(a) How much were your total earnings last year? (Count both wages and self-employment income. If none, write "None.") — Amount $_____

(b) How much have you earned so far this year? (If none, write "None.") — Amount $_____

(c) Did you receive any money from an employer(s) on or after the date in item 5(a) when you became unable to work because of your disability? (If "Yes," give amounts and explain in "Remarks" on page 3.)

☐ Yes   ☐ No   Amount $_____

(d) Do you expect to receive any additional money from an employer such as sick pay, vacation pay, other special pay? (If "Yes," please give amounts and explain in "Remarks" on page 3.)

☐ Yes   ☐ No   Amount $_____

PART II — INFORMATION ABOUT THE DEPENDENTS OF THE DISABLED WORKER

15. Have you ever been married?
(If "Yes," answer item 16) (If "No," go on to item 17.) → ☐ Yes ☐ No

16. (a) Give the following information about your current marriage. If not currently married, show your last marriage below.

To whom married		When (Month, day, year)	Where (Name of City and State)
Your current or last marriage	How marriage ended (If still in effect, write "Not ended.")	When (Month, day, year)	Where (Name of City and State)
	Marriage performed by: ☐ Clergyman or public official ☐ Other (Explain in Remarks)	Spouse's date of birth (or age)	If spouse deceased, give date of death
	Spouse's Social Security Number (If none or unknown, so indicate) ___ ___ ___ / ___ ___ / ___ ___ ___ ___		

(b) Give the following information about each of your previous marriages. **(If none, write "None.")**

To whom married		When (Month, day, year)	Where (Name of City and State)
Your previous marriage	How marriage ended	When (Month, day, year)	Where (Name of City and State)
	Marriage performed by: ☐ Clergyman or public official ☐ Other (Explain in Remarks)	Spouse's date of birth (or age)	If spouse deceased, give date of death
	Spouse's Social Security Number (If none or unknown, so indicate) ___ ___ ___ / ___ ___ / ___ ___ ___ ___		

(Use a separate statement for information about any other marriages.)

17. If your claim for disability benefits is approved, your children (Including natural children, adopted children, and stepchildren) or dependent grandchildren (including stepgrandchildren) may be eligible for benefits based on your earnings record.

List below FULL NAME OF ALL such children who are now or were in the past 12 months UNMARRIED and:
- UNDER AGE 18   ● AGE 18 TO 19 AND ATTENDING SECONDARY SCHOOL
- DISABLED OR HANDICAPPED (age 18 or over and disability began before age 22)

(IF THERE ARE NO SUCH CHILDREN, WRITE "NONE" BELOW AND GO ON TO ITEM 18.)

18. Do you have a dependent parent who was receiving at least one-half support from you when you became unable to work because of your disability? (If "Yes," enter name and address in "Remarks.")   ☐ Yes   ☐ No

REMARKS (You may use this space for any explanation. If you need more space, attach a separate sheet.)

Form **SSA-16-F6** (1-85) Page 3

30

IMPORTANT INFORMATION ABOUT DISABILITY INSURANCE BENEFITS —
PLEASE READ CAREFULLY

I. **SUBMITTING MEDICAL EVIDENCE:** I understand that as a claimant for disability benefits, I am responsible for providing medical evidence showing the nature and extent of my disability. I may be asked either to submit the evidence myself or to assist the Social Security Administration in obtaining the evidence. If such evidence is not sufficient to arrive at a determination, I may be requested by the State Disability Determination Service to have an independent examination at the expense of the Social Security Administration.

II. **RELEASE OF INFORMATION:** I authorize any physician, hospital, agency or other organization to disclose to the Social Security Administration, or to the State Agency that may review my claim or continuing disability, any medical record or other information about my disability.

I also authorize the Social Security Administration to release medical information from my records, only as necessary to process my claim, as follows:

- Copies of medical information may be provided to a physician or medical institution prior to my appearance for an independent medical examination if an examination is necessary.
- Results of any such independent examination may be provided to my personal physician.
- Information may be furnished to any contractor for transcription, typing, record copying, or other related clerical or administrative service performed for the State Disability Determination Service.
- The State Vocational Rehabilitation Agency may review any evidence necessary for determining my eligibility for rehabilitative services.

THIS MUST BE ANSWERED ➡ 19. DO YOU UNDERSTAND AND AGREE WITH THE AUTHORIZATIONS GIVEN ABOVE? ☐ Yes ☐ No (If "No,", explain why)

_____

_____

_____

_____

_____

_____

III. **REPORTING RESPONSIBILITIES:** I agree to promptly notify Social Security if:
- My MEDICAL CONDITION IMPROVES so that I would be able to work, even though I have not yet returned to work.
- I GO TO WORK whether as an employee or a self-employed person.
- I apply for or receive a decision on benefits under any WORKERS' COMPENSATION law or plan (including Black Lung benefits from the Department of Labor.) or other public benefit based on disability.
- I am imprisoned for conviction of a felony.

The above events may affect my eligibility to disability benefits as provided in the Social Security Act, as amended.

I know that anyone who makes or causes to be made a false statement or representation of material fact in an application or for use in determining a right to payment under the Social Security Act commits a crime punishable under Federal law by fine, imprisonment or both. I affirm that all information I have given in this document is true.

SIGNATURE OF APPLICANT	Date (Month, day, year)
Signature (First name, middle initial, last name) (Write in ink) SIGN HERE ➤	Telephone Number(s) at which you may be contacted during the day. (Include the area code)

Mailing Address (Number and street, Apt. No., P.O. Box, or Rural Route) (Enter resident address in "Remarks" if different)

City and State	ZIP Code	Enter Name of County (if any) in which you now live

Witnesses are required ONLY if this application has been signed by mark (X) above. If signed by mark (X), two witnesses to the signing who know the applicant must sign below, giving their full addresses. Also, print the applicant's name in the Signature block.

1. Signature of Witness	2. Signature of Witness
Address (Number and street, City, State, and ZIP Code)	Address (Number and street, City, State, and ZIP Code)

Form **SSA-16-F6** **(1-85)** Page 4

FOR YOUR INFORMATION

An agency in your State that works with us in administering the Social Security disability program is responsible for making the disability decision on your claim. In some cases, it is necessary for them to get additional information about your condition or to arrange for you to have a medical examination at Government expense.

RECEIPT FOR YOUR CLAIM FOR SOCIAL SECURITY DISABILITY INSURANCE BENEFITS

PERSON TO CONTACT ABOUT YOUR CLAIM	SSA OFFICE	DATE CLAIM RECEIVED
TELEPHONE NUMBER (INCLUDE AREA CODE)		

Your application for Social Security disability benefits has been received and will be processed as quickly as possible.

You should hear from us within _____ days after you have given us all the information we requested. Some claims may take longer if additional information is needed.

In the meantime, if you change your address, or if there is some other change that may affect your claim, you - or someone for you - should report the change. The changes to be reported are listed below.

Always give us your claim number when writing or telephoning about your claim.

If you have any questions about your claim, we will be glad to help you.

CLAIMANT	SOCIAL SECURITY CLAIM NUMBER

CHANGES TO BE REPORTED AND HOW TO REPORT
FAILURE TO REPORT MAY RESULT IN OVERPAYMENTS THAT MUST BE REPAID

► You change your mailing address for checks or residence. To avoid delay in receipt of checks you should ALSO file a regular change of address notice with your post office.

► You go outside the U.S.A.

► Any beneficiary dies or becomes unable to handle benefits.

► Custody Change — Report if a person for whom you are filing or who is in your care dies, leaves your care or custody, or changes address.

► You are confined to jail, prison, penal institution, or correctional facility for conviction of a felony.

► Change of Marital Status — Marriage, divorce, annulment of marriage.

► You return to work (as an employee or self-employed) regardless of amount of earnings.

► Your condition improves.

► If under age 65, you begin to receive workers' compensation or another public disability benefit (including Black Lung benefits) or the amount of your present Workers' compensation or public disability benefit changes.

HOW TO REPORT

You can make your reports by telephone, mail, or in person, whichever you prefer.

If you are awarded benefits, and one or more of the above changes occur, the change(s) should be reported by calling

_____

(Telephone Number—Include Area Code)

Collection and Use of Information From Your Application — Privacy Act Notice/Paperwork Act Notice

The Social Security Administration is authorized to collect the information on this form under sections 202(b), 202(c), 205(a), and 1872 of the Social Security Act, as amended (42 U.S.C. 402(b), 402(c), 405(a), and 1395ii). While it is VOLUNTARY, except in the circumstances explained below, for you to furnish the information on this form to Social Security, no benefits may be paid unless an application has been received by a Social Security office. Your response is mandatory where the refusal to disclose certain information affecting your right to payment would reflect a fraudulent intent to secure benefits not authorized by the Social Security Act. The information on this form is needed to enable Social Security to determine if you and your dependents are entitled to insurance coverage and/or monthly benefits. Failure to provide all or part of this information could prevent an accurate and timely decision on your claim or your dependent's claim, and could result in the loss of some benefits or insurance coverage. Although the information you furnish on this form is almost never used for any other purpose than stated in the foregoing, there is a possibility that for the administration of the Social Security programs or for the administration of programs requiring coordination with the Social Security Administration, information may be disclosed to another person or to another governmental agency as follows: 1. to enable a third party or an agency to assist Social Security in establishing rights to Social Security benefits and/or coverage; 2. to comply with Federal laws requiring the release of information from Social Security records (e.g., to the General Accounting Office and the Veterans Administration); and 3. to facilitate statistical research and audit activities necessary to assure the integrity and improvement of the Social Security programs (e.g., to the Bureau of the Census and private concerns under contract to Social Security).

Form SSA-16-F6 (1-85) Page 6

☆ U.S. GOVERNMENT PRINTING OFFICE 1984 461-398/10024

The regulations implementing the Social Security Act specifically prescribe that if you are able to perform any gainful work at all, you are not disabled for Social Security purposes. If the disability examiners judge that you could do some work, you are not disabled. You may protest that you do not know how to do the work the examiners believe you can do, that you have no chance of getting any training for it, and that the only shop that does that kind of work is in Shanghai. No matter. Practical difficulties like this aren't considered — only your state of body and mind. The definition leads to paradoxes: persons likely to live a long time, but not "able-bodied" in any sense, are denied benefits.

There is obviously a large subjective component to an examiner's determination as to whether or not a person is disabled in the sense the SSA law requires. There is no exact medical standard that determines, for example, that a person who has only partial use of one hand is capable or incapable of running a telephone answering service from home. The task is made harder because some disabled persons have achieved more than the vast majority of the nondisabled: Some who have only the use of their eyes and mouth have written novels and painted; a quadriplegic who has lost the ability to speak, but can still make sounds, is one of the world's leading astrophysicists. Usually such individuals have a good deal of support (for buying special equipment and hiring assistants). Disabled persons who have this level of support and the drive to make use of it are rare. But the fact that they exist makes it all the easier for examiners to deny benefits to disabled applicants.

Examiners in the same office, to say nothing of examiners in different parts of the country, arrive at completely opposite judgments about whether or not specific persons meet the requirements for disability benefits. And politics seems to enter the picture as well. Different presidential administrations have placed great emphasis on strict applications of the rules; others have not. Courts in different **federal judicial districts** have made different decisions about disability cases, and the **Department of Health and Human Services**, which includes the Social Security Administration and Medicare, is picking and choosing among them in an effort to keep costs down. Your chance of being found eligible for benefits on the basis of disability depends, unfortunately, on the luck of the draw: what your doctor says, which examiner you get, which federal judicial district you live in, and which **Administrative Law Judge (ALJ)** hears your appeal.

If you are denied benefits because you are found not disabled, we strongly urge you to appeal. At the same time, you should realize that time and costs will be involved and that you will probably need the help of a lawyer. We cover how to appeal decisions in chapter 8.

If All Else Fails, You Don't Have to Be Eligible to Buy It: What You Can Buy from Medicare

Persons 65 years old who do not otherwise qualify for Medicare can purchase Medicare coverage just like private insurance. The 1989 premium for the combined Part A (hospitalization insurance), Part B (doctor bill coverage), and catastrophic care coverage is $189.10 per month. If you purchase Medicare, you will still have to purchase supplemental insurance to have a package that really protects you against the financial effects of illness. You may find that it is cheaper to purchase individual coverage from a health maintenance organization (HMO), which offers very comprehensive benefits for one fixed price. We have a lot more to say on this in chapter 4.

You are permitted to purchase Part B of Medicare (insurance for doctor bills) if you are a resident of the United States, are 65 or over, and are either a citizen or an alien lawfully admitted for permanent residence who had resided in the United States for the last five years. (It is under this rule that everyone enrolls in Part B.) If you are not eligible for Part A of Medicare, enrolling for Part B entitles you to purchase it, so you have to buy Part B to get Part A.

Examples:

Victoria Smith-Jones's brother Cedric is entranced by Victoria's letters about life in the United States and decides to move here in late 1990. He is lawfully admitted for permanent residence. Being independently wealthy, he decides not to work. He loses most of his fortune in the 1994 stock market crash and can no longer afford his extremely expensive medical insurance. He is 65 in early 1995 and discovers that he is not automatically eligible for Medicare because he has never worked (anywhere, anytime). He decides to purchase Medicare. He calls his local Social Security office, establishes that he is not eligible but will meet the requirements for purchase, requests that an application to purchase Part B and Part A be sent to him, and signs up.

Marge's sister, Amber Smith Citron, aged 66, was married to her former husband, Harold Citron, for nine years and 361 days. She would have been eligible for Medicare on his earnings record had she been married to him for ten years. She has been working, and will have worked for six out of the last thirteen quarters, counting from the last quarter of 1989. But she is worried about medical expenses now. She meets the requirements of age (65 or over), citizenship, and current U.S. residence, and, like Cedric, signs up to purchase Medicare. Unlike Cedric, she will be eligible in early 1991. When she is eligible, she will no longer pay the Part A premium and will pay a reduced Part B premium.

How and When to Apply

Once more, being between ages 62 and 65 does not *entitle* you to Medicare. Being 65 or over does not *enroll* you for Medicare. It may take action on your part when you turn 65. Some people are automatically enrolled; others are given notices that they need to enroll. Automatic enrollment and notification are administrative actions of the Social Security Administration, not requirements of the law. The categories of those who are enrolled automatically have changed, and they could change again. *If you want Medicare, apply for it.* The worst that can happen is that you'll find out your enrollment is already taken care of.

As this is being written in mid-1988,

- If you are 65 or over and have been receiving Social Security benefits, you will automatically be enrolled for participation in Parts A and B (the hospital and doctor insurance portions of Medicare). You will receive a notice and your card (shown on page 37) about three to four months before your sixty-fifth birthday. Your card will not be valid until you turn 65. You are covered for Medicare even if you do not have your card; the hospital can bill under your Social Security number even if you do not have the card. You can obtain a Temporary Notice of Medicare Eligibility from your Social Security office.

- If you are 65 or over when you apply for Social Security benefits, you will automatically be enrolled as part of the application process for Social Security. Your card will be sent to you in the mail automatically. You are covered for Medicare even if you do not have your card if you are over 65 and have been found eligible for Social Security.

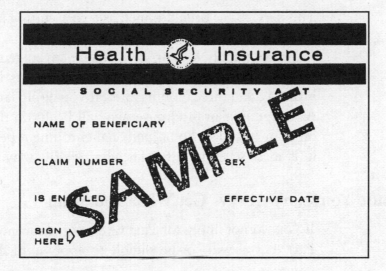

- End-stage-renal-disease patients are automatically enrolled if they are receiving Social Security disability benefits; otherwise, they must apply.

Your card also shows your health insurance claim number. Sometimes this claim number is referred to as your Medicare number. The claim number has nine digits and a letter. On some cards, there may also be another number after the letter. Your full claim number must always be included on all Medicare claims and correspondence. When a husband and wife both have Medicare, each will receive a separate card and claim number. Each spouse must use the exact name and claim number shown on his or her card.

It is important that you remember to

1. Always show your Medicare card when you receive services that Medicare can help you pay for.
2. Always write your health insurance claim number (including the letter) on any bills you send in and on any correspondence about Medicare. Also, you should have your Medicare card available when you make a telephone inquiry.
3. Carry your card with you whenever you are away from home. If you ever lose it, immediately ask your Social Security office to get you a new one.
4. Use your Medicare card only after the effective date shown on it.
5. Never permit someone else to use your Medicare card.

If you enrolled for Social Security and began receiving benefits before you were 65, *you must take action to enroll in Medicare.* Formerly, people were notified by mail when they were eligible to enroll.

This service has been dropped as a cost-cutting measure. You will have to keep track of the time yourself.

You can apply for Part B Medicare coverage *to begin on your sixty-fifth birthday* anytime between three months before your sixty-fifth birthday and three months after. If you apply later than this, your Part A (hospital insurance) coverage will begin on the date you apply, not on your birthday. Your "personal enrollment period," as the SSA calls it, is these seven months. The chart below may help.

Get It, Because You Can't Always Get What You Want

If you do not apply for Part B (doctor insurance) when you apply for Part A, you will not be eligible to apply until the next **general enroll-**

MONTH IN WHICH 65TH BIRTHDAY OCCURS	EARLIEST MONTH TO APPLY	LATEST MONTH TO APPLY
April 1989	January 1989	July 1989
May 1989	February 1989	August 1989
June 1989	March 1989	September 1989
July 1989	April 1989	October 1989
August 1989	May 1989	November 1989
September 1989	June 1989	December 1989
October 1989	July 1989	January 1990
November 1989	August 1989	February 1990
December 1989	September 1989	March 1990
January 1990	October 1989	April 1990
February 1990	November 1989	May 1990
March 1990	December 1989	June 1990
April 1990	January 1990	July 1990
May 1990	February 1990	August 1990
June 1990	March 1990	September 1990
July 1990	April 1990	October 1990
August 1990	May 1990	November 1990
September 1990	June 1990	December 1990
October 1990	July 1990	January 1991
November 1990	August 1990	February 1991
December 1990	September 1990	March 1991
January 1991	October 1990	April 1991
February 1991	November 1990	May 1991
March 1991	December 1990	June 1991

ment period, which runs from January 1 to March 31 of each year. Your premium will be raised 10 percent for each year you wait to apply. In addition, your coverage will not begin until July 1 of the year you enroll.

We recommend that you apply for Part B coverage at the same time you apply for Part A, if you can afford it. Failure to take Part B will make any supplemental insurance you buy harder to obtain, will make your premium higher, and may make supplemental insurance harder to get. The Part B premium is tax-deductible, just like any other medical insurance premium.

Application Forms and Process

Whether or not you are receiving Social Security, you should apply for Medicare three months before your sixty-fifth birthday. This will allow ample time for all the paperwork to be processed, any questions about your eligibility to be cleared up, and the like so that you obtain coverage as soon as you are eligible.

The first step is to telephone your local **Social Security office.** These offices are commonly listed under the federal government section in the blue pages of your local phone directory, and under "United States Government" in the white pages. If you can't find a listing, call the information operator and ask for any Social Security office. Calling any Social Security office will enable you to find out which one you should go to.

Call that office. Tell them you want to apply for Medicare (and Social Security, if you are not already receiving it). The SSA is making a determined effort to carry out as much business as possible over the phone. This is generally more efficient, and it saves you a visit to the Social Security office. At the same time, if you have trouble dealing with matters like this over the phone (if, for example, you have trouble hearing and don't have an amplified phone), you can insist on a face-to-face visit.

Whichever way you apply, the Social Security office representative will fill out most of the forms for you. This is done to ensure that the type of answers the SSA needs to make a decision are obtained on the forms involved. After the representative has filled out the forms, you should read them — and insist on the correction of any errors — before you sign them. If you need special assistance (if, for example, you are blind, deaf, or illiterate) special help will be made available to you. You may have to go to another Social Security office to find the right person to help you. The representative at the first Social Security Office you go to will give you instructions. If you think you will need special help, you should mention this when you first call.

The representative will ask you to bring certain documents when you come to the Social Security office, usually, the following:

- Proof of age
- Records of earnings, such as W-2 forms (or tax returns for the self-employed) for the past two years
- Your Social Security card

If you are applying because you think you are disabled, you will be asked to bring some documents relating to your medical problems. The Social Security office representative will tell you what they are.

Keep your originals. Keep your originals. Keep your originals. Need we say more?

The form of proof of age that the Social Security office wants is a birth certificate or a hospital birth record. If you can't obtain either of these, don't worry:

- The census records of 1910, 1920, or 1930 are accepted.
- Any school record that gives your age and was recorded before you were 21 is acceptable.
- Newspaper birth announcements are accepted.
- **Immigration and naturalization records** are acceptable.
- If all else fails, **notarized affidavits** from people who are in a position to know your age are acceptable.

The SSA will accept a number of other varieties of proof.

There are three reasons for asking you to bring in proof of earnings. First, it lets the representative at the Social Security office determine quickly, between the earnings on your Social Security earnings record and the proofs of earnings that you bring in, whether or not you have the required quarters of coverage. If you're close, having this information when you apply can eliminate a lot of worry and another phone call or trip. Second, your Social Security benefit is supposed to be based on the highest five years of your earnings, and having current information avoids having to give you a smaller benefit now, and a catch-up check and bigger benefits later, when the SSA computers get fed the information. Third, you may be receiving reduced Social Security. Suppose you chose to retire at age 62, applied for reduced benefits, and then took a job, or continued to work after 65 and earned enough to have your benefits reduced. In these cases, you are supposed to have your benefits recomputed periodically to take into account your additional earnings.

You also need not worry if you have lost your Social Security card. If you can remember the number, you can apply for a duplicate. If you can't remember the number, it is likely to be on a number of other documents around your house, such as payroll stubs, credit card bills, and insurance policies. If all else fails, the Social Security office has access to a computer system that will retrieve your name or any that sound like it from the Social Security computer system. This considerably narrows the search for your real number.

The forms you will face when you get to the Social Security office, and instructions for filling them out, are shown on pages 42–63. We also provide copies of some forms that are used for requesting reconsideration of denials of coverage and payment. The use of these forms is explained in chapters 6 and 8.

What Medicare Covers and What It Doesn't

A common misconception about Medicare is that it has a wide scope of coverage, comparable with the best private insurance plans. It doesn't. In fact, if Medicare were sold as private insurance at the current buy-in premium, it is doubtful that there would be many takers. Most health maintenance organizations offer much better coverage — in fact, unlimited coverage on most services — to individuals, and

Supplemental Premium Rates and Maximum Premium Rates for Beneficiaries Meeting or Exceeding Income Limits

	1988	1989	1990	1991	1992	1993
Premium rates for each $150 of income tax liability	$0	$22.50	$27.14	$30.17	$30.55	$29.55
Prescription drug premium	$0	$0	$10.36	$ 8.83	$ 9.95	$12.45
Total Premium per $150 of tax	$0	$22.50	$37.50	$39.00	$40.50	$42.00
Maximum Premium per taxable year	$0	$800	$850	$900	$950	$1050

The Secretary of the Treasury will direct the development of Premium Tables indexed for income tax liability. This premium will be collected at income tax time each year. It **is not** paid on a monthly basis.

SOURCE: Medicare Catastrophic Coverage Act of 1988, Report 100-661, page 161.

(Do not write in this space)

APPLICATION FOR RETIREMENT INSURANCE BENEFITS

I apply for all insurance benefits for which I am eligible under Title II (Federal Old-Age, Survivors, and Disability Insurance) and Title XVIII (Health Insurance for the Aged and Disabled) of the Social Security Act, as presently amended.

☐ Supplement. If you have already completed an application entitled "APPLICATION FOR WIFE'S OR HUSBAND'S INSURANCE BENEFITS", you need complete only the circled items. All other claimants must complete the entire form.

1. **(a)** PRINT your name — FIRST NAME, MIDDLE INITIAL, LAST NAME

(b) Enter your name at birth if different from item (a) — FIRST NAME, MIDDLE INITIAL, LAST NAME

(c) Check (✓) whether you are ⟶ ☐ Male ☐ Female

2. Enter your Social Security Number ⟶ _ _ _ / _ _ / _ _ _ _

3. **(a)** Enter your date of birth ⟶ MONTH, DAY, YEAR

(b) Enter name of State or foreign country where you were born. ⟶

If you have already presented, or if you are now presenting, a public or religious record of your birth established before you were age 5, go on to item 4.

(c) Was a public record of your birth made before you were age 5? ☐ Yes ☐ No ☐ Unknown

(d) Was a religious record of your birth made before you were age 5? ☐ Yes ☐ No ☐ Unknown

4. **(a)** Have you (or has someone on your behalf) ever filed an application for Social Security benefits, a period of disability under Social Security, supplemental security income, or hospital or medical insurance under Medicare? ⟶
☐ Yes *(If "Yes," answer (b) and (c).)*   ☐ No *(If "No," go on to item 5.)*

(b) Enter name of person on whose Social Security record you filed other application. ⟶ (First name, middle initial, last name)

(c) Enter Social Security Number of person named in (b). *(If unknown, so indicate)* ⟶ _ _ _ / _ _ / _ _ _ _

Do not answer 5 if you are age 66 and 5 months, or older. Go on to question 6.

5. **(a)** Are you so disabled that you cannot work or was there some period during the last 14 months when you were so disabled that you could not work? ⟶ ☐ Yes ☐ No

(b) If "Yes," enter the date you became disabled. ⟶ MONTH, DAY, YEAR

6. **(a)** Were you in the active military or naval service (including Reserve or National Guard *active* duty or active duty for training) after September 7, 1939 and before 1968? ⟶
☐ Yes *(If "Yes," answer (b) and (c).)*   ☐ No *(If "No," go on to item 7.)*

(b) Enter dates of service. ⟶ From: (Month, year)   To: (Month, year)

(c) Have you *ever* been (or will you be) eligible for a monthly benefit from a military or civilian Federal agency? (include Veterans Administration benefits *only* if you waived military retirement pay) ☐ Yes ☐ No

7. Have you or your spouse worked in the railroad industry for 7 years or more? ☐ Yes ☐ No

| 8. | (a) | Have you ever engaged in work that was covered under the social security system of a country other than the United States? ⟶ | ☐ Yes ☐ No *(If "Yes," answer (b).) (If "No," go on to item 9.)* |
| | (b) | If "Yes," list the country(ies). ⟶ | |

| 9. | Have you ever been married? ⟶ | ☐ Yes ☐ No *(If "Yes," answer item 10) (If "No," go to item 12.)* |

10.

(a) Give the following information about your current marriage. If not currently married, show your last marriage below.

To whom married		When *(Month, day, year)*	Where *(Name of City and State)*
Your current or last marriage	How marriage ended *(If still in effect, write "Not ended.")*	When *(Month, day, year)*	Where *(Name of City and State)*
	Marriage performed by: ☐ Clergyman or public official ☐ Other *(Explain in Remarks)*	Spouse's date of birth (or age)	If spouse deceased, give date of death
	Spouse's Social Security Number (If none or unknown so indicate) __ __ __ / __ __ / __ __ __ __		

(b) Give the following information about each of your previous marriages. **(IF NONE, WRITE "NONE")**

To whom married		When *(Month, day, year)*	Where *(Name of City and State)*
Your previous marriage (Use a separate statement for information about any other marriages)	How marriage ended	When *(Month, day, year)*	Where *(Name of City and State)*
	Marriage performed by: ☐ Clergyman or public official ☐ Other *(Explain in Remarks)*	Spouse's date of birth (or age)	If spouse deceased, give date of death
	Spouse's Social Security Number (If none or unknown so indicate) __ __ __ / __ __ / __ __ __ __		

11. If you are currently married, answer this question only if your spouse is within 3 months of age 62 or older, or has a child-in-care who is eligible on your earnings record.
Do you wish this application to protect your spouse's right to Social Security benefits? ☐ Yes ☐ No

12. List below FULL NAME OF ALL your children (including natural children, adopted children, and stepchildren) or dependent grandchildren (including stepgrandchildren) who are now or were in the past 6 months UNMARRIED and.
 • UNDER AGE 18 • AGE 18 TO 19 AND ATTENDING SECONDARY SCHOOL
 • DISABLED OR HANDICAPPED (age 18 or over and disability began before age 22)
Also list any student who is between the ages of 18 to 23 if such student was both: 1. Previously entitled to Social Security benefits on any Social Security record for August 1981, and 2. Was also in full-time attendance at a post-secondary school prior to May 1982.
(IF THERE ARE NO SUCH CHILDREN, WRITE "NONE" BELOW AND GO ON TO ITEM 13.)

13. Enter below the names and addresses of all the persons, companies, or government agencies for whom you have worked this year, last year, and the year before last.
IF NONE, WRITE "NONE" BELOW AND GO ON TO ITEM 15.

(a) NAME AND ADDRESS OF EMPLOYER *(If you had more than one employer, please list them in order beginning with your last (most recent) employer)*	Work Began		Work Ended *(If still working, Show "Not ended")*	
	Month	Year	Month	Year

(b) Are you an officer of a corporation, or are you related to an officer of a corporation? ⟶	☐ Yes ☐ No

14. May we ask your employers for wage information needed to process your claim? ⟶ ☐ Yes ☐ No

15 (a)	THIS ITEM MUST BE COMPLETED, EVEN IF YOU ARE AN EMPLOYEE Were you self-employed this year, last year, or the year before? ➞	☐ Yes *(If "Yes," answer (b).)* ☐ No *(If "No," skip to item 16.)*

(b) Check the year or years in which you were self-employed	In what kind of trade or business were you self-employed? *(For example, storekeeper, farmer, physician)*	Were your net earnings from your trade or business $400 or more? *(Check "Yes" or "No")*
☐ This year		
☐ Last year		☐ Yes ☐ No
☐ Year before last		☐ Yes ☐ No

16. (a) How much were your total earnings last year? ➞ $ _____

(b) Place an "X" in each block for EACH MONTH of last year in which you did not earn more than * $ _____ in wages, and did not perform substantial services in self-employment. These months are exempt months. If no months were exempt months, place an "X" in "NONE". If all months were exempt months, place an "X" in "ALL".

* Enter the appropriate monthly limit after reading the instructions, "How Your Earnings Affect Your Benefits".

NONE		ALL	
Jan.	Feb.	Mar.	Apr.
May	Jun.	Jul.	Aug.
Sept.	Oct.	Nov.	Dec.

17. (a) How much do you expect your total earnings to be this year? ➞ $ _____

(b) Place an "X" in each block for EACH MONTH of this year in which you did not or will not earn more than * $ _____ in wages, and did not or will not perform substantial services in self-employment. If no months are or will be exempt months, place an "X" in "NONE". If all months are or will be exempt months, place an "X" in "ALL".

* Enter the appropriate monthly limit after reading the instructions, "How Your Earnings Affect Your Benefits".

NONE		ALL	
Jan.	Feb.	Mar.	Apr.
May	Jun.	Jul.	Aug.
Sept.	Oct.	Nov.	Dec.

18. Answer this item ONLY if you are now in the last 4 months of your taxable year (Sept., Oct., Nov., and Dec., if your taxable year is a calendar year).

(a) How much do you expect to earn next year? ➞ $ _____

(b) Place an "X" in each block for EACH MONTH of next year in which you do not expect to earn more than * $ _____ in wages, and do not expect to perform substantial services in self-employment. These months will be exempt months. If no months are expected to be exempt months, place an "X" in "NONE". If all months are expected to be exempt months, place an "X" in "ALL".

* Enter the appropriate monthly limit after reading the instructions, "How Your Earnings Affect Your Benefits".

NONE		ALL	
Jan.	Feb.	Mar.	Apr.
May	Jun.	Jul.	Aug.
Sept.	Oct.	Nov.	Dec.

An ANNUAL REPORT of earnings must be filed with the Social Security Administration within 3 months and 15 days after the end of any taxable year in which you earn more than the yearly limit, if you are under age 70 for at least 1 full month of that year and receive some benefits during the taxable year. I AGREE TO FILE AN ANNUAL REPORT OF EARNINGS. THE ANNUAL REPORT IS REQUIRED BY LAW AND FAILURE TO REPORT MAY RESULT IN A MONETARY PENALTY.

19. If you use a fiscal year, that is, a taxable year that does not end December 31 (with income tax return due April 15), enter here the month your fiscal year ends. ➞ (Month) _____

IF YOU ARE AGE 65 AND 6 MONTHS, OR OLDER, DO NOT ANSWER ITEM 20. GO ON TO ITEM 21.

PLEASE READ CAREFULLY THE INFORMATION ON THE OPPOSITE PAGE AND ANSWER ONE OF THE FOLLOWING ITEMS. ➞

20. (a) I want benefits beginning with the earliest possible month that will be the most advantageous. ➞ ☐

(b) I am age 65 (or will be age 65 within 4 months) and I want benefits beginning with the earliest possible month that will be the most advantageous providing there is no permanent reduction in my ongoing ➞ ☐
monthly benefit.

(c) I want benefits beginning with _____ . I understand that either a higher initial payment or a higher continuing monthly benefit amount may be possible, but I choose not to take it. ➞ ☐

Form **SSA-1-F6** (1-86) Page 3   **(Turn to Page 4)**

If this claim is approved and you are still entitled to benefits at age 65, you will automatically have hospital insurance protection under Medicare at age 65. If you are not also eligible for automatic enrollment in the Supplementary Medical Insurance Plan, this application may be used for voluntary enrollment.

COMPLETE THIS ITEM ONLY IF YOU ARE WITHIN 3 MONTHS OF AGE 65 OR OLDER

ENROLLMENT IN MEDICARE'S SUPPLEMENTARY MEDICAL INSURANCE PLAN: The medical insurance benefits plan pays for most of the costs of physicians' and surgeons' services, and related medical services which are not covered by the hospital insurance plan. Coverage under this SUPPLEMENTARY MEDICAL INSURANCE PLAN does not apply to most medical expenses incurred outside the United States. Your Social Security district office will be glad to explain the details of the plan and give you a leaflet which explains what services are covered and how payment is made under the plan.

Once you are enrolled in this plan, you will have to pay a monthly premium to cover part of the cost of your medical insurance protection. The Federal Government contributes an equal amount or more toward the cost of your insurance. Premiums will be deducted from any monthly Social Security, railroad retirement, or civil service benefit checks you receive. If you do not receive such benefits, you will be notified about when, where, and how to pay your premiums. If you are eligible for automatic enrollment, you will be automatically enrolled unless you indicate, by checking the "NO" block below, that you do not want to be enrolled.

21.	DO YOU WISH TO ENROLL IN THE MEDICARE SUPPLEMENTARY MEDICAL INSURANCE PLAN? ⟶	☐ Yes	☐ No

Answer question 22 ONLY if you were born January 2, 1924, or later. Otherwise, go on to question 23.

22.	(a)	Are you entitled to, or do you expect to become entitled to, a pension or annuity based on work after 1956 not covered by Social Security?	☐ Yes (If "Yes," answer (b) and (c).)	☐ No (If "No," go on to item 23.)
	(b) ☐	I became entitled, or expect to become entitled, beginning ⟶	MONTH	YEAR
	(c) ☐	I became eligible, or expect to become eligible, beginning ⟶	MONTH	YEAR

I agree to notify the Social Security Administration if I become entitled to a pension or annuity based on employment after 1956 not covered by Social Security, or if such pension or annuity stops.

It is possible for your Social Security monthly payments to be forwarded directly to your bank, savings and loan, credit union, or other financial organization for deposit to your account. This method of payment is known as direct deposit. If you wish direct deposit you will have to contact your financial organization to complete the necessary form. We will advise you when your direct deposit request is processed. If you do not wish direct deposit your benefits will be paid by check to your mailing address.

23.	Do you plan to file a form through your financial organization to begin direct deposit payments? ⟶	☐ Yes	☐ No

It is possible that your claim will be ready to be paid before the direct deposit form is returned by your financial organization. Your claim will be processed and any payments due will be sent to you until your direct deposit request is received.

REMARKS *(You may use this space for any explanations. If you need more space, attach a separate sheet.)*

_____
_____
_____
_____
_____

I know that anyone who makes or causes to be made a false statement or representation of material fact in an application or for use in determining a right to payment under the Social Security Act commits a crime punishable under Federal law by fine, imprisonment or both. I affirm that all information I have given in this document is true.

SIGNATURE OF APPLICANT	Date *(Month, day, year)*
Signature *(First name, middle initial, last name) (Write in ink)*	Telephone number (s) at which you may be contacted during the day
SIGN HERE ⟶	_____ _____ _____ Area Code

Mailing Address *(Number and street, Apt. No., P.O. Box, or Rural Route) (Enter Resident Address in "Remarks", if Different.)*

City and State	ZIP Code	Enter Name of County (if any) in which you now live

Witnesses are required ONLY if this application has been signed by mark (X) above. If signed by mark (X), two witnesses who know the applicant must sign below, giving their full addresses. Also, print the applicant's name in the Signature block.

1. Signature of Witness	2. Signature of Witness
Address *(Number and street, City, State and ZIP Code)*	Address *(Number and street, City, State and ZIP Code)*

CHANGES TO BE REPORTED AND HOW TO REPORT

Failure to report may result in overpayments that must be repaid, and in possible monetary penalties

▶ You change your mailing address for checks or residence. To avoid delay in receipt of checks you should ALSO file a regular change of address notice with your post office.

▶ You go outside the U.S.A.

▶ Any beneficiary dies or becomes unable to handle benefits.

▶ Work Changes-On your application you told us you expect total earnings for 19___ to be $_____ .

You (are) (are not) earning wages of more than $_____a month.

You (are) (are not) self-employed rendering substantial services in your trade or business.

(Report AT ONCE if above work pattern changes)

▶ You are confined to jail, prison, penal institution, or correctional facility for conviction of a felony.

▶ You become entitled to a pension or annuity based on employment after 1956 not covered by Social Security, or if such pension or annuity stops.

▶ Custody Change—Report if a person for whom you are filing or who is in your care dies, leaves your care or custody, or changes address.

▶ Change of Marital Status—Marriage, divorce, annulment of marriage.

HOW TO REPORT

You can make your reports by telephone, mail, or in person, whichever you prefer.

WHEN A CHANGE OCCURS AFTER YOU RECEIVE A NOTICE OF AWARD, YOU SHOULD REPORT BY CALLING THE APPROPRIATE TELEPHONE NUMBER SHOWN NEAR THE TOP OF PAGE 6.

In addition, an annual report of earnings must be filed with the Social Security Administration within 3 months and 15 days after the end of any taxable year in which you earned more than the annual exempt amount.

THE ANNUAL REPORT OF EARNINGS IS REQUIRED BY LAW AND FAILURE TO REPORT MAY RESULT IN A MONETARY PENALTY.

PLEASE READ THE FOLLOWING INFORMATION CAREFULLY BEFORE YOU ANSWER QUESTION 20.

Benefits may be payable for some months prior to the month in which you file this claim (but not for any month before the first month you will be age 62 for the entire month) if:

(1) you have a child or spouse entitled to unreduced benefits based on your earnings during any of the past 6 months;

—OR—

(2) you will earn over the exempt amount this year. (For appropriate exempt amount, see the instructions, "How Your Earnings Affect Your Benefits".

If your first month of entitlement is prior to age 65, your benefit rate will be reduced. However if you do not actually receive your full benefit amount for one or more months before age 65 because benefits are withheld due to your earnings, your benefit will be increased at age 65 to give credit for this withholding. Thus, your benefit amount at age 65 will be reduced only if you receive one or more full benefit payments prior to the month you are 65.

Form SSA-1-F6 (1-86) Page 5

RECEIPT FOR YOUR CLAIM FOR SOCIAL SECURITY RETIREMENT INSURANCE BENEFITS

| TELEPHONE NUMBER(S) TO CALL IF YOU HAVE A QUESTION OR SOMETHING TO REPORT | **BEFORE** YOU RECEIVE A NOTICE OF AWARD | SSA OFFICE | DATE CLAIM RECEIVED |
| | **AFTER** YOU RECEIVE A NOTICE OF AWARD | | |

Your application for Social Security benefits has been received and will be processed as quickly as possible.

You should hear from us within____ days after you have given us all the information we requested. Some claims may take longer if additional information is needed.

In the meantime, if you change your address, or if there is some other change that may affect your claim, you—or someone for you—should report the change. The changes to be reported are listed on page 5.

Always give us your claim number when writing or telephoning about your claim.

If you have any questions about your claim, we will be glad to help you.

| CLAIMANT | SOCIAL SECURITY CLAIM NUMBER |
| | |

Collection and Use of Information From Your Application — Privacy Act/Paperwork Act Notice

The Social Security Administration is authorized to collect the information on this form under sections 202(a), 205(a) and 1872 of the Social Security Act, as amended (42 U.S.C. 402(a), 405(a), and 1395ii). While it is voluntary, except in the circumstances explained below, for you to furnish the information on this form to Social Security, no benefits may be paid unless an application has been received by a Social Security office. Your response is mandatory where the refusal to disclose certain information affecting your right to payment would reflect a fraudulent intent to secure benefits not authorized by the Social Security Act. The information on this form is needed to enable Social Security to determine if you and your dependents are entitled to insurance coverage and/or monthly benefits. Failure to provide all or part of this information could prevent an accurate and timely decision on your claim or your dependent's claim, and could result in the loss of some benefits or insurance coverage. Although the information you furnish on this form is almost never used for any other purpose than stated in the foregoing, there is a possibility that for the administration of the Social Security programs or for the administration of programs requiring coordination with the Social Security Administration, information may be disclosed to another person or to another governmental agency as follows: 1. to enable a third party or an agency to assist Social Security in establishing rights to Social Security benefits and/or coverage; 2. to comply with Federal laws requiring the release of information from Social Security records (e.g., to the General Accounting Office and the Veterans Administration); and 3. to facilitate statistical research and audit activities necessary to assure the integrity and improvement of the Social Security programs (e.g., to the Bureau of the Census and private concerns under contract to Social Security).

APPLICATION FOR ENROLLMENT IN MEDICARE
THE MEDICAL INSURANCE PROGRAM

(TID) SMI

1. SOCIAL SECURITY CLAIM NUMBER

(CAN) ☐ ☐ ☐ — ☐ ☐ — ☐ ☐ ☐ ☐

2. FOR AGENCY USE ONLY

(BIC) ☐ ☐ ☐

3. DO YOU WISH TO ENROLL FOR MEDICAL INSURANCE UNDER MEDICARE?

(DEC) YES ☐

4. CLAIMANT'S NAME

(CLN)

Last name   First name   Middle initial

5. PRINT SOCIAL SECURITY NUMBER HOLDER'S NAME IF DIFFERENT FROM YOURS

6. MAILING ADDRESS (NUMBER AND STREET, P.O. BOX, OR ROUTE)

IF THIS IS A CHANGE OF ADDRESS, CHECK HERE ☐

7. CITY, STATE, AND ZIP CODE

8. TELEPHONE NUMBER

9. WRITTEN SIGNATURE (DO NOT PRINT)

SIGN HERE ➡

10. DATE SIGNED

(DOF) _ _ / _ _ / _ _
　　　MONTH　DAY　YEAR

IF THIS APPLICATION HAS BEEN SIGNED BY MARK (X), A WITNESS WHO KNOWS THE APPLICANT MUST SUPPLY THE INFORMATION REQUESTED BELOW

11. SIGNATURE OF WITNESS

12. DATE SIGNED

13. ADDRESS OF WITNESS

14. REMARKS

(TOA) 1

TO: (Circle one)

(1) NEPSC	(2) MATPSC	(3) SEPSC	(4) GLPSC	(5) WNPSC	(6) MAMPSC	(7) ODO	(8) DIO

FORM HCFA-40B (3/86)

PRIVACY ACT NOTICE

The following information is given pursuant to the Privacy Act of 1974. The Social Security Administration is authorized to collect information about your medical insurance enrollment. While completing this form is voluntary, failure to provide all or part of this information will result in your not being enrolled for medical insurance under Medicare. The routine uses for information obtained are fully explained and published annually in the Federal Register. The Social Security Administration will further explain these uses upon request.

SPECIAL MESSAGE FOR INDIVIDUAL APPLYING
FOR MEDICAL INSURANCE UNDER MEDICARE

This form is your application for the medical insurance part of Medicare. It can be used either during your personal enrollment period or during any general enrollment period.

Your personal enrollment period lasts for 7 months. It begins 3 months before the month you reach age 65 (or 3 months before the 25th month you have received social security disability benefits) and it ends 3 months after you reach age 65 (or 3 months after the 25th month you have received social security disability benefits). To have medical insurance start in the month you are 65 (or the 25th month of disability insurance benefits), you must sign up in the first 3 months of your personal enrollment period. If you sign up in any of the remaining 4 months, your medical insurance starting date will be later.

If you do not file during your personal enrollment period, you can file any time after that during a general enrollment period which is the first 3 months of every year. If you sign up in a general enrollment period, your medical insurance begins July 1 of that year. However, when you file in a general enrollment period, your premium may be subject to a penalty increase. For each 12 month period elapsing between the end of your personal enrollment period and the general enrollment period in which you file, your premium will be increased 10 percent.

☆ U.S.G.P.O.: 1986-491-258/53764

Form Approved
OMB No. 72-R0705

(Do not write in this space)

APPLICATION FOR HOSPITAL INSURANCE

(This application form may also be used to
enroll in Supplementary Medical Insurance)

I apply for entitlement to Medicare's hospital insurance under Part A of title XVIII of the Social Security Act, as presently amended, and for any cash benefits to which I may be entitled under title II of that Act.

1.	(a) Print your name ⟶	(First name, middle initial, last name)
	(b) Enter your sex (check one) ⟶	☐ Male ☐ Female
	(c) Enter your Social Security Number ⟶	__ __ __/__ __/__ __ __ __
2.	Enter your name at birth if different from item 1 ⟶	
3.	(a) Enter your date of birth (Month, day, year) ⟶	
	(b) Enter name of State or foreign country where you were born ⟶ If you have already submitted a public or religious record of your birth made before you were age 5, go on to item 4)	
	(c) Was a public record of your birth made before you were age 5?	☐ Yes ☐ No ☐ Unknown
	(d) Was a religious record of your birth made before you were age 5?	☐ Yes ☐ No ☐ Unknown
4.	(a) Have you (or has someone on your behalf) ever filed an application for social security benefits, a period of disability under social security, supplemental security income, or hospital or medical insurance under Medicare? ⟶	☐ Yes ☐ No If "Yes," answer (If "No," go on (b) and (c).) to item 5.)
	(b) Enter name of person on whose social security record you filed other application. ⟶	
	(c) Enter Social Security Number of person named in (b). (If unknown, so indicate) ⟶	__ __ __/__ __/__ __ __ __
5.	(a) Were you in the active military or naval service (including Reserve or National Guard *active* duty or active duty for training) after September 7, 1939? ⟶	☐ Yes ☐ No If "Yes," answer (If "No," go on (b) and (c).) to item 7.
	(b) Enter dates of service ⟶	From: (Month, year) | To: (Month, year)
	(c) Have you *ever* been (or will you be) eligible for a monthly benefit from a military or civilian Federal agency? (Include Veterans Administration benefits *only* if you waived military retirement pay) ⟶	☐ Yes ☐ No
6.	Did you work in the railroad industry any time on or after January 1, 1937? ⟶	☐ Yes ☐ No

| 7. | (a) Have you ever engaged in work that was covered under the social security system of a country other than the United States? ⟶ | ☐ Yes   ☐ No |
| | (b) If "Yes," list the country(ies). ⟶ | |

| 8. | (a) How much were your total earnings last year? ⟶ *(If none, write "None")* | Earnings
$ |
| | (b) How much do you expect your total earnings to be this year? ⟶ *(If none, write "None")* | Earnings
$ |

| 9. | Are you a resident of the United States? ⟶ *(To reside in a place means to make a home there.)* | ☐ Yes   ☐ No |

| 10. | (a) Are you a citizen of the United States? ⟶ *(If "Yes," go on to item 11.) (If "No," answer (b) and (c) below.)* | ☐ Yes   ☐ No |
| | (b) Are you lawfully admitted for permanent residence in the United States? ⟶ | ☐ Yes   ☐ No |

(c) Enter below the information requested about your place of residence in the last 5 years:

ADDRESS AT WHICH YOU RESIDED IN THE LAST 5 YEARS (Begin with the most recent address. Show actual date residence began even if that is prior to the last 5 years.)	DATE RESIDENCE BEGAN			DATE RESIDENCE ENDED		
	Month	Day	Year	Month	Day	Year

(If you need more space, use the "Remarks" space on the third page or another sheet of paper)

| 11. | Are you currently married? ⟶ | ☐ Yes   ☐ No |

(If "Yes," give the following information about your current marriage.) (If "No," go on to item 12.)

YOUR CURRENT MARRIAGE

To whom married *(Enter your wife's maiden name or your husband's name)*	When *(Month, day, year)*
Spouse's date of birth (or age)	Spouse's Social Security Number *(If none or unknown, so indicate)* ___ ___ ___ / ___ ___ / ___ ___ ___ ___

12. If you had a previous marriage and your spouse died, OR if you had a previous marriage which lasted 10 or more years, give the following information. *(If you had no previous marriage (s), enter "NONE.")*

YOUR PREVIOUS MARRIAGE

To whom married *(Enter your wife's maiden name or your husband's name).*	When *(Month, day, year)*
Spouse's date of birth (or age)	Spouse's Social Security Number *(If none or unknown, so indicate)* ___ ___ ___ / ___ ___ / ___ ___ ___ ___
If spouse deceased, give date of death ⟶	

(Use "Remarks" space on page 3 for information about any other marriages.)

Form **SSA-18 F5** (3-80) Page 2

13.	Is or was your spouse a railroad worker, railroad retirement pensioner, or a railroad retirement annuitant? ⟶	☐ Yes	☐ No
14.	(a) Were you or your spouse a civilian employee of the Federal Government after June 1960? ⟶ (If "Yes," answer (b).) (If "No," omit (b), (c), and (d).)	☐ Yes	☐ No
	(b) Are you or your spouse now covered under a medical insurance plan provided by the Federal Employees Health Benefits Act of 1959? ⟶ (If "Yes," omit (c) and (d).) (If "No," answer (c).)	☐ Yes	☐ No
	(c) Are you **and** your spouse barred from coverage under the above Act because your Federal employment, or your spouse's was not long enough? ⟶ (If "Yes," omit (d) and explain in "Remarks" below.) (If "No," answer (d).)	☐ Yes	☐ No
	(d) Were either you or your spouse an employee of the Federal Government after February 15, 1965? ⟶	☐ Yes	☐ No

Remarks:

_____

_____

_____

_____

_____

_____

| 15. | If you are found to be otherwise ineligible for hospital insurance under Medicare, do you wish to enroll for hospital insurance on a monthly premium basis (in addition to the monthly premium for supplementary medical insurance)? ⟶
 (If "Yes," you MUST also sign up for medical insurance.) | ☐ Yes | ☐ No |

INFORMATION ON MEDICAL INSURANCE UNDER MEDICARE

Medical insurance under Medicare helps pay your doctor bills. It also helps pay for a number of other medical items and services not covered under the hospital insurance part of Medicare.

If you sign up for medical insurance, you must pay a premium for each month you have this protection. If you get monthly social security, railroad retirement, or civil service benefits, your premium will be deducted from your benefit check. If you get none of these benefits, you will be notified how to pay your premium.

The Federal Government contributes to the cost of your insurance. The amount of your premium and the Government's payment are based on the cost of services covered by medical insurance. The Government also makes additional payments when necessary to meet the full cost of the program. (Currently, the Government pays about two-thirds of the cost of this program.) You will get advance notice if there is any change in your premium amount.

If you have questions or would like a leaflet on medical insurance, call any Social Security office.

> SEE OTHER SIDE TO SIGN UP FOR MEDICAL INSURANCE

Form **SSA-18 F5** (3-80) Page 3   (Over)

If you become entitled to hospital insurance as a result of this application, you will be enrolled for medical insurance automatically unless you indicate below that you do not want this protection. If you decline to enroll now, you can get medical insurance protection later only if you sign up for it during specified enrollment periods. Your protection may then be delayed and you may have to pay a higher premium when you decide to sign up.

The date your medical insurance begins and the amount of the premium you must pay depend on the month you file this application with the Social Security Administration. Any social security office will be glad to explain the rules regarding enrollment to you.

16.	**DO YOU WISH TO ENROLL FOR SUPPLEMENTARY MEDICAL INSURANCE?** ⟶ *(If "Yes," answer question 17.)*	☐ Yes ☐ No ☐ Currently Enrolled

17.	Are you or your spouse receiving an annuity under the Federal Civil Service Retirement Act, or other law administered by the Office of Personnel Management ? ⟶	☐ Yes ☐ No
	(If "Yes," enter Civil Service annuity number here. Include the prefix "CSA" for annuitant, "CSF" for survivor.)	Your No. _____ Spouse's No. _____
	If you entered your spouse's number, is he (she) enrolled for supplementary medical insurance under social security? ⟶	☐ Yes ☐ No

I know that anyone who makes or causes to be made a false statement or representation of material fact in an application or for use in determining a right to payment under the Social Security Act commits a crime punishable under Federal law by fine, imprisonment or both. I affirm that all information I have given in this document is true.

SIGNATURE OF APPLICANT	Date *(Month, day, year)*
Signature *(First name, middle initial, last name) (Write in ink)* **SIGN HERE** ▶	Telephone Number(s) at which you may be contacted during the day

Mailing Address *(Number and street, Apt. No., P.O. Box, or Rural Route)*

City and State	ZIP Code	Enter Name of County (if any) in which you now live

Witnesses are required ONLY if this application has been signed by mark (X) above. If signed by mark (X), two witnesses to the signing who know the applicant must sign below, giving their full addresses.

1. Signature of Witness	2. Signature of Witness
Address *(Number and street, City, State, and ZIP Code)*	Address *(Number and street, City, State, and ZIP Code)*

A REMINDER TO APPLICANTS FOR THE SOCIAL SECURITY HOSPITAL INSURANCE

NAME OF PERSON TO CONTACT ABOUT YOUR CLAIM	SSA OFFICE	DATE
TELEPHONE NO.		

RECEIPT FOR YOUR CLAIM

Your application for the hospital insurance has been received and will be processed as quickly as possible.

You should hear from us within   days after you have given us all the information we requested. Some claims may take longer if additional information is needed.

In the meantime, if you change your mailing address, you should report the change.

Always give us your claim number when writing or telephoning about your claim.

If you have any questions about your claim, we will be glad to help you.

CLAIMANT	SOCIAL SECURITY CLAIM NUMBER

COLLECTION AND USE OF INFORMATION FROM YOUR APPLICATION — PRIVACY ACT NOTICE

PRIVACY ACT NOTICE: The Social Security Administration (SSA) is authorized to collect the information on this form under sections 226 and 1818 of the Social Security Act, as amended (42 U.S.C. 426 and 1395-17) and section 103 of Public Law 89-97. The information on this form is needed to enable social security and the Health Care Financing Administration (HCFA) to determine if you and your dependents may be entitled to hospital and/or medical insurance coverage and/or monthly benefits. While you do not have to furnish the information requested on this form to social security, no benefits or hospital or medical insurance can be provided until an application has been received by a social security office. Failure to provide all or part of the information requested could prevent an accurate and timely decision on your claim or your dependent's claim, and could result in the loss of some benefits or hospital or medical insurance. Although the infor-

mation you furnish on this form is almost never used for any other purpose than stated above, there is a possibility that for the administration of the social security or HCFA programs or for the administration of programs requiring coordination with SSA or HCFA, information may be disclosed to another person or to another governmental agency as follows: 1) to enable a third party or an agency to assist social security or HCFA in establishing rights to social security benefits and/or hospital or medical insurance coverage; 2) to comply with Federal laws requiring the release of information from social security and HCFA records (e.g., to the General Accounting Office and the Veterans Administration); and 3) to facilitate statistical research and audit activities necessary to assure the integrity and improvement of the social security and HCFA programs (e.g., to the Bureau of the Census and private concerns under contract to social security and HCFA).

Form **SSA-18 F5** (3-80) Page 5

DEPARTMENT OF HEALTH, EDUCATION AND WELFARE
Health Care Financing Administration

FORM APPROVED
OMB NO 66-R0123

APPLICATION FOR HEALTH INSURANCE BENEFITS
UNDER MEDICARE FOR INDIVIDUAL
WITH CHRONIC RENAL DISEASE

I hereby request that my right to health insurance benefits be determined under Section 226 (A) of the Social Security Act.

1.	Print Your Full Name *(First name, middle initial, last name)*	Enter your Social Security Number
		___ __ — __ __ — __ __ __ __

2.	Check (✓) whether you are: ☐ Male ☐ Female	Enter your maiden name *(if applicable)*

3.	Enter your date of birth (Month, day, year) ───▶	

4.	(a) Have you received regularly scheduled dialysis? ───▶ *(If "Yes," answer (b).)* *(If "No," go to 6.)*	☐ Yes ☐ No
	(b) Enter beginning date(s) and ending date(s) (if applicable) of all periods of regularly scheduled dialysis *(month, year)* ───▶	Dialysis Began: Ended:

5.	(a) Have you participated (or do you expect to participate) in a self-dialysis training program? ───▶ *(If "Yes," answer (b).)* *(If "No," go to 6.)*	☐ Yes ☐ No
	(b) Enter date self-dialysis training began (or is expected to begin) *(month, year)* ───▶	

6.	(a) Have you received a kidney transplant? ───▶ *(If "Yes," answer (b).)* *(If "No," go to (e).)*	☐ Yes ☐ No
	(b) Enter date(s) of transplant(s) *(month, year)* ───▶	
	(c) Were you in a hospital for transplant surgery or for necessary procedures preliminary to transplant before the month you actually received the transplant? ───▶ *(If "Yes," answer (d).)* *(If "No," go to 7.)*	☐ Yes ☐ No
	(d) Enter dates of hospitalization for 6(c) *(month, day, year)* ───▶	From: To:
	(e) If you are scheduled to receive a transplant, enter date *(month, year)* ───▶	

7. ENROLLMENT IN THE SUPPLEMENTARY MEDICAL INSURANCE PLAN: The medical insurance benefits plan pays for most of the costs of physicians' and surgeons' services, and other covered medical services such as OUTPATIENT MAINTENANCE DIALYSIS TREATMENTS, which are not covered by the hospital insurance plan. This plan covers outpatient treatment provided in a hospital or a facility which meets prescribed conditions. It also COVERS HOME DIALYSIS, including the rental or purchase of home dialysis machine, and the purchase of disposable equipment and supplies needed for the dialysis.

Coverage under this SUPPLEMENTARY MEDICAL INSURANCE PLAN does not apply to most medical expenses incurred outside the United States. Your social security district office will be glad to explain the details of the plan and give you a leaflet which explains what services are covered and how payment is made under the plan.

Once you are enrolled in this plan, you will have to pay a monthly premium to cover part of the cost of your medical insurance protection. The Federal Government contributes an equal amount or more toward the cost of your insurance. Premiums will be deducted from any monthly social security, railroad retirement, or civil service benefit checks you receive. If you do not receive such benefits, you will be notified about when, where, and how to pay your premiums.

YOU WILL BE AUTOMATICALLY ENROLLED IN THIS PLAN UNLESS YOU INDICATE, BY CHECKING THE "NO" BLOCK BELOW, THAT YOU DO NOT WANT TO BE ENROLLED.

(a) DO YOU WISH TO ENROLL IN THE SUPPLEMENTARY MEDICAL INSURANCE PLAN? *(If "No", go to 8.)*   ☐ Yes   ☐ No

(b) If your application is processed within 5 months after the first month in which you meet all the requirements for your Medicare entitlement, your coverage will begin with that first month.
If your application is processed more than 5 months after your first possible month of entitlement, you may choose one of the following for your first month of coverage. (Please check one):

*The earliest possible month of entitlement, if you are willing and able to pay all premiums for past months of coverage   ☐

OR

*The month in which this application is filed, if it is the same as, or later than, your first possible month of entitlement   ☐

OR

*The month in which this enrollment will be processed   ☐

ITEMS 8 THROUGH 16 REQUEST INFORMATION NEEDED TO DETERMINE INSURED STATUS FOR MEDICARE ENTITLEMENT.

8. (a) Have you (or has someone on your behalf) ever filed an application for social security benefits, a period of disability under social security, or hospital or medical insurance under Medicare?   ☐ Yes   ☐ No
(If "Yes," answer (b) and (c).)
(If "No," go to 9.)

(b) Enter name of person(s) on whose social security record(s) you filed other application(s)   *(First, middle initial, last)*

(c) Enter social security number(s) of person(s) named in (b). *(If unknown, so indicate.)*

9. (a) Have you (or has someone on your behalf) ever filed an application for monthly benefits or hospital or medical insurance under Medicare with the Railroad Retirement Board?   ☐ Yes   ☐ No
(If "Yes," answer (b) and (c).)
(If "No," go to 10.)

(b) Enter the name of person(s) on whose railroad record you filed other application(s)   *(First, middle initial, last)*

(c) Enter Railroad Number of person named in (b). *(If unknown, so indicate.)*

Form **HCFA-43** (11-78) (Page 2)

IF YOU ARE ALREADY ENTITLED TO A MONTHLY SOCIAL SECURITY BENEFIT OR A MONTHLY RAILROAD ANNUITY, DO NOT COMPLETE ITEMS 10 THROUGH 16.

10.	(a) Were you in the active military or naval service (including Reserve or National Guard active duty or active duty for training) after September 7, 1939? ———————————▶ *(If "Yes," answer (b).) (If "No," go to 11.)*	☐ Yes ☐ No

	(b) Enter dates of service ————————————————▶	FROM: *(Month, year)*	TO: *(Month, year)*

11.	Have you worked in the railroad industry any time on or after January 1, 1937? ———————————▶	☐ Yes ☐ No

12.
- Enter below the names and addresses of all the persons, companies, or Government agencies for whom you worked during the last 12 months.
- If you worked in agricultural employment, give this information for this year and last year.
- If neither of the above applies, write "None" below and go to 14.

Name and address of employer *(If you had more than one employer, please list them in order beginning with your last (most recent) employer.)*	Work began		Work ended *(If still working, show "Not Ended")*	
	Month	Year	Month	Year
(If you need more space, use "Remarks" space on back page.)				

13.	May we ask your employers for wage information needed to process your claim? ———————————▶	☐ Yes ☐ No

14.	(a) Were you self-employed this year, last year, or the year before? *(If "Yes," answer (b).) (If "No," go to 15.)* ———————▶	☐ Yes ☐ No

(b) Check the year or years in which you were self-employed.	In what kind of trade or business were you self-employed? *(For example, storekeeper, farmer, physician)*	Were your net earnings from your trade or business $400 or more? *(Check "Yes" or "No")*
☐ This year		
☐ Last year		☐ Yes ☐ No
☐ Year before last		☐ Yes ☐ No

Form **HCFA-43** (11-78) (Page 3)

IF YOU HAVE BEEN CONTINUALLY EMPLOYED FOR 2 OR MORE YEARS IN THE LAST 3 YEARS, DO NOT COMPLETE ITEMS 15 AND 16.

15. (a) **Check your Marital Status.** *(If single, go to 16.)*

☐ MARRIED   ☐ WIDOWED   ☐ DIVORCED   ☐ SINGLE

(b) Enter your wife's maiden name or your husband's name	Date of marriage	Date of divorce *(if divorced)*	Date of death *(if deceased)*	Your wife's or your husband's Social Security or Railroad Number *(If none or unknown, so indicate.)*

(c) **Check (✓) whether your marriage was performed by:**
☐ Clergyman or authorized public official, or   ☐ Other *(Explain in Remarks)*

(d) **Were you married before your present marriage?**
(If "Yes," give the following information about each of your previous marriages. If you need more space, use "Remarks" section below or attach a separate sheet.)   ☐ Yes   ☐ No

YOUR PREVIOUS MARRIAGE	To Whom Married	When *(Month, day, and year)*	Where *(Enter name of city & State)*
	How Marriage Ended	When *(Month, day, and year)*	Where *(Enter name of city & State)*

16. Complete the following if you are single.

MOTHER'S NAME	MOTHER'S SOCIAL SECURITY OR RAILROAD NUMBER
FATHER'S NAME	FATHER'S SOCIAL SECURITY OR RAILROAD NUMBER

REMARKS: _____

_____

_____

_____

IMPORTANT: Medicare coverage based on kidney failure will end with either:

a. The last day of the 36th month after the month in which a kidney transplant is received, or

b. The last day of the 12th month after the month in which a regular course of dialysis is discontinued, unless another course of dialysis is initiated or another transplant is received before the last day of

I AGREE TO NOTIFY THE SOCIAL SECURITY ADMINISTRATION IF THE COURSE OF DIALYSIS ENDS OR A KIDNEY TRANSPLANT IS RECEIVED.

I know that anyone who makes or causes to be made a false statement or representation of material fact in an application or for use in determining a right to payment under the Social Security Act commits a crime punishable under Federal law by fine, imprisonment or both. I affirm that all information I have given in this document is true.

SIGNATURE OF APPLICANT	Date *(Month, day, year)*
Signature *(First name, middle initial, last name) (Write in ink)* SIGN HERE ▶	Telephone Number(s) at which you may be contacted during the day

Mailing Address *(Number and street, Apt. No., P.O. Box, or Rural Route)*

City and State	ZIP Code	Enter Name of County (if any) in which you now live

Witnesses are required ONLY if this application has been signed by mark (X) above. If signed by mark (X), two witnesses to the signing who know the applicant must sign below, giving their full addresses.

1. Signature of Witness	2. Signature of Witness
Address *(Number, Street, City, State, and ZIP Code)*	Address *(Number, Street, City, State, Zip Code)*

Form **HCFA-43** (11-78) (Page 4)   ☆U.S. G.P.O. 1980-311-171/3015

PLEASE DETACH THIS PAGE AND KEEP FOR YOUR RECORDS

APPLICATION FOR HEALTH INSURANCE BENEFITS
UNDER MEDICARE FOR INDIVIDUAL
WITH CHRONIC RENAL DISEASE
Collection and Use of Information from Your Application

The Privacy Act of 1974 requires the Social Security Administration to give the following facts to individuals from whom information about themselves is requested:
- the statutory authority for the request,
- whether it is mandatory or voluntary to give the information,
- the principal purpose(s) for which the information is needed,
- the effects of not providing the information, and
- the routine uses which may be made of the information.

These items are explained in the following sections. If you have any questions about your rights under the Privacy Act, you may contact any social security office.

I.   The Social Security Administration is authorized to collect the information on this form under 205(a), 226(A), and 1872 of the Social Security Act, as amended (42 U.S.C. 405(a), 426, and 1395ii).

II. While it is not mandatory, except in the circumstances explained below, for you to furnish the information on this form to social security, health insurance entitlement cannot be established unless an application has been received by a social security office. Your response is mandatory where the refusal to disclose certain information affecting your entitlement would reflect a fraudulent intent to secure benefits not authorized by the Social Security Act.

III. The information on this form is needed to enable social security to determine if you are entitled to health insurance coverage.

IV. Failure to provide all or part of this information could prevent an accurate and timely decision on your claim, and could result in the loss of some insurance coverage.

V.   Although the information you furnish on this form is almost never used for any other purpose than stated in Part III, above, there is a possibility that for the administration of the social security programs or for the administration of programs requiring coordination with the Social Security Administration, information may be disclosed to another person or to another governmental agency as follows:

1. To enable a third party or an agency to assist social security in establishing rights to health insurance coverage.

2. To comply with Federal laws requiring the release of information from social security records (e.g., to the General Accounting Office and the Veterans' Administration).

3. To facilitate statistical research and audit activities necessary to assure the integrity and improvement of the social security programs (e.g., to the Bureau of the Census and private concerns under contract to social security.)

Form **HCFA-43** (11-78)

PLEASE DETACH THIS PAGE AND KEEP FOR YOUR RECORDS

DEPARTMENT OF HEALTH, EDUCATION, AND WELFARE
HEALTH CARE FINANCING ADMINISTRATION

Form Approved.
OMB No. 086-R-0067

REQUEST FOR RECONSIDERATION OF PART A HEALTH INSURANCE BENEFITS

INSTRUCTIONS: *Please type or print firmly.* Leave the block empty if you cannot answer it. Take or mail the WHOLE form to your
Social Security office which will be glad to help you. Please read the statement on the reverse side of page 2.

1. BENEFICIARY'S NAME	2. HEALTH INSURANCE CLAIM NUMBER

3. REPRESENTATIVE'S NAME, IF APPLICABLE

☐ RELATIVE ☐ ATTORNEY ☐ OTHER PERSON) ☐ PROVIDER FILING

4. PLEASE ATTACH A COPY OF THE NOTICE(S) YOU RECEIVED ABOUT YOUR CLAIM TO THIS FORM.

5. THIS CLAIM IS FOR

☐ INPATIENT HOSPITAL   ☐ SKILLED NURSING FACILITY (SNF)   ☐ HEALTH MAINTENANCE
☐ EMERGENCY HOSPITAL   ☐ HOME HEALTH AGENCY (HHA)   ORGANIZATION (HMO)

6. NAME AND ADDRESS OF PROVIDER (Hospital, SNF, HHA, HMO)	CITY AND STATE	PROVIDER NUMBER

7. NAME OF INTERMEDIARY	CITY AND STATE	INTERMEDIARY NUMBER

8. DATE OF ADMISSION OR START OF SERVICES	9. DATE(S) OF THE NOTICE(S) YOU RECEIVED

10. I DO NOT AGREE WITH THE DETERMINATION ON MY CLAIM. PLEASE RECONSIDER MY CLAIM BECAUSE

11. YOU MUST OBTAIN ANY EVIDENCE (For example, a letter from a doctor) YOU WISH TO SUBMIT.

☐ I HAVE ATTACHED THE FOLLOWING EVIDENCE:

☐ I WILL SEND THIS EVIDENCE WITHIN 10 DAYS:

☐ I HAVE NO ADDITIONAL EVIDENCE OR OTHER INFORMATION TO SUBMIT WITH MY CLAIM.

13. ONLY ONE SIGNATURE IS NEEDED. THIS FORM IS SIGNED BY:
☐ BENEFICIARY ☐ REPRESENTATIVE ☐ PROVIDER REP.

SIGN HERE ▶

14. STREET ADDRESS

12. IS THIS REQUEST FILED WITHIN 60 DAYS OF THE DATE OF YOUR NOTICE?

☐ YES ☐ NO

IF YOU CHECKED "NO" ATTACH AN EXPLANATION OF THE REASON FOR THE DELAY TO THIS FORM.

CITY, STATE, ZIP CODE

TELEPHONE	DATE

15. If this request is signed by mark (X), TWO WITNESSES who know the person requesting reconsideration must sign in the space provided on the reverse side of this page of the form.

DO NOT FILL IN BELOW THIS LINE — FOR SOCIAL SECURITY USE — THANK YOU

16. ROUTING

☐ INTERMEDIARY

☐ HCFA, RO-MEDICARE

☐ BSS, ODR

18. SSA OR INTERMEDIARY DATE STAMP

17. ADDITIONAL INFORMATION

FORM HCFA-2649 (8-79 FORMERLY SSA-2649)
DESTROY PRIOR EDITIONS

INTERMEDIARY

Page 1 of 4

DEPARTMENT OF HEALTH,
EDUCATION, AND WELFARE
SOCIAL SECURITY ADMINISTRATION
BUREAU OF HEARINGS AND APPEALS

REQUEST FOR HEARING
PART A HEALTH INSURANCE BENEFITS
Take or mail original and all copies to your local Social Security office.

CLAIMANT'S NAME

WAGE EARNER'S NAME (Leave blank if same as above)

HI CLAIM NUMBER

NAME AND ADDRESS OF INTERMEDIARY

CLAIM FOR
☐ Hospital Services
☐ Extended Care Facility Services
☐ Home Health Agency Services
☐ Emergency Services

PERIOD IN QUESTION
FROM: TO:

NAME AND ADDRESS OF PROVIDER

I disagree with the determination made on the above claim and request a hearing before a hearing examiner of the Bureau of Hearings and Appeals. My reasons for disagreement are: (additional pages may be added if necessary.)

Check one of the following:

☐ I have additional evidence to submit.
(Attach such evidence to this form or forward to the Social Security Office within 10 days.)

☐ I have no additional evidence to submit.

Check ONLY ONE of the statements below.

☐ I wish to appear in person before the hearing examiner.

☐ I waive my right to appear and give evidence, and hereby request a decision on the evidence before the hearing examiner.

Signed by: (Either the claimant or representative should sign-Enter addresses for both. If claimant's representative is not an attorney, complete Form SSA-1696)

SIGNATURE OR NAME OF CLAIMANT'S REPRESENTATIVE
☐ ATTORNEY ☐ NON-ATTORNEY

CLAIMANT'S SIGNATURE

ADDRESS

ADDRESS

CITY, STATE, AND ZIP CODE

CITY, STATE, AND ZIP CODE

TELEPHONE NUMBER | DATE:

TELEPHONE NUMBER

Claimant should not fill in below this line

Is this request filed within 6 months of the reconsideration determination?   ☐ Yes   ☐ No
If "No" is checked: (1) attach claimant's explanation for delay, (2) attach any pertinent letter, material, or information in the Social Security Office.

ACKNOWLEDGMENT OF REQUEST FOR HEARING
Your request for a hearing was filed on_____at _____
The hearing examiner will notify you of the time and place of the hearing at least 10 days prior to the date which will be set for the hearing.

Hearing Examiner Copy

TO:
☐ Hearing Examiner _____ (Location)

Claim File Copy

TO:
☐ BHI, Reconsideration Branch

☐ BHI, Regional Office _____
(Only emergency services in other than Federal Hospitals)

For the Social Security Administration

By: _____
(Signature)   (Title)

_____
(Street Address)

_____
(City)   (State)   (ZIP Code)

Interpreter Needed _____
(Language)

Servicing District Office Code_____

Form HA 501.1
(2-72)

HEARING EXAMINER

61

DEPARTMENT OF HEALTH AND HUMAN SERVICES
HEALTH CARE FINANCING ADMINISTRATION

Form Approved
OMB No. 0938-0033

REQUEST FOR REVIEW OF PART B MEDICARE CLAIM
Medical Insurance Benefits - Social Security Act

NOTICE—Anyone who misrepresents or falsifies essential information requested by this form may upon conviction be subject to fine and imprisonment under Federal Law.

Carrier's Name and Address

The name and address of the Carrier for your state will be listed in this space.

1 Name of Patient

2 Health Insurance Claim Number

3 I do not agree with the determination you made on my claim as described on my Explanation of Medicare

Benefits dated:

4 MY REASONS ARE: *(Attach a copy of the Explanation of Medicare Benefits, or describe the service, date of service, and physician's name—NOTE.—If the date on the Notice of Benefits mentioned in item 3 is more than six months ago, include your reason for not making this request earlier.)*

_____

_____

_____

_____

_____

_____

_____

5 ☐ I have additional evidence to submit. *(Attach such evidence to this form)*

☐ I do not have additional evidence.

COMPLETE ALL OF THE INFORMATION REQUESTED. SIGN AND RETURN THE FIRST COPY AND ANY ATTACHMENTS TO THE CARRIER NAMED ABOVE. IF YOU NEED HELP, TAKE THIS AND YOUR NOTICE FROM THE CARRIER TO A SOCIAL SECURITY OFFICE, OR TO THE CARRIER. KEEP THE DUPLICATE COPY OF THIS FORM FOR YOUR RECORDS.

6
SIGNATURE OF **EITHER** THE CLAIMANT **OR** HIS REPRESENTATIVE

Representative	Claimant
➤	➤
Address	Address
City, State, and ZIP Code	City, State, and ZIP Code
Telephone Number	Date	Telephone Number	Date

Form **HCFA-1964** (1-78) (Formerly SSA-1964)   **CARRIER'S COPY**   (over)

62

Form Approved
OMB No. 0938-0034

REQUEST FOR HEARING - PART B MEDICARE CLAIM
Medical Insurance Benefits - Social Security Act

NOTICE—Anyone who misrepresents or falsifies essential information requested by this form may upon conviction be subject to fine and imprisonment under Federal Law.

Carrier's Name and Address	**1** Name of Patient
The name and address of the Carrier for your state will be listed in this space.	**2** Health Insurance Claim Number

3 I disagree with the review determination on my claim, and request a hearing before a hearing officer of the insurance carrier named above.

MY REASONS ARE: *(Attach a copy of the Review Notice. NOTE.—If the review decision was made more than 6 months ago include your reason for not making this request earlier)*

_____

_____

_____

_____

4 Check one of the Following:

☐ I have additional evidence to submit.
(Attach such evidence to this form or forward it to the carrier within 10 days.)

☐ I do not have additional evidence.

Check <u>Only One</u> of the Statements Below:

☐ I wish to appear in person before the Hearing Officer.

☐ I do not wish to appear and hereby request a decision on the evidence before the Hearing Officer.

5 EITHER THE CLAIMANT OR REPRESENTATIVE SHOULD SIGN IN THE APPROPRIATE SPACE BELOW:

Signature or Name of Claimant's Representative ➡	Claimant's Signature ➡
Address	Address
City, State, and ZIP Code	City, State, and ZIP Code
Telephone Number / Date	Telephone Number / Date

(Claimant should not write below this line)

ACKNOWLEDGMENT OF REQUEST FOR HEARING

Your request for a hearing was received on _____. You will be notified of the time and place of the hearing at least 10 days before the date of the hearing.

Signed	Date

Form **HCFA-1965** (8-79) (Formerly SSA-1965)

CARRIERS COPY

Proposed Premium Rates for Medicare Part B, Catastrophic Insurance and Prescription Drug Benefit 1988–1993

	1988	1989	1990	1991	1992	1993
Part B	$24.80	$27.90	$28.10*	$29.60*	$30.80*	$32.40*
Catastrophic	—	$ 4.00	$ 4.90	$ 5.46	$ 6.75	$ 7.18
Prescription Drugs	—	—	—	$ 1.94	$ 2.45	$ 8.02
Total Monthly Premium	$24.80	$31.90	$33.00**	$37.00**	$40.00**	$42.60**

*Actual figures will be determined by the Department of Health and Human Services based upon current program costs and that portion of program costs to be paid for by the beneficiaries.

The new premiums rates will be announced in September of the year preceding their implementation.

**Approximate monthly premium.

SOURCE: Medicare Catastrophic Coverage Act of 1988. Report 100-661, page 54.

sometimes to families, for less than the 1989 combined Part A/Part B/ Catastrophic Coverage buy-in premium of $189.90 per month.[1]

The Meaning of "Coverage"

Coverage under Medicare is limited three ways, first by the services that are covered at all. By "covered" we mean that Medicare is willing to pay something for the service — not necessarily the full amount the **provider** wants, not necessarily enough to relieve you of all the burden of payment, not necessarily enough to attract enough providers to make the service routinely available, but something. (A provider is a person or institution of a sort for whose services Medicare makes payments. Some providers are people; some are institutions, such as hospitals.) Services for which Medicare will pay nothing are "not covered." The chart on page 65 provides a brief summary of what is covered and what is not.

[1]For 1989, the Part A premium will be approximately $158.00; the Part B premium, $27.90; and the Catastrophic Coverage premium, $4.00 per month — a total of $2278.80 per year. The 40 percent of Medicare beneficiaries with the highest incomes will also pay an additional, income-related premium, with a maximum of $800 in 1989. This amount will rise annually until it hits $1,050 in 1993, where it will be capped. (Note: The figures quoted here on Part A are working figures as of publication date. They may vary by a few dollars when finalized by HCFA. If you have any questions contact your Social Security office.)

THE MEDICARE PROGRAM . . . .
WHAT IT PAYS . . . . WHAT YOU PAY

Program services, as well as deductibles and copayments, are subject to change on a yearly basis.
For the most current information, consult the latest edition of *Your Medicare Handbook,* available
at most Social Security Administration offices.

SCHEDULE OF BENEFITS

Medicare Part A: Hospital Insurance	Benefits Effective Through December 31, 1988	Changes Effective January 1, 1989
Hospital Deductibles	$540 initial deductible; 61–90 days $135 per day copayment; 91–150 days $270 per day copayment	Unlimited hospital days after a one-time yearly deductible of $560.
Skilled Nursing Facility	100 days total benefit; 1–20 days no cost; 21–100 days $67.50 per day copayment; 3-day prior hospitalization	150 days/year Copayment of $22.00 in 1989 on days 1 through 8 after which Medicare covers all costs for days 9–150. Beginning in 1990 the copayment will be adjusted to equal 20% of the average charge for one day in a skilled nursing facility. No prior hospitalization required.
Hospice (Care for the terminally ill)	(2) 90-day periods (1) 30-day period Beneficiary responsible for deductible and copayment on out-patient drugs and inpatient respite care.	Unlimited days as medically necessary
Blood (Whole blood or packed red cells)	As needed. Beneficiary pays deductible equal to the first 3 pints of blood. Any deductible paid under Part B does not apply.	As needed. Beneficiary pays a single yearly deductible equal to the cost of the first 3 pints of blood. Any deductible paid under the Part B benefit is also applied.
Additional Part A Services	**Benefits Effective Through December 31, 1989**	**Changes Effective January 1, 1990**
Home Health Care	5 days per week for 21 days.	7 days/week up to 38 consecutive days. May under certain conditions be extended.
Respite Care (In-home services for the chronically disabled. Provides a rest for the care giver)	Part of hospice care through 1989. Limited to no more than 5-day inpatient stay. Beneficiary pays 5% of outpatient drug costs or $5; 5% of inpatient costs up to the Part A deductible.	Benefit includes up to 80 hours/year of services to include: nursing, homemaker and personal care. Beneficiaries are eligible after they meet the Part B copayment limit or the prescription drug deductibles.
Medicare Part B: Medical Insurance	**Benefits Effective Through December 31, 1989**	**Changes Effective January 1, 1990**
Part B Deductibles Coverage of physician's services, outpatient hospital care, outpatient therapy, home health care and other services not covered by Hospital insurance.	As needed. After beneficiary pays $75 annual deductible. Medicare pays 80% of approved charges.	Yearly limit on out-of-pocket expenses on Part B covered services. Beneficiary pays deductible of $75/year after which Medicare pays 80% of all approved charges. Out-of-pocket expenses are limited to $1370 in 1990; $1530 in 1991; $1700 in 1992; and $1900 in 1993. After which Medicare pays 100% of approved charges. Physician fees and other charges that exceed the Medicare approved charges do not count toward the out-of-pocket limit.
Mammography Screening	No benefit	Provides for biannual (every-other-year) screening. Medicare pays 80% of the costs up to $50 the first year.
Home Health Care	5 days per week for 21 days	7 days/week up to 38 consecutive days. May under certain conditions be extended.
Respite Care (In-home services for the chronically disabled. Provides a rest for the care giver)	Part of hospice care through 1989. Limited to no more than 5-day inpatient stay. Beneficiary pays 5% of outpatient drug costs or $5; 5% of inpatient costs up to the Part A deductible.	Benefit includes up to 80 hours/year of services to include: nursing, homemaker and personal care. Beneficiaries are eligible after they meet the Part B copayment limit or the prescription drug deductible.

Medicare Part B: Medical Insurance	Benefits Effective Through December 31, 1989	Changes Effective January 1, 1990
IV Drug Therapy (In-home service)	No benefit	80% of all costs after deductible of $550 in 1990; 50% of all costs after deductible of $600 in 1991; 60% of all costs after deductible of $652 in 1992 and 80% of all costs after deductible in 1993. Deductibles and copayments may be waived if therapy was started as a result of hospital inpatient service.
Immunosuppressive Drugs	Medicare covers one year of drugs used in immunosuppressive therapy after transplantation, with the beneficiary paying the 20% copayment.	Medicare pays 50% of the cost of these drugs after a deductible of $550 in 1990; 50% of the costs after a deductible of $600 in 1991; and 60% of the costs after a deductible of $652 in 1992. Beginning in 1993 Medicare pays 80% of all costs after the deductible.

Additional Services	Benefits Effective Through December 31, 1990	Changes Effective January 1, 1991
Outpatient Prescription Drug Service (Coverage for prescriptions which are written independent of any stay in the hospital)	No benefit	50% of all costs after meeting deductible of $600 in 1991; 60% of all costs after deductible of $652 in 1992 and 80% of all costs after deductible to be determined for 1993 and beyond.

Nursing Homes Are Partially Covered

Medicare does not cover what we usually think of as "nursing home care." There are three levels of nursing home care:

- **Skilled nursing facilities** (SNFs) offer care delivered by registered and licensed practical nurses on the orders of an attending physician. They offer services such as oxygen therapy, intravenous and tube feedings, care of catheters and wound drains, and physical, occupational, and speech therapy.

- **Intermediate Care Facilities** (ICFs) provide less intensive care than skilled nursing facilities. Patients are generally more mobile, and rehabilitation therapies are stressed.

- **Sheltered, or custodial, care** is nonmedical. Residents do not require constant attention from nurses and aides but need assistance with one or more daily activities or no longer want to be bothered with keeping up a house. The social needs of residents are met in a safe, secure environment free of as many anxieties as possible.

Medicare covers nursing home care at the **skilled nursing facility** (SNF, pronounced *sniff*) level only. Further, Medicare will pay for skilled nursing facility services *only* if the following conditions are met:

- The nursing home must be a skilled nursing facility, and it must be certified to participate in the Medicare program.
- No prior hospitalization is required, but a physician must certify that the person requires skilled care.
- There must be ongoing utilization review to determine if the person is receiving skilled nursing services.
- If a determination is made that skilled care is no longer required, Medicare coverage ceases.

You should be aware that Medicare is not a long-term solution to paying for nursing home care, because it does not cover intermediate or sheltered care (the two most common levels of care required). Medicare coverage for skilled care in 1989 is as follows:

TIME IN DAYS	MEDICARE PAYS	YOU PAY
1–8	Balance of cost after $22.00 per day copayment	$22.00 per day copayment
9–150	All costs	Nothing
151+	Nothing	All costs

NOTE: In 1990 and beyond, the copayment will be set to equal 20 percent of the average daily rate at a skilled nursing facility.

Let's consider an example:

The Smith family's aged grandmother, Iphigenia, has had a stroke and broken her hip when falling down. She had to have the hip replaced with an artificial one and has been in and out of the hospital with infections and failure of the bone to solidify around the hip. The last stay in the hospital seems to have finally fixed her hip, but she is currently unable to walk and has trouble with bowel and bladder control, and tends to get dehydrated very easily. She needs a long stay in a nursing home for recuperation, with almost constant nursing attention to make sure that her wound does not get reinfected and her fluid intake is adequate, and occupational and speech therapy. As things turn out, she has to stay in the nursing home for an entire year after her last discharge from the hospital.

Let's see what Medicare paid: The nursing home charged $110.00 per day for skilled nursing facility services. (This figure included the room charge plus estimated ancillary charges, for items such as medicine, equipment, and the like.) Medicare paid for the first 8 days, less the $22.00 copayment, and for the next 142 days in full. That leaves 210 days to pay for.

What's the proportion paid by Medicare, and what's the proportion paid by the Smiths?	
Total cost: $110.00 × 365 =	$40,150
Medicare payment for first 8 days:	
8 × $(110.00 − $22.00) =	$ 704
Smiths' copayment for the first 8 days:	
8 × $22.00 =	$ 176
Medicare payment for days 9–150:	
142 × $110 =	$15,620
Smiths' payment for days 9–150:	$0
Medicare payment for days 151–365:	$0
Smiths' payment for days 151–365:	
215 × $110 =	$23,650
Medicare pays:	$16,324 (40.7%)
The Smiths paid: $40,150 − $16,324 =	$23,826 (59.3%)

In 1990, suppose the *average* charge for skilled nursing facility services is $120 per day (regardless of what the Smiths are actually charged by the nursing home Iphigenia is in). What happens then?

```
Total cost: $110 × 365 =                          $40,150
Medicare payment for first 8 days:
    8 × $(110 − $[20% of $120] = $24) =        $    688
Smiths' copayment = 8 × $24 =                  $    192
Medicare payment for days 9–150:
    142 × $110 =                                  $15,620
Smiths' payment for days 9–150:                   $0
Smiths' payment for days 151–365:
    215 × $120 =                                  $23,650
Medicare payment for days 151–365:                $0

Medicare pays:                                    $16,308 (40.6%)
The Smiths paid: $40,150 − $16,308 =              $23,842 (59.4%)
```

Note that even though the Smiths' nursing home has not increased its prices, the charge to the Smiths has gone up. Medicare is paying less because the national average charge for skilled nursing facility services has risen.

Another common misconception is that "Medicare will take care of you until you're well." This is not true. Most Medicare recipients recover sufficiently to leave the hospital, but they are discharged when they no longer need hospital services — not when they are completely well. Some never get completely well. Some never recover sufficiently to leave a skilled nursing facility. In recognition of this, Medicare imposes a cutoff point for skilled nursing facility services. Longer-term needs are taken care of by federal/state programs such as **Medicaid** and **Supplemental Security Income** (SSI). There is a growing recognition on the part of policy makers that some of the needs of the elderly, such as the need for help in eating and dressing, are not medical needs. They're not medical because medicine can't do anything for them. They are social problems that ought to be handled outside the medical model. The federal government has sponsored a few experiments with **social health maintenance organizations** (SHMOs) to test ways to provide care outside the medical model, but this sort of work is still in its infancy. For the moment, don't assume that Medicare will take care of any need you have for long-term care. It won't.

What options are available when Medicare runs out? The chief one is Medicaid, a program that is jointly funded by the states and the federal government. States have a wide range of latitude in whom they cover, what services they cover, and the income and resource limits they use. For these reasons, it is hard to be too specific with numerical examples. It is possible to state the general principles.

The Medicaid program does cover nursing home care, but Medicaid is intended for the *very* poor who have nowhere else to turn. Not all of the very poor are covered. Medicaid is a state-run program that receives federal funds. States make most of the rules, and the trend in recent years has been to make requirements more stringent. The old law virtually guaranteed that the spouse who stayed at home would have to impoverish himself or herself to pay for the care of the spouse in the nursing home.

The new Medicare catastrophic coverage provisions greatly reduce the burden but can still lead to a substantial loss of assets. Beginning January 1, 1989,

- In any month in which a married person is in a nursing home, no income of the at-home spouse is to be considered available to the spouse in the nursing home.

- Income is considered the property of the person to whom it is paid. Income paid to both spouses is attributed 50 percent to each.

- The home, household goods, and personal effects of both spouses are not counted in considering Medicaid eligibility.

- All assets other than these will be counted and divided in two. If the at-home spouse has less than $12,000, the spouse in the nursing home may transfer assets to him or her to make up to $12,000 available to the at-home spouse. (States may, at their option, raise this figure to any amount less than $60,000. The $12,000 amount will be indexed to inflation.)

- The assets that remain in the name of the spouse in the nursing home are considered available to pay for his or her nursing home care. All assets in excess of $60,000 are attributed to the spouse in the nursing home and are considered available to pay for nursing home care.

- States must allow nursing home residents to retain certain sums for medical expenses not covered by Medicare or Medicaid before contributing to the expense of their nursing home care. The states may place "reasonable limits" on the amounts spent.

- Starting September 30, 1989, the states must allow the at-home spouse sufficient income from the other spouse to bring total household income of the at-home spouse to at least 122 percent of the federal poverty level for a two-person household. In 1989, this will be $789 per month. On July 1, 1991, it will be raised to 133 percent of the poverty level, and to 150 percent on July 1, 1992. States will not be required to allow more than $1,500 per month, except by court order or change in regulations.

One very important point: your spouse and parents do not *actually* have to give anything toward the cost of your care, but your *eligibility* is determined as though they are. Even though the catastrophic coverage laws make things much more uniform across the nation than they were, the exact requirements, as well as the exact amount of liquid assets and income you may retain and still be eligible, will vary from state to state because of the range ($12,000–$60,000) in which Congress allows states to set the level. Check the list of Medicaid state offices in appendix N to find out where to call to determine the exact eligibility requirements for your state.

You are *automatically* eligible for Medicaid if you are eligible for, or receiving, **Supplemental Security Income** (SSI) payments for the aged, blind, and disabled, but you must apply at a state welfare office. If you meet the requirements for SSI, there is little chance that you would have to give up additional income or assets to qualify for Medicaid.

If your income, less certain deductions and medical bills, is within certain (low) limits, you may be eligible for Medicaid as **medically needy.** You must "spend down" (deduct medical bills from income) to the point at which you are eligible. If you have low enough income, high enough medical bills, and meet certain other tests, Medicaid pays for all of them. You can contact your state Medicaid agency, listed in appendix N, to find out about application procedures and eligibility requirements in your state.

The new catastrophic coverage offers a third way to qualify for some assistance, although not necessarily for all services offered by the state Medicaid program. Whether or not you are eligible under the regular or medically needy provisions,

- If you have income below the federal poverty limit ($5,700 for individuals in 1988, and resources less than twice the SSI standard ($3,800 in 1988), your state will be required to pay all of your Medicare-related deductibles, coinsurance, and premiums.

- Note that this coverage will be phased in. Individuals with incomes less than 85 percent of the poverty level will be covered beginning

January 1, 1989; the full 100 percent standard will not apply until 1992.

- If you live in Hawaii, Illinois, North Carolina, or Ohio, which have had more restrictive standards, you may have to wait an additional year for coverage, depending on your income. These states will be required to cover only those with incomes less than 80 percent of the federal poverty level in 1989, and will lag behind the rest of the nation by a year in reaching the full 100 percent standard.

What Medicare Means by "Services"

Medicare covers "hospital services," but not all of them. **Private rooms, private duty nursing,** radios, televisions, and telephones are among the services offered by hospitals, but Medicare does not automatically pay for them the way it does, say, for operating room charges. Medicare doesn't pay for private rooms unless they are prescribed by doctors or no other room is available. The same is true for private duty nursing. Radios, televisions, and telephones are never covered. Medicare will not pay for the first three pints of blood used in blood transfusions in a year, but it will pay for all blood used after those first three. Any blood deductible paid under Part A *or* Part B applies, so you will have to pay for no more than three pints of blood in any year. The deductible is waived if you or someone else replaces the blood. Check with the local blood bank or the hospital blood bank on how to have a pint credited to your deductible.

Drugs administered in the hospital are normally covered, but those that have not been judged "safe and effective" by the Food and Drug Administration are not covered.

All insurance plans have reserved the right, from their inception, to pay for what the carrier defines as covered, not anything a doctor may choose to prescribe or a patient may want. So, too, with Medicare. As the cost of medical care rises, limitations on payment by insurance companies and Medicare will increase, not decrease. Medicare and private insurers are likely to insist on more, rather than less, proof of safety and effectiveness before paying for a new service.

In the following sections, we discuss what is covered and what is not for each type of service. Chapter 3 explains the **copayments** and **deductibles** that are involved. These are charges that you or your insurance company have to cover. Depending on the details of your supplemental insurance for Medicare (if you own such a policy), only part of the copayment or deductible may be paid. You pay the remainder. (See chapter 4 for a discussion of insurance to supplement Medicare.)

Services Covered: Hospitals

Medicare covers the following services for **inpatient hospital care:**

- Semiprivate room (no more than two beds to a room)
- All meals, including any special diets that are needed, plus **hyperalimentation**
- Nursing services regularly provided by the unit you are in (Medicare pays for nursing services in the **intensive care unit**, even though they are more expensive than those on the **general medical/surgical floors.**)
- Intensive care, intensive care units, and care in other **special care units** (for example, a brain surgery unit)
- Drugs furnished in the hospital, unless they are excluded because the Food and Drug Administration has not found them "safe and effective"
- Blood transfusions, except for the cost of the first three pints of blood (As we noted before, the cost of the blood can be met under the Part A or Part B deductible, and will be waived if the blood is replaced.)
- Hospital charges for lab tests
- Hospital charges for **X rays** and **radiotherapy**
- Medical supplies, such as dressing, casts, splints, **catheters,** and **intravenous (IV) lines**
- Use of **durable medical equipment**, such as wheelchairs and crutches, while in the hospital
- All hospital **operating room** and **recovery room** charges
- Rehabilitation services, such as physical therapy, speech pathology, and the like, provided during the inpatient stay

The charges of **hospital-based physicians,** such as **pathologists, radiologists, physiatrists, nuclear medicine** and **pulmonary specialists,** to name a few, are not covered under the hospital insurance portion of Medicare but are paid by Part B, doctor insurance. This splitting of charges between the hospital and the physician for what looks like a hospital-provided service can often be confusing. The Claims Log we provide for you (see appendix B) will help you keep all of this straight and make sure that you pay no more than you absolutely have to.

Medicare now pays for an unlimited number of hospital days after a once-per-year deductible, as long as the care is a **medical necessity.** The deductible is estimated at $560 in 1989. Someone who has an unbroken stay — even one of years — need pay the deductible only once. If you are discharged and then return to the hospital in the same calendar year, you do not have to pay the deductible again. If you are readmitted in the next calendar year, you must pay it. You do *not* have to pay an additional deductible if your hospital stay starts in one calendar year and continues into another.

Before the coming of catastrophic care coverage and the **diagnosis-related groups (DRG) system,** limitations on days paid for by Medicare could have affected your hospital stay. The diagnosis-related groups system provides a set payment for each condition. In addition, there is a process that allows the hospital to apply for more money if your case is unusually expensive. Now you can be discharged only when hospital care is no longer medically necessary. The deal between the hospital and Medicare under the DRG system requires that the hospital provide as much service as Medicare patients' doctors' deem necessary for their care.

You may think that Medicare pays for care anywhere in the world. It doesn't. Only care in hospitals in the fifty states and the District of Columbia, Puerto Rico, and the last two U.S. territories — Guam and the Virgin Islands — is paid for. Care you receive in Europe, Canada, Mexico, and the rest of the world is *not* covered. The only exception is if you are close to the Canadian or Mexican border and in need of emergency care, and the nearest hospital is a Canadian or Mexican one. In this situation, Medicare will pay for services in a Canadian or Mexican hospital.

Another limitation on hospital services, mentioned briefly earlier, is **medical necessity**. We'll discuss this more in chapter 8. For the moment, the general idea is this: Medicare will not pay for anything it does not consider dictated by the needs of good, professional medicine as applied to your case. Sometimes, for example in certain types of surgery that are often abused, the **medical necessity determination** is made before you go into the hospital or have the operation. In other instances, it is made after Medicare-mandated reviewers of coverage, such as the **peer review organizations (PROs),** review your chart and decide that your case has not been handled as it should have been.

Medicare has been experimenting with ways to hold down costs ever since the program began to cost much more than anticipated, in the late 1960s. The peer review organizations are the latest example. Peer review organizations are groups of doctors who contract with Medicare to make sure that the care given to Medicare beneficiaries is of acceptable quality and is really needed. The requirement that care be "reasonable and necessary" has always been in the law. The peer review organizations are just the latest means of enforcing it. They review some cases before care is given, if local or national evidence indicates a high level of inappropriate use. In these situations, approval is required before Medicare pays. In other cases, they look at charts after the patient has been discharged and make decisions about the appropriateness of what was done. Finally, they review requests from hospitals for extra payment (over and above the amount the diagnosis-related groups system pays) and extra days of care.

Unless you have received an official notice that a service is not considered medically necessary before you have it done, or that additional hospital days are not necessary before you decide to stay, you never have to pay for medically unnecessary care. We discuss in chapter 8 what to do when you receive such notices.

Physicians and Related Services

Medicare pays for most services of physicians — holders of the degrees of **Doctor of Medicine** (**M.D.**) or **Doctor of Osteopathy** (**D.O.**) — and some of the services of **podiatrists** (foot doctors) some of the services of **chiropractors,** and dental surgery performed by **dentists** in a hospital. Some services of **optometrists** (those licensed to prescribe eyeglasses and contact lenses) are covered as well.

Most **outpatient treatments** and tests, such as **electrocardiograms** (**EKGs**), X rays, and physical therapy, are covered. When the Medicare law was passed, most such services were performed in the outpatient departments of hospitals. Now most of them are available in physicians' offices and are covered by Medicare.

For coverage of nonhospital services (or Medicare services in general), the usual rule is that routine services, such as annual physicals, that are not aimed at treating a specific illness are not covered, and that services designed to improve appearance or bodily function, such as cosmetic surgery, are not covered unless they are needed to restore a state of health that existed before illness or injury.

Outpatient psychiatric services are covered, but only to a total of $1,100 per year, starting in 1989. The limit on total lifetime inpatient psychiatric hospital days has been raised to 190.

At present (until December 31, 1989, for some drugs and December 31, 1990, for all other drugs), drugs and **biologicals** (**hormones, serums, vaccines,** and such) are covered only if administered by the treating professional. They are not covered if they are prescribed for self-administration. Prescription drugs that the doctor prescribes for you to administer to yourself are generally not covered. The only exceptions are immunosuppressive drugs, such as cyclosporine, an antirejection drug prescribed for kidney transplant patients under the end stage renal disease portion of Medicare.

Beginning January 1, 1990, Medicare will cover at-home administration of **intravenous antibiotics**. Other intravenous drugs for at-home administration may be added later. In 1990 these drugs for at-home administration will be covered after a deductible of $550 is paid. You must pay 20 percent of the cost after that. These drugs will then be covered under the prescription drug program that starts in 1991. After January 1, 1991, the drug deductible will not apply to these drugs if their administration was started in the hospital and continued at home. Supplies, equipment, nursing services, and pharmacy services will be covered beginning in 1990. The drugs themselves will be covered in 1991.

Immunosuppressive drugs used for transplant patients will be covered at the following rates:

- In 1990, 50 percent copayment after a $550 deductible
- In 1991, 50 percent copayment after a $600 deductible
- In 1992, 40 percent copayment after a $652 deductible
- In 1993 and later years, 20 percent copayment after a deductible if premiums have been enough to cover the costs

Outpatient prescription drugs that are prescribed by a physician for self-administration will be covered in 1991, with an initial deductible of $600. After that is met, Medicare will pay for 50 percent of the cost in 1991, 60 percent in 1992, and 80 percent in 1993 and thereafter. At present, HCFA plans a nationwide computer network linking Medicare-participating pharmacies. Instant access to a central computer will ensure that pharmacists will know when the deductible is met and will not overcharge recipients. Pharmacies will be forbidden to charge more than Medicare will pay or to charge Medicare beneficiaries more than they charge the general public.

While the drug benefit is certainly a help, only a few Medicare recipients will need as much as $600 worth of outpatient drugs. The statistical pattern is for the great majority of recipients to use less than this in most years. Even if you use $599.99 worth of drugs, there will be no Medicare coverage.

Services Covered: Nursing Homes

As we discussed earlier, Medicare payment for nursing home treatment is limited to 150 days in a skilled nursing facility, with full payment for the days 9–150 and a copayment for the first 8 days (the copayment will be $22.00 in 1989). *Medicare simply does not pay for nursing home care that is needed because you can no longer care for yourself.* The limited payment for skilled nursing facility services actually functions as a money-saver: if you need skilled nursing services to recover, but can safely have them outside a hospital, it makes sense for the government to cover them in a lower-cost setting like a nursing home.

The enormous expense of nursing home services — $40 billion in 1988 — indicates that they have certainly helped many people who could not care for themselves. But the care given in many nursing homes is, frankly, of uncertain quality. Quality of nursing home care is not well monitored. Medicare has only recently decided to require that some sort of nurse (a **registered nurse** [R.N.], or a **licensed practical nurse** [L.P.N.] or **licensed vocational nurse** [L.V.N.]) be available on all shifts in all nursing homes. We have much more to say about nursing homes in chapter 7.

Other Covered Services

Home Health Care: Home health care is covered for up to thirty-eight consecutive visits; there is no limit on the total number of visits. The major restriction is that the visits must be for medical care only. Homemaker-type services, such as cooking, cleaning, and shopping, are not included. After a series of thirty-eight consecutive visits, there must be a break of at least one day before another series will be paid for.

Durable Medical Equipment: A number of pieces of **durable medical equipment,** such as wheelchairs, hospital beds for home use, and oxygen tanks, are covered. If a doctor prescribes it, Medicare will usually pay for all of the cost of it if it is provided under Part A, and 80 percent of the cost of it under Part B. Regardless of the part of Medicare under which it is paid, Medicare pays 100 percent of the costs for used equipment.

Eyeglasses, Contact Lenses, and Hearing Aids: Eyeglasses and contact lenses are covered only if needed following eye surgery, or as a result of eye disease other than normal visual defects such as astigmatism and myopia.

How to Maximize Your Medicare Benefits

In this section, we talk about some of the ways to get more out of Medicare that are emerging. Most are the results of experiments by the federal government to make market forces play a bigger role in health care, experiments in health care cost containment, or making approaches to paying for health care that have worked well for people under 65.

Medicare Supplemental Insurance

One of the most effective ways to maximize the value of your Medicare dollar is to purchase Medicare supplemental insurance. Since what Medicare will cover and how much it will pay are known in advance, as is the amount of various services used by Medicare recipients, designing a policy that will afford protection against more than minor out-of-pocket expenses ought to be easy. Unfortunately, insurance companies have seldom chosen to do this.

Rather, they have treated the pricing of Medicare insurance as a great mystery. They have also made the classic insurance boner of protecting people from what they can afford to pay, and not protecting them from what they can't afford, such as long nursing home stays. Add to this the use of scare tactics in selling — envelopes that look like official U.S. government correspondence — and the history of Medicare supplemental insurance is not a particularly happy one.

The new Medicare catastrophic coverage law contains a number of restrictions on sellers of Medicare supplemental insurance *who want their policies certified by the federal government. These restrictions do not apply to insurers who do not seek this certification:*

- You must now be given a free-look period, of at least thirty days, during which you can decide to cancel a policy and receive a refund of all premiums paid.
- Expected payout of benefits must equal 60 percent of premiums for individual policies and 75 percent for group policies.
- Certified insurers are required to follow ethical practices, including submitting advertising to state insurance commissioners for review.

We suggest that, at a minimum, you purchase a policy that covers *all* the deductibles and copayments for hospital and doctor bills. This means that you will have to pay only what Medicare does not reimburse, and it limits your expense to relatively minor items (with the exception of nursing home care). You should also check for coverage of amounts charged by physicians in excess of the Medicare approved charge. Policies that cover this expense typically do not pay unlimited amounts to doctors, but they will further limit your out-of-pocket expenses. The policy should also cover the copayment for the first eight days of skilled nursing facility care.

The new Medicare catastrophic coverage law limits your out-of-pocket liability for charges under Medicare Part B (*not* your total out-of-pocket expenses) to $1,370 beginning January 1, 1990. You have no out-of-pocket protection in 1989, and no protection at any time against charges from nonparticipating doctors who are permitted to charge more than the Medicare-approved amounts. Your out-of-pocket protection applies *only* to Part B charges of Medicare-participating doctors. The out-of-pocket limit is also scheduled to rise so that only 7 percent of beneficiaries hit the cap. This, in effect, leaves 93 percent with no cap. The estimated limits are as follows:

- $1,530 in 1991
- $1,700 in 1992
- $1,900 in 1993

Your Medicare supplemental policy should provide *more* protection than this; and it should cover charges of doctors in excess of the Medicare-approved amounts.

Here are some other features to look for:

- Guaranteed renewability
- No restrictions on payment for preexisting conditions
- No limitations to single diseases, such as cancer
- Payment for services in full, rather than payment of fixed money amounts
- No waiting periods for coverage

In chapter 4, we explain more about supplemental insurance and give you a means of comparing policies.

Negotiating with Your Doctor

Another way to make the most of Medicare is to talk with your doctor about your care. We go into great depth in this area in chapter 5. Among the reasons you should negotiate your care (and his or her fees) with your doctor(s) are these:

- Most Americans experience their first serious illness only when they are over 50 or thereabouts. Yuppies can arrange heart attacks in their 30s, but serious illness, for most people, comes with age.
- Because of this, the most expensive illnesses will come when people have reduced incomes, and when they are dependent on Medicare for health coverage.
- Medicare pays, on average, only about half of the health care expenses of elderly and disabled people, and that percentage is falling each year.
- Almost no form of supplementary insurance covers everything that people will need.

- The cost of treatment, the physical and psychological burdens of treatment, and the effect on relatives are *all* determined mostly by the doctor.
- The doctor, in large measure, determines how and when people die.

You should fight the tendency — which is forced on Americans by their culture — to think of Medicare as some sort of charity. Medicare beneficiaries paid premiums for Part A through their work in the past and are paying premiums for Part B now. In dealing with your doctor, think of Medicare as just like any other insurance. Medicare may not pay everything that the doctor might like, but the doctor's prices, which are largely unaffected by market forces, are a sort of wish list to begin with. It's probable that *no* insurance company is paying the doctor everything he or she wants.

Even better, don't think of the insurance issue at all. Doctors make their living by selling their services, and the satisfaction of their customers should be a big concern to them. When it comes right down to it, if a doctor loses you as a patient, any and all fees he or she might have gotten from you are lost. If the doctor keeps you as a patient and accepts Medicare **assignment** to help you pay only a bearable portion of your income for medical expenses, all that is lost is the difference between the doctor's wishes and the Medicare payment. If you have to point this out, do so. Your doctor may learn something.

Health Maintenance Organizations (HMOs)

Health Maintenance Organizations (**HMOs**) are a proven approach to medical care delivery. When they were first started, they were bitterly opposed by doctors and medical organizations, because they either required the doctors to become employees and accept a salary, or because they limited what doctors could charge. In the 1930s, a group of consumers in Washington, D.C., set up an HMO, which they owned and controlled (and still do). The doctors were hired by a board elected from the membership, and were actually (and still are) employees of their patients. The **American Medical Association** (**AMA**) sued them, and the case reached the Supreme Court. The Court said that if a group of people wanted to hire a group of doctors to take care of them, they could not be prevented from doing so.

Even though HMOs are growing rapidly, only about half of the Medicare beneficiaries in the nation live in the service areas of those with Medicare contracts. Because such organizations are new to many, we'll explain in some detail how they work with Medicare.

Most HMOs are not consumer-owned. Whether or not they are for-profit or nonprofit, they are "owned" by a self-perpetuating board of trustees, the same way **nonprofit voluntary hospitals** are. Regardless of who owns them, they usually make at least a pretense of seeking member involvement in the way the HMO is run.

The basic idea behind health maintenance organizations is that health care will, overall, be cheaper if preventive services are covered and if there is no need for people to worry about the cost before seeking care. This makes sense. HMOs have clearly demonstrated that they can save at least 25 percent over the cost of care provided in a **fee-for-service system,** like Medicare, in which doctors are paid something for each service they provide. It is thought that this provides a **perverse incentive** for the doctor to give care that is not really needed. Much research evidence suggests that this is true.

The opposite side of the coin, of course, is the risk that HMO doctors may be tempted to undertreat people to save money. This has happened, but rarely. Studies of HMO patients in general have found that their health is just as good as, and perhaps a little bit better than, the health of patients treated by doctors in private practice. Studies have also shown that the quality of care given in HMOs is, in the main, just as good as or just a little bit better than the care given by doctors in private practice.

As a Medicare patient in an HMO, you will have either no or far fewer forms to fill out than a Medicare patient being treated by private doctors. You will most likely get more services, at a lower cost, than you will as a patient of doctors in private practice. HMOs usually offer what those in the health insurance industry call a "Cadillac" package of services, with few or no copayments or deductibles, depending on the organization. Prescription drugs are often provided at no or low cost. This alone can make an HMO worth considering for someone who must take several expensive drugs. They do this both because they believe in the original ideal of supplying services to maintain health, rather than just cure illness, and because they need to attract patients.

Some people do not like certain features of health maintenance organizations, so HMOs compete in other ways, often by offering more benefits than do traditional insurance plans. The same features that deter some people often attract other people. For one thing, your choice of doctors is limited to doctors who are employees of the HMO (if it is a **staff model health maintenance organization**), to those who are in the **group practices** that the HMO has contracted with (if it is a **group model health maintenance organization**), or to doctors in private practice who have signed on as members of an **individual practice** association (IPA) model health maintenance organization. Opponents of HMOs make a big issue of the supposed denial of freedom of choice. It is little understood that Blue Shield, still the major supplier of insurance for doctors' services in the country, works on essentially the same principle: it will pay in full only for the services of doctors on the Blue Shield panel. The difference in HMOs is that no payment is made for services of doctors not on the HMO panel, unless an HMO doctor calls them in as a consultant or refers you to them.

A group or staff model HMO is far more convenient for a person, especially a moderately sick one, than seeing a physician in private practice. Usually, **primary care physicians** (**general practitioners, family practitioners,** general **internists, pediatricians,** and **obstetrician-gynecologists**) are located in the same building with **specialists**. Often, but not always, it is possible to see a specialist immediately if the primary care physician thinks one is needed. **Outpatient surgery** suites, **chemotherapy** rooms, X-ray departments, laboratories, and pharmacies are often located in the same building as the doctors' offices. HMOs pioneered "one-stop shopping" in medicine primarily as a means of cost control and as a convenience to their doctors, but it is a great convenience for patients as well. Some large HMOs even have their own emergency rooms, located in their clinics.

An IPA model HMO uses the offices of private physicians who have agreed to see HMO patients in addition to their private patients. Office care in an IPA model HMO feels just like going to a doctor in private practice. Otherwise, all the following comments regarding hospital care and the like apply.

On the negative side (and not all agree that it is a negative), your choice of hospitals as an HMO member will be limited to those that the HMO has contracted with. Since HMOs are looking to control costs, these often will not be what are perceived to be the best hospitals in the city. The HMO management will learn which hospitals are the cheapest and have the best records for particular diseases and types of patients. You may find that you are admitted to one hospital, treated for one condition, and then transferred to another hospital for treatment of a second. If you need specialized surgery, you may have the surgery in a university medical school hospital and be transferred to a small community hospital to recuperate. Saving money in this way enables HMOs to offer the Cadillac plan at a rate that employers, patients — and Medicare — are willing to pay.

Health maintenance organizations usually offer high-option and low-option plans. A typical high-option plan can include all physician services for any purpose, all drugs for any purpose with no or a small copayment, unlimited hospital care, all emergency care, and all outpatient care, as well as podiatric services, eyeglasses, and hearing aids. Low-option plans vary widely. An increasingly common one is one small copayment — $5 to $10 — for everything. This greatly simplifies the HMO's bookkeeping and billing operations. It can mean, however, that one owes $200–$300 for a heavy day that included a visit with the primary care physician, a referral to a specialist, a welter of lab tests, a special X-ray series, a visit to the HMO nurse for shots and treatment, and five or six prescriptions. Even so, this is a very small amount compared to the out-of-pocket expenses for a Medicare beneficiary with no supplemental insurance or a plan that imposes heavy copayments and deductibles.

In some HMOs, the low option is limited to only the services covered by Medicare, but with the HMO covering all of Medicare copayments and deductibles and imposing none of its own. This is like a Medicare supplemental insurance plan that covers all the gaps in Medicare coverage but adds nothing else.

Premiums vary greatly, depending on the package of services chosen, the HMO's experience with Medicare patients, how many Medicare beneficiaries are enrolled versus younger (and usually healthier) people, who are cheaper to care for, the hospitals the HMO contracts with, going rates for doctors in the area, and so on. HMO enrollment is growing rapidly, and HMOs are experimenting with ways to enroll and retain people, so shopping around, especially in urban areas, is possible. It is safe to say that you will always be able to obtain *all* of the care you need in a HMO more cheaply than with a supplemental insurance plan, and certainly more cheaply than the cost of Medicare Part B premiums plus the copayments and deductibles.

Some people think that joining a health maintenance organization requires turning over their Social Security check to it. This is not true. When you enroll in an HMO that accepts Medicare patients, Medicare makes a regular monthly payment to the HMO. You continue to pay the Part B premium and may also have to pay a premium to the HMO to pay for services which Medicare does not cover. This extra premium may be larger or smaller than the Part B premium. It is just like the premium you pay for supplemental medical insurance to an insurance company.

Some HMO patients on a low-option plan that imposes a copayment for each service who are very sick and use a large amount of outpatient services will find themselves spending thousands of dollars out of pocket. It may even be cheaper (for them, not the HMO) to be treated in the hospital. This, paradoxically, is something that HMOs were set up to avoid. Such situations are teaching HMOs something that providers of employee benefit plans have known for years — that it is important to provide a maximum **out-of-pocket limit**, or **stop-loss provision**, for persons who have **catastrophic illnesses.**

There are other aspects of being an HMO member that you may or may not find to your liking. Virtually all HMOs require that they approve **out-of-area care** before it is provided, except in life-threatening emergencies. This may leave you sitting in the emergency room in Dubuque while the emergency room doctor and your HMO doctor in Los Angeles argue about whether you really need to be admitted. This stressful situation, which HMOs pioneered, is becoming more common as private insurance plans and Medicare itself have started requiring the same sort of preapproval for many services.

Some, but not all, HMOs try to make maximum use of **physician extenders**, such as **nurse practitioners, medical technicians**, and **physicians' assistants.** They do this based on research that shows that persons with these sorts of training can do as well as, or better than, doctors for a limited range of situations and can be trusted to recognize situations they can't handle and call in the doctor. If you think of them as specialists in low-end routine care, you can be comforted by the evidence that they sometimes are better than M.D.'s. If your image of proper medical care is having one specialist to look at your eyes, another to listen to your heart, a third to talk about your arthritis, and a fourth to talk about your kidneys, a visit with the nurse practitioner will not make you happy. From the HMO's viewpoint, using physician extenders cuts costs, enables more people to be seen, gives them a sympathetic ear for problems that the doctor seems too busy to listen to, and makes the best use of expensive physicians' time.

Some HMOs have a lot of general internists on staff and have **protocols** that require the other primary physicians to refer patients to them as special situations develop. This may lead to having your horse switched in midstream for no apparent reason while you are assured that there is no need to refer you to a specialist. Others treat internists as specialists in the use of drugs to treat disease of the internal organs — their original self-definition as specialists, before they got turned into a species of generalists. Still others make no distinction at all between the types of primary care providers. Some are quite happy to let your gynecologist attend to all your medical needs. Others are very strict about limiting gynecologists to **gynecological problems** only.

It is safe to say three things about the kind of care you will receive in a health maintenance organization. First, no matter how friendly it is, it will appear a little more regimented and impersonal than care in a private physician's office. It will feel a bit like a clinic, no matter how hard the HMO works at atmosphere. Second, your choice of primary care doctor will be limited to those who have signed up with the HMO, either as employees of a staff model HMO, members of a group practice HMO, or individual practice association HMO doctors. Third, you will get more care for the dollar than in traditional insurance plans, and your out-of-pocket expenses will be less. Whether you like the trade-offs is up to you. The rate of withdrawal — dropping out after signing up — is quite low. Most of those who get as far as enrolling seem to think the trade-offs are worth it.

Conditions for HMO Enrollment as a Medicare Beneficiary

Health maintenance organization membership was not available for Medicare beneficiaries until recently. Now it is almost routine. To be an HMO member as a Medicare beneficiary,

- You must be enrolled in *both* Part A and Part B of Medicare.
- You can join only an HMO that has a contract with Medicare, not just any one.
- You must live in the **service area** of the HMO, that is, the geographical area from which the HMO is licensed to enroll members.
- You must enroll during the open enrollment period of the HMO you have chosen. This may be all year, or it may be limited to a few months.
- You can drop out at any time by notifying the HMO in writing, on a form it prescribes for this purpose. A letter will not do, unless the organization specifically allows withdrawal requests by letter. You must submit the withdrawal request by the tenth day of the month to be returned to the regular Medicare program on the first of the next month. Requests received after the tenth will result in return to the regular program on the first of the month after next. In either case, the HMO will continue to provide you with services.

You have certain protections as an HMO member. Medicare requirements for HMO beneficiaries may go beyond what the state requires to license an HMO.

- You cannot be denied enrollment because of your state of health. The HMO *is* allowed to deny *high-option* coverage to persons with some medical conditions.

- All Medicare-covered services must be available with reasonable promptness when needed. Emergency facilities must be available around the clock.
- The HMO cannot terminate your membership because of poor health or because of the cost of treating you.
- If the HMO ends its contract with Medicare — thereby dropping all Medicare beneficiaries — you must be given at least sixty days' notice.
- The HMO must have written procedures for resolving complaints.
- You have the same rights to appeal decisions about your care in an HMO as you do for regular services (see chapter 8).
- You can withdraw from the HMO at any time by notifying it in writing. If the HMO requires that a special form be used to withdraw, you must use it.

Since the absence of freedom of choice is the one big negative associated with HMOs, many are experimenting with **freedom of choice options**. Usually, this means that you can see any doctor you want, provided that he or she has credentials satisfactory to the HMO, but must pay a copayment to see one who is not on the HMO panel.

The HMO is required to maintain a certain ratio between Medicare and non-Medicare patients. It is almost impossible to avoid a situation in which the younger, healthier members of an HMO are partially subsidizing the care of older, sicker ones. (This is true in HMOs that do not enroll Medicare members. The healthier patients who use few services subsidize those who are sicker. If this were not the case, a different premium would have to apply to every individual, and sick people could not afford care. There is nothing shady about this; it's part of the basic concept of insurance.) Medicare payment to the HMO, which is based on the average Medicare expenditure per person in the region, may not cover the cost of all HMO services. Because of this, the HMO may have closed enrollment and will allow no more Medicare recipients to join until the ratio is adjusted.

A chart you can use to compare different HMOs is provided in chapter 4, on supplemental health insurance for Medicare beneficiaries.

Competitive Medical Plans

Competitive medical plans (CMPs) are insurance plans that contract with Medicare to provide all Medicare-covered services for a flat fee paid to them by Medicare. They can charge a premium, over and above the cost of Medicare, for services not covered by Medicare. Some competitive medical plans are health maintenance organizations, but they are not required to follow the HMO model.

The important thing to remember is that in a competitive medical plan, you do not immediately return to regular Medicare coverage when you withdraw unless you have submitted your request by the tenth of the month. If you have not done so, you are returned to the regular Medicare coverage *no earlier than* the first day of the first month following the month in which you request withdrawal. (If, for example, you request withdrawal on September 1, you would not be covered under the regular Medicare program until October 1.)

MIGs at Twelve O'Clock — Medicare Insured Groups

Congress has appropriated funds for three **Medicare insured groups,** or **MIGs.** These are experiments in which a purchaser of health insurance to those under 65, such as an employer or a union health plan, undertakes to provide health insurance to Medicare beneficiaries on the same basis, in return for a payment from the federal government. If the experimental MIGs work well, they will probably be written into the Social Security act as one more option for receiving health care under Medicare, along with health maintenance organizations and competitive medical plans.

Medicare has a pamphlet on various prepaid health coverage plans, "Medicare and Prepayment Plans," which can be obtained at your local Social Security office. If they have none, ask them to order HCFA publication number 02143.

In this chapter you will learn: What is covered by Medicare Part A hospital insurance ▪ What is covered by Medicare Part B medical insurance ▪ What is meant by deductibles and copayments ▪ When new services become effective ▪ When you *are not* responsible for the cost of services received ▪ When you *are* responsible for the cost of services received ▪ How to read an Explanation of Medicare Benefits ▪ How the Diagnosis-Related Groups system affects hospital payment and you ▪ What your rights are while a hospital patient

3. What Medicare Does (and Doesn't) Pay For

The purpose of this chapter is to explain, in terms that are as clear as the complexity of the program permits, exactly what Medicare pays for and what you (or your insurer, or both) have to pay for.

Medicare pays in full for only a few items. Even if you have insurance that supplements Medicare, the insurance plan may require you to pay part of the cost. The same is true if you belong to a **Health Maintenance Organization** (HMO) through which you obtain Medicare services. The phrase "what you pay for" in this chapter should be understood to include what has to be paid, regardless of who pays it. You may have other sources of payment for what Medicare doesn't cover — payments made by your insurer or HMO (plus what you pay out-of-pocket).

What gets paid for, how much, and when, under Medicare, is an odd combination of the following:

- The *services* that providers agree to provide in their contracts with Medicare
- The *amount* of the services that Medicare covers
- Medicare's commitment to *cost-sharing* through copayment and deductibles

- *How* the law establishing Medicare (Title XVIII of the Social Security act) dictates that each type of **provider** be paid
- The *medical necessity* of the services you actually received

The regulations that govern Medicare are *not* set up this way. As a result, it is very hard to discover exactly what is paid, or not paid, under what conditions, by reading them. But the ways we have cut them up, above, really do cover all the issues that are involved in determining what you wind up paying for. In each of the sections that begin on page 94, we discuss what Medicare pays and what you pay under related headings:

- Covered Services
- Limitations on Services
- Cost-sharing
- How Payment Is Made
- Medical Necessity Determinations

When You Never Have to Pay

There are numerous situations in which Medicare decides not to pay a provider, or to pay less than the provider wanted. It's important to understand when you don't have to pay for something that Medicare has refused to pay a provider for: *You are never obligated to pay for a service unless you can reasonably have been expected to know that the service was not covered, or was not (medically) reasonable and necessary. You are never obligated to pay more than Medicare has decided to pay the provider if the provider has agreed to accept* **assignment**.

"Reasonably Have Been Expected to Know"

"Reasonably have been expected to know" is a legal phrase. What it means, basically, is this: if you have not been informed *in writing* by an appropriate review authority, the provider, a Medicare intermediary or carrier, or Medicare itself that a service is not covered or is not (medically) reasonable and necessary, and you could not be expected to know it from official sources (such as pamphlets that you were given when you signed up for Medicare, or from prior notices that such services were not covered), then you are protected from having to pay for it, even if Medicare doesn't. The key word is *reasonably*. What you can reasonably be expected to know is that which a reasonable person would expect an individual like you, in your situation, having received the information you received, to know. The working definition, as Medicare's **administrative law judges** and the courts use it, resides in **case law** and is continuously evolving. As it stated in the regulations, there are two important parts: you have to receive *a written notice*, and you have to receive it from *an appropriate source*.

Some examples may help here:

Example 1: *You go into the hospital for surgery. The operation (or procedure; we'll call all procedures "operations" for the sake of simplicity) is one that Medicare normally requires be done in an* **outpatient** *facility, because it has been proven that this can be done safely and at lower cost than in the hospital. Your doctor believes that he can show that your case required* **inpatient** *surgery. The* **Peer Review Organization (PRO)** *that reviews such cases disagrees. The hospital gets paid nothing. You do not have to pay anything. Why? Because you cannot reasonably have been expected to know exactly which operations are required to be done as outpatient operations, or to know the steps your doctor should have followed to check.*

Example 2: *You go into the hospital for surgery. The operation is one that Medicare normally requires be done only after the peer review organization has approved it. (This may be because there is disagreement among doctors about when the operation is needed or whether it works, or because there is wide variation across the country in the number of operations done on similar groups of people. It may also be because the peer review organization has determined that many of the operations performed in your area turn out to be unnecessary.) The hospital does not obtain approval. The hospital is paid nothing, but you are not required to pay anything. You could not reasonably have been expected to know which operations were on the preapproval list.*

Example 3: *You have carefully searched for a doctor who accepts* **assignment.** *The doctor you chose is on the list of* **Medicare-participating physicians** *that your local Social Security office provided you. You specifically ask her if she takes assignment. She says that she does. The old year passes, and the new one begins. You suddenly begin getting bills from her for more than 20 percent of Medicare's charge for her services. It turns out that she has not renewed her* **participating-physician agreement** *with Med-*

icare and has taken no steps to inform her patients. You call the office to complain, and find out that she no longer accepts assignment. You do not have to pay more than 20 percent of the Medicare-approved charge until you learn this. You are required to pay the extra costs for services received after you learn this.

Example 4: *You are discharged from the hospital but need further therapy before you can go home. You are admitted to a nursing home for some physical therapy and daily changing of a dressing. The peer review organization determines that you could have been treated at home, or at the doctor's office, so your stay is not* **medically necessary.** *The nursing home is paid nothing, but you do not have to pay anything.*

Don't worry if you didn't understand everything in the examples. What you need to understand is the general principle: when Medicare makes a payment, all sorts of wheels turn which you cannot reasonably be expected to know about. You are protected from the consequences of behind-the-scenes decisions if you are not informed of them. *The fact that Medicare has refused payment doesn't mean that you have to pay.*

On the other hand, there *are* situations in which you *can* "reasonably be expected to know" something or other, and you must act to make sure that you do not have to pay more than is necessary. Some examples, parallel to the ones above, should help make this clear:

Example 1: *You go into the hospital for surgery. The operation is one that Medicare normally requires be done in an* **outpatient** *facility, because it has been proven that this can be done safely and at lower cost than in the hospital. Your doctor believes that he can show that your case requires* **inpatient** *surgery. He checks with the appropriate personnel at the hospital. They advise him that your condition does not require hospitalization and can safely be done in an outpatient facility (a clinic, an* **ambulatory surgery** *center, or the doctor's office). You are informed of this in* writing. *You do not appeal. You decide to go to the hospital. As expected, the* Peer Review Organization (PRO) *will recommend that nothing be paid for the hospital stay. You are so informed,* in writing. *You do not appeal. You have to pay the hospital bill and any doctors' bills associated with doing the operation in the hospital. Why? You could reasonably have been expected to know that this operation was required to be done as an outpatient operation; you were informed in writing.*

Example 2: You go into the hospital for surgery. The operation is one that Medicare normally requires be done only after the peer review organization has approved it. The hospital does not obtain approval. Your doctor tells you this, in writing. *You do not insist that a formal determination be made, or one is made and you do not appeal it. You decide to go ahead with the operation. You have to pay the hospital bill plus any additional doctors' fees. Why? You could reasonably have been expected to know that Medicare would not pay for the operation; you were informed in writing.*

Example 3: You have carefully searched for a doctor who accepts **assignment***. The doctor you chose is on the list of* **Medicare-participating physicians** *that your local Social Security office provided you. You specifically ask her if she takes assignment. She says that she does. The old year passes, and the new one begins. The doctor informs all her patients,* in writing, *by letter, that she will no longer accept assignment for all Medicare patients. You suddenly begin getting bills from her for more than 20 percent of the Medicare charge for her services. You have to pay anything over the Medicare-paid amount — 80 percent of the Medicare-approved charge. You do not have to pay more than the Medicare* **maximum allowable actual charge** *for the services you received from the physician, less 80 percent of the Medicare-approved charge. Why? You could reasonably have been expected to know that the physician no longer takes assignment; you were informed in writing.*

The maximum allowable actual charge is established for each service provided by each individual physician, based on that physician's history of bills to Medicare patients. You can find out your doctor's maximum allowable actual charge by calling the Medicare carrier in your area (see the list in appendix A) and telling them who your doctor is and what service you received or will receive. The doctor is not permitted to charge any Medicare beneficiary more than the maximum allowable for the service.

Example 4: You are discharged from the hospital but need further therapy before you can go home. You are admitted to a nursing home for some physical therapy and daily changing of a dressing. The Peer Review Organization determines that you could have been treated at home, or at the doctor's office, so your stay is not medically necessary. You are informed of this in writing, *and you elect not to appeal the decision or you lose your appeal. You have to pay for the nursing home stay. Why? You* could *reasonably have been expected to know that Medicare would not pay; you were informed in writing.*

Again, don't worry about the technicalities here. We'll inform you about what you can appeal, and how to do it, below. Chapter 8 provides more detail about the appeal process. For the moment, remember three things:

- First, an oral notice to you isn't worth the paper it's printed on. Only *written* notifications have effect.
- Second, the written notice must come from an appropriate source: the Peer Review Organization, the Medicare intermediary or carrier, or the provider (doctor, hospital, nursing home official).
- Third, once you have been informed that a service is not covered, you are expected to know that it is not covered in the future.

Dealing with Claims, Bills, and Carriers

We aren't saying that hospitals and doctors are unethical, but — like most of us — they prefer getting money to not getting money. They do not see it as their job to determine exactly what has and hasn't been approved and bill you only for your share of the approved charges. The **intermediaries** or **carriers** who handle Medicare payments see it as their primary duty to get the checks and the bills out. The peer review organization is interested in making determinations of medical necessity, and arguing with Medicare to get more money in their next review contract. So *none of these parties has, as its main concern, making sure that you get billed for only what you really have to pay for. You have to look out for yourself.* Because the payment system under Medicare is so complicated, it is virtually certain that at least one of your encounters with a health care provider will result in a bill for something you don't really owe. Because of this same complexity, and because there can be a considerable time lag before your case is reviewed (if it needs it) or the hospital is audited, a long time can pass before who gets what, and who has to pay for what, is finally decided. This is why it is important for you to understand this chapter and, in particular, to use the Medicare Claims Log we provide in appendix B to keep track of the services you received, what you had to pay, and when you paid it. The **Explanation of Medicare Benefits** sent to you by the Medicare carrier, and the information you receive from your insurance company, should enable you to do this.

They *should*, but they often don't. Your Medicare carrier or intermediary is required, as part of its contract with Medicare, to maintain a mailing address you can write to about amounts that you think you don't owe. Most of them also provide a telephone number. Your Medicare Supplemental Insurance carrier should have such an address, and a telephone number, and is usually required by state insurance laws to have both. (Addresses and telephone numbers of the various Medicare intermediaries and carriers are provided in appendix A. Where to write with insurance complaints for each of the states is provided in appendix C.) Your health maintenance organization, if you belong to one, is required by both state and federal laws to have a procedure for resolving disputes and usually will maintain an address and a telephone number. Don't hesitate to call them. We can guarantee you that more than one of the explanations they send you won't make sense. (A sample Explanation of Medicare Benefits is shown on page 95.)

Hospitals

Covered Services

You may wish to skip ahead and read the section on the DRG system in "How Payment Is Made" before you read the discussion of limitations on services.

Medicare's discussion of covered services for hospitals is basically an attempt to describe, at length, the services that hospitals normally provide to all patients. Bed and board, nursing services, use of hospital facilities, medical social services, drugs, biologicals, use of supplies and equipment, diagnostic and therapeutic services, and the services of **house staff** (**interns** and **residents** in training) are covered.

Limitations on Services

Private rooms are not covered unless your medical condition requires you to be isolated or there are no semiprivate or ward rooms available. Medicare will pay until you no longer need the private room or until you could be transferred to a semiprivate room or ward. You do not have to pay for the private room unless it was requested by you or a member of your family who was told, at the time the request was made, that there would be an additional charge. (Please note that the notice here does not need to be a written one.)

Medicare will not pay for the services of a **private duty nurse** unless the hospital normally provides one for patients in your condition.

Medicare will pay only for drugs used in the hospital. The hospital

This is your Part B Carrier. If you suspect a mistake, contact this office.

YOUR EXPLANATION OF MEDICARE BENEFITS
Read this notice carefully and keep it for your records.
This is not a bill.

HEALTH CARE FINANCING ADMINISTRATION

Iphigenia Smith
4321 Edgar Allen Poe Drive
San Diego, CA 99110

Dec. 31, 1987
Need help? Contact:
TRANSAMERICA OCCIDENTAL
   LIFE INSURANCE
1149 South Broadway
Box 54905 Terminal Annex
Los Angeles, CA 90054
Phone: 213 Area: 748-2311
   Other Areas: 1-800-252-9020

This tells you if Assignment was taken and the dollar amount billed.

Assignment was taken on your claim for $45.00 from MIDWAY MEDICAL CLNC.
(See item 4 on back.)

This indicates the service and date provided.

		Billed	Approved
1 Office Service	Dec 05, 1987	$45.00	$40.00

Approved amount limited by item 5c on back.

This indicates amount Billed and Approved.

Total approved amount	$40.00
Medicare payment (80% of the approved amount minus 2.324%)	$31.26

This indicates the Approved amount and Medicare's 80 percent.

MIDWAY MEDICAL CLNC agreed to charge no more for the above approved services than the amount approved by Medicare. We are paying a total of $31.26 to MIDWAY MEDICAL CLNC.

This is what Medicare pays.

You are responsible to the physician / supplier for the difference of $8.00 between the approved amount and the Medicare payment. If you have other insurance, it may help with the part Medicare did not pay.

This explains what You pay.

A new law has reduced your Medicare payment by 2.324% for services from November 21, 1987 to March 31, 1988. You are not responsible for the 2.324% reduction on this assigned claim.

This explains any change in billing and what — if any — affect on you.

(You have met the deductible for 1987)

This indicates whether or not you have met the $75 deductible.

95

IMPORTANT: If you do not agree with the amounts approved you may ask for a ——This gives you the time
review. To do this you must *write* to us before *Jun 31, 1988.* (See item 1 on the   frame to file any appeal.
back.)

DO YOU HAVE A QUESTION ABOUT THIS NOTICE? If you believe Medicare
paid for a service you did not receive, or there is an error, contact us
immediately. Always give us the: Use these numbers
                                                                                        when making any inquiry
Medicare Claim No. 987 65 4321A   Claim Control No. 7350 316 290   on your claim.

may give you a limited supply of drugs to take with you if this will facilitate your discharge and the drug is needed until you can obtain a continuing supply. Beginning January 1, 1990, supplies, nursing services, and pharmacy services for home administration of intravenous antibiotics will be covered. The drugs will be covered, with a 20 percent copayment, after you have paid the first $550. In 1991 they will be covered under the regular Medicare drug program, with a 50 percent copayment after a deductible of $600. If they were initially prescribed for administration in the hospital and administration at home is a continuation of this therapy, you will not have to pay for drugs.

Medicare will pay for all supplies and equipment used in the hospital. It will pay for supplies taken out of the hospital for outpatient use only if use must continue after you leave (example: a heart pacemaker) or they are required to assist your departure (example: crutches.)

The chart on pages 98–99 should make it obvious that there is a good reason to have some Medicare Supplemental Insurance. The trick is to get what you need while paying no more than you have to. We discuss how to find good insurance in chapter 4.

There is a separate deductible for blood. You are responsible for paying for the first three units of whole blood or **packed red cells** received in a hospital or skilled nursing facility. You must either pay for the blood or have it replaced. You are considered to have it replaced if an acceptable donor offers to replace it in your behalf, whether or not the provider or its blood supplier accepts the offer. The blood deductible can be met under Part A or Part B.

How Payment Is Made

Payment for hospitals under Medicare was always complicated. It has recently gotten more so, because of changes to the Medicare law passed by Congress that established the **prospective payment system** for hospitals. Prospective payments to hospitals are made through the **diagnosis-related groups (DRG) system.**

Why Prospective Payment? Consider an example. Suppose you go to an auto dealer and ask whether or not you need a car. If the answer is yes, you want the dealer to decide what kind of car a person like you should have, get it for you, and bill you, without regard to price. The chances are you will get a Mercedes, with all the options. Consider another. You go to the car dealer and say, "I want a compact car with all-weather radial tires, a stereo cassette deck, and air conditioning. I want it in black. It has to have at least a 50,000-mile guarantee on all

THE MEDICARE PROGRAM . . . .
WHAT IT PAYS . . . . WHAT YOU PAY

Program services, as well as deductibles and copayments, are subject to change on a yearly basis. For the most current information, consult the latest edition of *Your Medicare Handbook,* available at most Social Security Administration offices.

SCHEDULE OF BENEFITS

Medicare Part A: Hospital Insurance	Benefits Effective Through December 31, 1988	Changes Effective January 1, 1989
Hospital Deductibles	$540 initial deductible; 61–90 days $135 per day copayment; 91–150 days $270 per day copayment	Unlimited hospital days after a one-time yearly deductible of $560.
Skilled Nursing Facility	100 days total benefit; 1–20 days no cost; 21–100 days $67.50 per day copayment; 3-day prior hospitalization	150 days/year Copayment of $22.00 in 1989 on days 1 through 8 after which Medicare covers all costs for days 9–150. Beginning in 1990 the copayment will be adjusted to equal 20% of the average charge for one day in a skilled nursing facility. No prior hospitalization required.
Hospice (Care for the terminally ill)	(2) 90-day periods (1) 30-day period Beneficiary responsible for deductible and copayment on out-patient drugs and inpatient respite care.	Unlimited days as medically necessary
Blood (Whole blood or packed red cells)	As needed. Beneficiary pays deductible equal to the first 3 pints of blood. Any deductible paid under Part B does not apply.	As needed. Beneficiary pays a single yearly deductible equal to the cost of the first 3 pints of blood. Any deductible paid under the Part B benefit is also applied.

Additional Part A Services	Benefits Effective Through December 31, 1989	Changes Effective January 1, 1990
Home Health Care	5 days per week for 21 days.	7 days/week up to 38 consecutive days. May under certain conditions be extended.
Respite Care (In-home services for the chronically disabled. Provides a rest for the care giver)	Part of hospice care through 1989. Limited to no more than 5-day inpatient stay. Beneficiary pays 5% of outpatient drug costs or $5; 5% of inpatient costs up to the Part A deductible.	Benefit includes up to 80 hours/year of services to include: nursing, homemaker and personal care. Beneficiaries are eligible after they meet the Part B copayment limit or the prescription drug deductibles.

Medicare Part B: Medical Insurance	Benefits Effective Through December 31, 1989	Changes Effective January 1, 1990
Part B Deductibles Coverage of physician's services, outpatient hospital care, outpatient therapy, home health care and other services not covered by Hospital insurance.	As needed. After beneficiary pays $75 annual deductible. Medicare pays 80% of approved charges.	Yearly limit on out-of-pocket expenses on Part B covered services. Beneficiary pays deductible of $75/year after which Medicare pays 80% of all approved charges. Out-of-pocket expenses are limited to $1370 in 1990; $1530 in 1991; $1700 in 1992; and $1900 in 1993. After which Medicare pays 100% of approved charges. Physician fees and other charges that exceed the Medicare approved charges do not count toward the out-of-pocket limit.
Mammography Screening	No benefit	Provides for biannual (every-other-year) screening. Medicare pays 80% of the costs up to $50 the first year.
Home Health Care	5 days per week for 21 days	7 days/week up to 38 consecutive days. May under certain conditions be extended.
Respite Care (In-home services for the chronically disabled. Provides a rest for the care giver)	Part of hospice care through 1989. Limited to no more than 5-day inpatient stay. Beneficiary pays 5% of outpatient drug costs or $5; 5% of inpatient costs up to the Part A deductible.	Benefit includes up to 80 hours/year of services to include: nursing, homemaker and personal care. Beneficiaries are eligible after they meet the Part B copayment limit or the prescription drug deductible.

Medicare Part B: Medical Insurance	Benefits Effective Through December 31, 1989	Changes Effective January 1, 1990
IV Drug Therapy (In-home service)	No benefit	80% of all costs after deductible of $550 in 1990; 50% of all costs after deductible of $600 in 1991; 60% of all costs after deductible of $652 in 1992 and 80% of all costs after deductible in 1993. Deductibles and copayments may be waived if therapy was started as a result of hospital inpatient service.
Immunosuppressive Drugs	Medicare covers one year of drugs used in immunosuppressive therapy after transplantation, with the beneficiary paying the 20% copayment.	Medicare pays 50% of the cost of these drugs after a deductible of $550 in 1990; 50% of the costs after a deductible of $600 in 1991; and 60% of the costs after a deductible of $652 in 1992. Beginning in 1993 Medicare pays 80% of all costs after the deductible.

Additional Services	Benefits Effective Through December 31, 1990	Changes Effective January 1, 1991
Outpatient Prescription Drug Service (Coverage for prescriptions which are written independent of any stay in the hospital)	No benefit	50% of all costs after meeting deductible of $600 in 1991; 60% of all costs after deductible of $652 in 1992 and 80% of all costs after deductible to be determined for 1993 and beyond.

major parts and the body. I know cars like this can be bought for no more than $7,500. Get me the car, and I will pay you that, but no more." Chances are that you will get what you want, for no more than $7,500. The dealer will try to get a higher price, and you will have to negotiate, but you will get the car you specified.

Any insurer — including Medicare — that makes **retrospective payments** to a health care provider is in the first situation. (Retrospective payments are made after a service has been rendered. It is the main way the medical system in the United States works now, although this is changing.) In this **fee-for-service system**, in which providers render whatever services they think necessary and then bill for them, there is a danger of getting much more than is needed and paying more than is really necessary. You are also in danger of being told that you need a car when you really don't. In the second situation, you are protected: you have made the decision that you want the car, and you will not buy it at more than the agreed-upon price. This is the benefit of prospective payment, especially with appropriate controls such as second opinions on surgery and the requirement of preapproval for some operations and hospital stays. Providers argue constantly about the evils of prospective payment, but there is considerable research evidence that shows that the quality of care need not suffer and that providers can make a good profit under it.

Congress required that Medicare pay for hospital services under Medicare via a prospective payment scheme because it was convinced that this step would help avoid unnecessary hospitalization and control costs. Prospective payment protects you.

The Diagnosis-Related Groups (DRG) System

The DRG system is Medicare's current method of prospective payment. It was developed originally by the Yale School of Organization and Management and became law for hospitals in the state of New Jersey before Congress made it nationwide for Medicare. Using sophisticated statistical techniques, Medicare cases were analyzed to see how payments should be set to cover as many cases as possible. This research showed that the main or **primary diagnosis** of the patient, **secondary diagnoses**, age, and operations performed predicted costs for the majority of patients quite well. The billions of possible combinations of these factors were reduced to 467 **diagnosis-related groups** (**DRGs**), which are best understood as the overall condition of a patient. Congress understood that these 467 groups would not cover every case, and they made provisions for **outliers** — people who needed more days in the hospital, or more expensive hospital stays, because they had illnesses, or needed operations, that fell outside the DRGs. Hospitals can be granted payment for cases that require more hospital days than predicted by the DRG, provided the continued stay is medically necessary. Cases that do not exceed the length of stay criteria, but are more costly than predicted by a certain amount, are paid more if the hospital applies for additional payment.

DRG, Hospitals, and You: The DRG system was phased in over several years, and as of October 1, 1987, virtually every general, acute-care hospital in the country was paid with DRGs. The way it works is as follows: You are admitted to the hospital as a Medicare patient. Your DRG cannot be assigned when you come in, because your diagnosis may be unknown or wrong. Also, the operation(s) that you will have cannot be predicted in advance, especially if you are admitted for a **diagnostic workup**. Once everything has been done, and you are ready to be discharged (dead or alive), the hospital prepares a **face sheet** for your hospital chart which indicates your DRG. The DRG will probably have been assigned by a computer program that was purchased by the hospital and designed to pick the highest-paid DRG possible, based on your combination of age, diagnoses, operations, and other factors. The Medicare **intermediary** pays the hospital the DRG rate, after a computer review of the hospital's DRG coding.

Note that the hospital couldn't assign the DRG when you came in, and therefore could not predict the cost of your care or how much it would be paid. The result is that on some admissions the hospital will lose money and on some admissions it will make money. On the average, hospitals that are generally as "good" — measured by their use of resources on patients, not by the results they produce — as the average hospital will break even. Those that are better, in this sense, will make money, and they are allowed to keep their profits. Those that are worse will lose money, and they will have to swallow their losses.

The important point is this: *there is no guarantee from Medicare that the hospital will not lose money, or make money, on your case. Its loss or gain, under the DRG system, is supposed to have nothing to do with your care.*

Let's look at some examples:

You are over 75 years old, have a minor heart attack, and fall down a flight of stairs as a result and break a hip. The surgeon decides that a total hip replacement is needed. You have the op-

eration. Much to everyone's surprise, there are no complications, and you quickly learn to walk with the artificial hip and are able to go home well before the DRG-assigned number of hospital days. The hospital makes money on your case and gets to keep it.

*Now imagine the same circumstances, but (as might be expected given this situation) your care is long and difficult, and complications arise. You develop **thrombophlebitis** in your legs and have to have more surgery and additional drugs. You have a bleeding episode as a result of the drugs and need a transfusion. You are very weak and take a long time to get to the point at which you can be discharged to a **skilled nursing facility** to learn to walk again. Even with outlier payments, the hospital loses a great deal of money on your case.*

In both of these situations, the hospital is supposed to give you care that is medically necessary, regardless of the amount it has to spend.

Results to date suggest that *hospital profits are at their highest level in history,* based largely on profits from Medicare patients. Some types of hospitals, such as rural hospitals, inner-city hospitals with large charity care burdens, and hospitals that are the sole hospital for large areas, seem to be losing money. Congress has required Medicare to watch hospital profits carefully and to report to it, through the Prospective Payment Assessment Commission, on any adjustments that should be made. For the most part, though, DRGs have been a financial boon to hospitals.

Another point that needs to be understood is this: Since DRG payments are based on national/regional averages, it is *planned* that some hospitals will make money and some will lose money. It's part of the concept. One of the objectives of the DRG system, in fact, was the closure of the nation's least efficient hospitals. It was hoped that they would lose so much money that they would have to close. Patients would then go to the more efficient hospitals, and overall costs would be reduced. This is another reason that losses (or profits) made by the hospital under the DRG system should have nothing to do with your care. *These losses (or profits) are a result of the overall efficiency of the hospital, not your particular medical needs. No one case is going to break (or make) a hospital.*

During the early days of the DRG system, there were a number of instances of abuse. Patients were told that they had to leave the hospital "because your DRG has run out" or something similar. Discharging any patient who still needs hospital care because of financial considerations is a total violation of the hospital's contract with Medicare. The hospital has agreed to provide services to you as long as they are medically necessary.

Because of the abuses that were observed, the **People's Medical Society (PMS)** and the **American Association of Retired Persons (AARP)** joined forces to ask Medicare to require hospitals to "mirandize" Medicare patients: just as persons being arrested are told of their constitutional rights. Medicare now requires *all* hospitals to provide Medicare beneficiaries with an *Important Message from Medicare* upon admission for *any* inpatient hospital care. It appears on pages 104–106.

To sum up: the only reasons that you can be discharged from a hospital under Medicare are *medical* ones.

Medical Necessity Determinations

Medicare does not pay for services that are not medically "reasonable and necessary."

Who makes this determination? The first one, obviously, is your doctor. If your doctor suggests that you are ready to go home, you are likely to comply. If you feel you need more time, discuss it with him or her. The real issue comes when you want to stay in the hospital and the hospital's **utilization review committee (URC)** wants you to leave, or the Peer Review Organization wants you to leave. In either case, you will receive a written notice that a decision has been made, and that you have the right to appeal it. How to appeal it is covered in chapter 8.

If you win the appeal, you stay. If you lose, you may be required to pay for up to one day of hospital stay after the original cutoff date. It's important to understand that there are two tracks here, as described in the information on requesting a review given a few pages back. If you are asking the Peer Review Organization to review the hospital's decision, you are not responsible for services received before you get the notice of the Peer Review Organization's decision. If you are asking the Peer Review Organization to rethink its own decision, the hospital may start billing you beginning with the third calendar day after you received the Notice of Noncoverage. If the Peer Review Organization does not reverse its position and you decide not to stay in the hospital, you may have to pay for the third day. If you decide to stay, you are responsible for the further cost of your care.

AN IMPORTANT MESSAGE FROM MEDICARE

YOUR RIGHTS WHILE YOU ARE A MEDICARE HOSPITAL PATIENT

- You have the right to receive all the hospital care that is necessary for the proper diagnosis and treatment of your illness or injury. According to Federal law, **your discharge date must be determined solely by your medical needs,** not by "DRGs" or Medicare payments.

- You have the right to be fully informed about decisions affecting your Medicare coverage and payment for your hospital stay and for any post-hospital services.

- You have the right to request a review by a Peer Review Organization of any written Notice of Noncoverage that you receive from the hospital stating that Medicare will no longer pay for your hospital care. Peer Review Organizations (PROs) are groups of doctors who are paid by the Federal Government to review medical necessity, appropriateness and quality of hospital treatment furnished to Medicare patients. The phone number and address of the PRO for your area are:

  _____

  _____

  _____

TALK TO YOUR DOCTOR ABOUT YOUR STAY IN THE HOSPITAL

You and your doctor know more about your condition and your health needs than anyone else. Decisions about your medical treatment should be made between you and your doctor. **If you have any questions about your medical treatment, your need for continued hospital care, your discharge, or your need for possible post-hospital care, don't hesitate to ask your doctor.** The hospital's patient representative or social worker will also help you with your questions and concerns about hospital services.

IF YOU THINK YOU ARE BEING ASKED TO LEAVE THE HOSPITAL TOO SOON

- Ask a hospital representative for a written notice of explanation immediately, if you have not already received one. This notice is called a "Notice of Noncoverage." You must have this Notice of Noncoverage if you wish to exercise your right to request a review by the PRO.

- The Notice of Noncoverage will state either that your doctor or the PRO agrees with the hospital's decision that Medicare will no longer pay for your hospital care.

  + If the hospital and your doctor agree, the PRO does not review your case before a Notice of Noncoverage is issued. But the PRO will respond to your request for a review of your Notice of Noncoverage and seek your opinion. You cannot be made to pay for your hospital care until the PRO makes its decision, if you request the review by noon of the first work day after you receive the Notice of Noncoverage.

+ If the hospital and your doctor disagree, the hospital may request the PRO to review your case. If it does make such a request, the hospital is required to send you a notice to that effect. In this situation the PRO must agree with the hospital or the hospital cannot issue a Notice of Noncoverage. You may request that the PRO reconsider your case after you receive a Notice of Noncoverage but since the PRO has already reviewed your case once, you may have to pay for **at least one day of hospital care** before the PRO completes this reconsideration.

IF YOU **DO NOT** REQUEST A REVIEW, **THE HOSPITAL MAY BILL YOU** FOR ALL THE COSTS OF YOUR STAY BEGINNING WITH THE THIRD DAY AFTER YOU RECEIVE THE NOTICE OF NONCOVERAGE. THE HOSPITAL, HOWEVER, CANNOT CHARGE YOU FOR CARE UNLESS IT PROVIDES YOU WITH A NOTICE OF NONCOVERAGE.

HOW TO REQUEST A REVIEW OF THE NOTICE OF NONCOVERAGE

- If the Notice of Noncoverage states that your **physician agrees** with the hospital's decision:
  + You must make your request for review to the PRO by **noon of the first work day** after you receive the Notice of Noncoverage by contacting the PRO by phone or in writing.
  + The PRO must ask for your views about your case before making its decision. The PRO will inform you by phone and in writing of its decision on the review.
  + If the PRO agrees with the Notice of Noncoverage, you may be billed for all costs of your stay beginning at noon of the day **after** you receive the PRO's decision.
  + Thus, you will **not** be responsible for the cost of hospital care before you receive the PRO's decision.

- If the Notice of Noncoverage states that the PRO agrees with the hospital's decision:
  + You should make your request for reconsideration to the PRO **immediately** upon receipt of the Notice of Noncoverage by contacting the PRO by phone or in writing.
  + The PRO can take up to three working days from receipt of your request to complete the review. The PRO will inform you in writing of its decision on the review.
  + Since the PRO has already reviewed your case once, prior to the issuance of the Notice of Noncoverage, the hospital is permitted to begin billing you for the cost of your stay beginning with the third calendar day after you receive your Notice of Noncoverage **even if the PRO has not completed its review.**
  + Thus, if the PRO continues to agree with the Notice of Noncoverage, **you may have to pay for at least one day of hospital care.**

NOTE: The process described above is called "immediate review." If you miss the deadline for this immediate review while you are in the hospital, you may still request a review of Medicare's decision to no longer pay for your care at any point during your hospital stay or after you have left the hospital. The Notice of Noncoverage will tell you how to request this review.

POST-HOSPITAL CARE

When your doctor determines that you no longer need all the specialized services provided in a hospital, but you still require medical care, he or she may discharge you to a skilled nursing facility or home care. The discharge planner at the hospital will help arrange for the services you may need after your discharge. Medicare and supplemental insurance policies have limited coverage for skilled nursing facility care and home health care. Therefore, you should find out which services will or will not be covered and how payment will be made. Consult with your doctor, hospital discharge planner, patient representative and your family in making preparations for care after you leave the hospital. **Don't hesitate to ask questions.**

ACKNOWLEDGEMENT OF RECEIPT — My signature only acknowledges my receipt of this Message from (name of hospital) on (date) and does not waive any of my rights to request a review or make me liable for any payment.

_____

Signature of beneficiary or
person acting on behalf of beneficiary.

Skilled Nursing Facilities

Covered Services

Care in a **Skilled Nursing Facility** (**SNF**) is care that is less intense than that you receive in a hospital, but more intense than the custodial care provided in an intermediate care facility or custodial care nursing home. Basically, all of the services listed under hospitals are covered under skilled nursing facilities. The exceptions are services that skilled nursing facilities do not normally provide, such as operating rooms. Medicare permits hospitals with fewer than one hundred beds that have empty beds to run a skilled nursing facility within their walls, using beds that have been designated as **swing beds**. Swing beds are used as skilled nursing facility beds when there is a need for skilled nursing facility services, and as hospital beds when there is a need for hospital services. In effect, the hospital uses part of its capacity as a skilled-nursing-facility-type nursing home.

Many people think that Medicare pays for long-term nursing home care. There are sometimes tragic results from confusion about this. *Medicare does not pay for "custodial" or "personal care" services in nursing homes, only for rehabilitative care. This care is limited to 150 days per year.*

Limitations on Services and Cost-Sharing

You are entitled to 150 days of skilled nursing facility care during each calendar year. For the first 8 days, you must pay a coinsurance equal to one-fifth of the average national charge for SNF services, starting at $22.00 in 1989. An example:

After a long and complicated hospital stay, Victoria Smith-Jones is sent to a skilled nursing facility. She does not improve as rapidly as everyone hoped, and has to spend 135 days there. For the first 8 days, she has to pay $22.00 per day. For days 9–135, Medicare pays for everything. Her total charge for the stay in the nursing home is $176.00.

How Payment Is Made

The skilled nursing facility (or the hospital that provides skilled nursing facility care in a swing bed) is paid a daily amount by the intermediary, less your coinsurance.

Medical Necessity Determinations

Medical necessity is *the* key issue in payment for skilled nursing facility services. (The skilled nursing facility regulations go to great lengths to define what is and is not skilled nursing facility care. The key is that care complex enough to require the services of a nurse or skilled rehabilitation personnel is covered; care that you could handle by yourself is not. But complications may require skilled-nursing-facility-level care, even for situations that would normally not be covered. Basically, skilled nursing facility care is rehabilitation; if your condition cannot be expected to improve as a result of skilled nursing facility care *and* you do not need observation by skilled personnel, your care will not be covered. Obviously, what your doctor writes in the chart makes a big difference in what gets covered. If you are worried about coverage of skilled nursing facility services, discuss this with your doctor.

If you receive a written notice from the skilled nursing facility's or the hospital's utilization review committee, or from the peer review organization, that your condition no longer requires skilled nursing facility services, you can appeal. If you win the appeal, your care is paid for as long as it is medically necessary. If you lose, you pay for all care after the cutoff date. Chapter 8 explains how to appeal decisions regarding coverage related to medical necessity.

Home Health Services

Covered Services

Medicare covers medical services that are needed to allow you to live at home. The scope of benefits includes part-time or intermittent nursing care; physical, occupational, or speech therapy; medical social services; part-time or intermittent services of a home health aide; medical supplies; **durable medical equipment**; and the services of interns and residents if the **home health agency** (HHA) is affiliated with a teaching hospital. If the patient needs occupational therapy alone, that is not covered, but if occupational therapy is started as part of a program of rehabilitation that includes physical or speech therapy, continuing services are paid for even after the physical or speech therapy is over.

Beginning in 1990, pharmacy services, nursing services, and supply costs for the intravenous administration of antibiotics at home are covered. The drugs themselves are covered in 1990, with a copayment of 20 percent after a deductible of $550. In 1991, they will be covered just like other prescription drugs — 50 percent after a $600 deductible. Your cost will shrink to 40 percent, and then to 20 percent, during the next two years. If the drugs are a continuation of therapy started in the hospital, you pay nothing. Intravenous drugs other than antibiotics will be added as the secretary of health and human services finds them useful and safe for home administration.

As with skilled nursing facilities, personal care services are not covered. Housekeeping and transportation are not included. To receive home health services, you must be confined to your home or to an institution that is not a nursing home. Being able to take trips to see the doctor or to go to the hospital does not mean that you are not homebound.

Home health care (HHC) is covered under both Part A (hospital insurance) and Part B (doctor insurance) of Medicare. For coverage, all the following conditions must exist:

- You are confined to your home.
- You need part-time skilled nursing or physical or speech therapy.
- A doctor prescribes home health care.
- The **Home Health Agency** is approved by Medicare.

Limitations on Services

Home health care limited to thirty-eight consecutive visits.

Cost-Sharing

There is no cost-sharing under home health care except for the $75 Part B deductible for services furnished under Part B, and 20 percent of the reasonable charge for durable medical equipment supplied by home health care. The home health agency will charge patients for any services provided by it that are not covered under Medicare. You should ask the doctor and the HHA if any services not covered under Medicare are provided, and ask what the charges will be. Based on what you hear, you may want to discuss your plan of care with your doctor.

How Payment Is Made

Home health agencies bill the Medicare intermediary directly and bill you for any noncovered services.

Medical Necessity Determinations

Your need for continuing home health care must be reviewed periodically by a physician. You will be notified in writing if a finding is made that home health care is no longer medically necessary, and you have appeal rights, which are discussed in chapter 8.

Doctors' Services Under Part B of Medicare

Covered Services

Medicare was designed around the Blue Cross/Blue Shield model, which has one part paying for hospital services and another paying for everything else. "Everything else" is the job of Part B of Medicare, formally called supplemental medical insurance, or SMI. The scope of benefits as described in the regulations is as follows:

Medical and other health services such as physicians' services, outpatient hospital services, diagnostic tests, outpatient physical therapy and speech pathology services, rural health clinic services and outpatient renal dialysis services . . . services furnished by ambulatory surgical centers (ASCs), Home Health Agencies, (HHAs), and comprehensive outpatient rehabilitation facilities (CORFs) . . . other medical supplies, equipment, and supplies that are not covered under Medicare Part A hospital insurance.

Again, it's easier to talk about what is not covered than what is.

Limitations on Services

The following is a laundry list of what is not covered:

- Chiropractor's services are limited to manual manipulation of subluxation of the spine demonstrated by X ray. The X rays cannot be taken by the chiropractor. Only twelve treatments by the chiropractor are covered, unless more are determined to be medically necessary.
- Optometrists' services are limited to testing and examination needed to fit artificial lenses to treat aphakia (absence of the lens of the eye, whether natural or caused by the removal of a cataract).
- Dentists' and dental surgeons' services are covered only if they would have been covered if performed by a doctor.
- Podiatrists' services are covered only if they would have been covered if they had been performed by a doctor.
- Any prescription drug that can be self-administered (until January 1, 1991).
- More than $1,100 worth of outpatient psychiatric services in a calendar year.

Cost-Sharing

Part B is modeled on basic Blue Cross/Blue Shield plans as they existed in the mid-1960s. You are responsible for a $75 annual deductible and 20 percent of the "reasonable cost" of all services. An out-of-pocket limit applies for the services of **Medicare-participating physicians.** These limits are as follows:

- $1,370 in 1990
- An estimated $1,530 in 1991
- An estimated $1,700 in 1992
- An estimated $1,900 in 1993

These amounts are estimated because they are determined by a formula based on the percentage of Medicare beneficiaries who actually hit the limit.

How Payment Is Made

Now the fun begins. We get to talk about the usual, customary, and reasonable (UCR) process for determining doctors' payments under Medicare, and about assignment. One of the things that doctors insisted on in the formulation of the original Blue Shield plans was that they get paid, in essence, what they wanted. This approach was unlikely to sit well with those who paid the premiums — employers and employees — or with state governments that chartered the Blues. The process that was developed as a compromise is called the **usual, customary, and reasonable (UCR) reimbursement system**. It survives today in Medicare's notion of **approved charges**.

The approved charge for a physician service is the *lowest* of the following:

- The amount you were actually charged for the service
- The midpoint of all the charges that your doctor made for this service during the period from July 1, two years ago, to June 30, last year
- An amount large enough to cover 75 percent of the bills submitted for this service by all the doctors in the relevant locality

Example: Let's say that you were charged $200 for the service. The midpoint of all of the doctor's charges for the period specified is $183. An amount large enough to cover 75 percent of all bills submitted by all physicians is $275. The Medicare approved charge is $183. If the physician takes assignment, he is not allowed to charge you any more than that. Medicare will pay 80 percent of this ($146.40); you have to pay the remainder ($36.60). There is an extensive discussion of assignment, and the limits placed on physicians who do not participate in Medicare, with more examples, in chapter 5.

It is important to note here that your doctor has an incentive to jack up his or her fees from a median of $183 for this service to $275. If this is done, your doctor can painlessly raise prices to $275, still accept assignment, and obtain an extra $73.60 from Medicare free, even without billing you for the higher copayment. Medicare has attempted to provide some incentives for accepting assignment which we discuss in chapter 5. It should be clear to you that the doctor has no incentive to lower his or her prices or hold them stable under this system. Why? The doctors wanted it this way.

Recently, Medicare has started to impose a **maximum allowable actual charge (MAAC)** for each service provided by each physician. This is the maximum amount that the physician can charge any Medicare beneficiary, regardless of the approved charge. You can find out both the approved charge for what your doctor wants to do as well as the maximum allowable annual charge by calling or writing the Medicare intermediary or carrier for your area. These are listed in appendix A at the back of this book. To get the information, you need to have your doctor's name and address, the name or description of the medical service needed, and the Medicare code number for it, which you can get from your doctor.

Asking you to have a code number seems extreme. The need for it arises because services that have various names in the medical community but that are sometimes in fact the same, and services called by the same name, are sometimes different. Please keep in mind, when you call, that small differences in digits can make a big difference in payment. Suppose your doctor plans to do a 50725 and tells you so, but does a 50726 instead, with a $300 price difference. This does not necessarily mean that the doctor misled you. It may simply mean that once into the operation and having exposed the tissue that needed work, your doctor found that a more complicated operation than originally planned was needed, and altered course accordingly.

Another advantage of assignment, discussed in chapter 5, is related to paperwork. A doctor who accepts assignment files the claim with the Medicare carrier and bills you for the 20 percent copayment. You then either pay the doctor's bill or send it on to your Medicare supplemental insurance carrier (if you have supplemental insurance). Otherwise, you have to deal with both yourself.

Medical Necessity Determinations

Physician services under Medicare are reviewed just like other services. Actual and proposed operations are reviewed most stringently. If payment is denied to the physician on the grounds that the operation was unnecessary, you are protected from having to pay for it, because you could not have been expected to know this at the time.

Summing Up

As you have seen, Medicare covers quite a bit. The problem is with the limitations on the amount of services you can receive, the requirements for receiving them, and the copayments and deductibles. For Part B, for example, Medicare beneficiaries pay about 43 percent of the actual bill, not the 20 percent that Congress intended. It should be clear to you that insurance to supplement Medicare would be nice to have; we'll discuss that in chapter 5.

The big exclusions, those you should be most concerned about, are as follows:

- All chiropractic services, except for treatment of **subluxation of the spine**
- Purely custodial care — nursing homes
- Most dental care, and dentures
- **Over-the-counter drugs**
- Most eyeglasses and eye exams
- Hearing aids and fittings
- Full-time nursing care in the home
- Routine physical exams

Also, services paid for by Workers' Compensation, automobile or other liability insurance, employer health plans (for retirees *or* current employees, whichever you happen to be), and other government programs are not covered to the extent that these programs pay for the services you receive. Depending on the circumstances and the service, Medicare may pay the difference between what these programs paid and what you owe, but Medicare pays nothing unless you are obligated to make a payment.

In this chapter you will learn: The role of Medicare supplemental insurance ▪ How to provide for nursing home coverage that Medicare doesn't ▪ How to compare supplemental policies and what to look for ▪ Shopping tips to help you select the right policy ▪ How and why to check the product of insurance companies ▪ How health maintenance organizations may be a viable alternative

4. How to Pay for What Medicare Doesn't Cover

Medicare, as we've noted in other chapters, is an exercise in ambivalence. Congress wanted protection for senior citizens but did not want anything resembling national health insurance. It wanted to keep costs down and to give the **American Medical Association (AMA)** and the hospitals everything they wanted. It wanted cost-sharing by beneficiaries and wanted to sharply reduce the 15 percent of their income that the elderly were spending on health care.

If this last desire is taken as the standard, Medicare is a failure. Senior citizens once again spend 15 percent of their income on health care, and that proportion will rise sharply over the next few years, if cost trends for the under-65 population are any indication. On the other hand, Medicare has increased access to health care for the elderly and eliminated many of the abuses found in the old systems of charity care. (It all but eliminated charity care in the process, leaving us with other problems, but that's another story. . . .)

The dream of having guaranteed health care for Americans over 65, supplemented by modest amounts out of their own pockets, has not been realized. What this means, in practical terms, is that you have to buy insurance to supplement Medicare if you want the degree of protection that the original program was supposed to give you. This chapter is about how to buy the best insurance for the least money.

It's not easy. Elderly Americans spent $6.2 billion on Medicare supplemental insurance in 1986 — an average of $277 each. And many question their value. Policies that return only 25 cents of each premium dollar in benefits are not unusual, according to the General Accounting Office, an arm of Congress. John Gilmore, an insurance agent who has testified before Congress about sales practices, said "The goal is to take advantage of what the seniors don't know. And believe me, most seniors don't know very much about Medicare." Robert Hunter, head of the National Insurance Consumer Organization, which Ralph Nader helped establish, said, "We think that the vast bulk of Medigap policies are rip-offs. . . . Good health insurance pays out 85% to 90%" (*Journal of Commerce* (August 25, 1987): 9A).

Some Insurance Concepts

Insurance is, from your angle, a gamble. Some religious groups object to it on that basis. The insurance company is betting that you will stay relatively healthy. If you do, the premiums you pay while you are insured will at least equal your actual costs of medical care, plus the costs of running the company, plus a prudent reserve for unforeseen circumstances, plus a profit. If the company is a privately held, or stock, company, the profit will be distributed to the owners or shareholders, or reinvested. If it is a mutual company, the profits will be returned to the members (invisibly, in the form of low premiums, or visibly, in the form of dividends or rebates.) This is a little bit of an oversimplification, but enough to give the flavor.

You, on the other hand, are betting that you will get sick and that the company will have to pay much more to doctors and hospitals than you put in. (If you weren't making this bet and didn't believe this would happen, you would be better off just to start a savings account for future medical bills. There would be no advantage in insurance.)

Insurance can also be looked at as **risk pooling,** a process whereby *all* the insured cover the expenses that only a *few* of them will have in any given year. (Example: Depending on the age group, 12–20 percent of a population will have a hospital stay in a given year. This leaves the hospital insurance premiums of the other 80–88 percent to cover the costs.) In practice, there's more to it than this. Insurance companies, particularly health insurers, do a great variety of things, such as contracting with hospitals for guaranteed rates, fixing fee schedules for doctors, reviewing use of hospitalization and surgery, and so on. But what we've told you is the essence.

Insurance companies engage in awesome statistical exercises to make sure that the claims that are paid will stay in line with the premiums that are paid in. One of the insights that emerges is that protection against *all* risks is too expensive for any insurance company to offer. So all policies have *exclusions,* most have *deductibles,* many have *benefit maximums,* and a great number have a sliding scale of premiums based on the amount of risk the insured is willing to assume. Since most claims under most types of insurance are small, an insured's willingness to assume a small risk (via, say, a deductible of $200 rather than $100) is worth far more to the insurer than high-end limitations. Assuming an additional risk of $100 at the low end is worth far more to the company than a reduction of the maximum amount paid from $1,000,000 to $999,900.

So total coverage for all hazards is too expensive to offer. What happens instead is bargaining between the insured and the insurance company. This takes the form of the insured person's picking and choosing among high-option plans, low-option plans, and everything in between, adjusting the amount of risk the insured person is willing to assume versus the premium he or she has to pay until satisfied.

So goes the theory, anyway. In fact, there are pitfalls to buying insurance. The greatest of them is not knowing what it is that you want to buy in the way of protection, which is what insurance is all about.

The Dark Side: Catastrophic Illness and Nursing Home Care

So insurance sounds like a good thing, but all is not rosy. There has been a persistent tendency in the health insurance industry to insure people against the things most can perfectly well afford — such as the $75 Medicare Part B deductible, or a copayment of more than $2 per prescription under an employer's health benefit plan — and not to insure them against what they can't afford. Since the latter is the whole purpose of insurance, something is wrong. This is what led to the recent passage of the so-called Medicare catastrophic coverage act — which really doesn't provide coverage in catastrophic situations, although it dramatically expands the scope of Medicare coverage.

Medicare has eliminated all payments for covered hospital services except for the annual deductible, but Part B out-of-pocket caps apply only to the services of Medicare-participating doctors. Although the limits are relatively low — $1,370 in 1990, $1,530 in 1991, $1,700 in 1992, and $1,900 in 1993 — they still permit impoverishment if you can't find participating doctors.

"Catastrophic" can be variously defined, but any illness that leaves you with medical expenses you can't pay is usually a catastrophe for you, whether the amount involved is $100 or $100,000. An illness that forces you into a nursing home for a long period of time can be a catastrophe. (Remember, Medicare pays only for **Skilled Nursing Facility** (**SNF**) services, not custodial care, and only at the rate of 150 days per calendar year. You may need nursing home care for the rest of your life, but Medicare will pay for a maximum of 150 SNF days per year. On the bright side, only about 5 percent of older people are in nursing homes, but this proportion is expected to grow as the overall population ages and the number of the "oldest old" (those 85 and over) grows.

Tragic stories of those who were forced to sell their homes in order to qualify for **Medicaid** payments to keep a spouse in a nursing home are all too true. The catastrophic coverage legislation eliminates the possibility of total impoverishment of the spouse, but, for a (relatively) wealthy couple, most assets over $60,000 may still go to pay for nursing home care. The new provisions are these:

Beginning January 1, 1989,

- In any month in which a married person is in a nursing home, no income of the at-home spouse is to be considered available to the spouse in the nursing home.

- Income is considered the property of the person to whom it is paid. Income paid to both spouses is attributed 50% to each.

- The home, household goods, and personal effects of both spouses are not counted in considering Medicaid eligibility.

- All assets other than these will be counted and divided in two. If the at-home spouse has less than $12,000, the spouse in the nursing home may transfer assets to him or her to make up to $12,000 available to the at-home spouse. (States may, at their option, raise this figure to any amount less than $60,000. The $12,000 amount will be indexed to inflation.)

- The assets that remain in the name of the spouse in the nursing home are considered available to pay for his or her nursing home care. All assets in excess of $60,000 are attributed to the spouse in the nursing home and are considered available to pay for nursing home care.

- States must allow nursing home residents to retain certain sums for medical expenses not covered by Medicare or Medicaid before contributing to the expense of their nursing home care. The states may place "reasonable limits" on the amounts spent.

Beginning September 30, 1989,

- The states must allow the at-home spouse sufficient income from the other spouse to bring the total household income of the at-home spouse to at least 122 percent of the federal poverty level for a two-person household. In 1989, this will be $789 per month. On July 1, 1991, it will be raised to 133 percent of the poverty level, and to 150 percent on July 1, 1992. States will not be required to allow more than $1,500 per month, except by court order or change in regulations.

Outpatient Care: The Real Catastrophe

If you are a Medicare beneficiary in reasonable health, your biggest potential for catastrophic costs in the immediate future lies with the failure of Part B of Medicare — doctor insurance — to pick up more than about 52 percent of total expenses. Doctors are doing increasingly more work outside the hospital, pressure to keep people out of the hospital is mounting, and there is a (too) slowly growing realization among doctors that hospitals are dangerous places that should be reserved for the very sick. The result is that a growing percentage of your medical expenses is being forced into the area of Medicare — Part B — that affords you the least protection. The out-of-pocket limits that will be effective starting in 1990 are these: $1,370 in 1990, $1,530 in 1991, $1,700 in 1992, and $1,900 in 1993. Remember that these apply only to Medicare-approved charges. Doctors who do not participate in Medicare may charge more, and these amounts do not come under the limits.

Medication, which until 1991 Medicare does not cover at all when you are outside a hospital or skilled nursing facility, is another problem area. Dramatic progress in the development of effective drugs has been made in the last decade. Many medical problems that could be treated only poorly a few years ago now yield to new drugs. The problem is that these new drugs usually carry high research and development costs. To make matters worse, many drug patents have recently expired, which lowers their profitability and makes drug companies jack up the price of new drugs even more.

An increasing amount of care is shifting to the outpatient arena. Neither Medicare nor private insurance has caught up with the trend. Tests and treatments formerly given only to inpatients — and covered 100 percent — are being done on an outpatient basis, subject to cost-sharing. While over 1,400 procedures are now covered at 100 percent if performed on an outpatient basis, still more adjustment is needed to make Medicare reflect current realities.

The average savings account in America contains $9,733. This would cover 88 days of skilled nursing facility at $110 per day (remember that Medicare covers only 150 days per year, and does not cover custodial care). Most people do not have savings to cover more than a small fraction of medical expenses.

Doctors, of course, are not required to take **assignment** — to accept Medicare's approved charge as their total payment. It is perfectly possible for the balance of your bill from a doctor who does not take assignment to be two or three times the total amount Medicare pays. Supplemental insurance for Medicare is a good idea.

Assignment

What does "taking assignment" mean? It's a very important concept. A doctor who agrees to take assignment agrees to accept the payment that the Medicare carrier has decided is appropriate for the service rendered. This does not mean that the doctor has agreed to accept it as payment in full. He or she is supposed to charge you 20 percent of the Medicare price; Medicare pays the other 80 percent. The doctor handles all the paperwork with Medicare and is the recipient of the check. You just have to deal with the doctor's bill and your insurance company.

Buying Insurance to Supplement Medicare

Unfortunately, all too many insurance companies are aware of the fear of being bankrupted by health care costs that older people have. Insurance policies are not famous for being written in clear English, and when one is dealing with insurance to supplement a program as complex as Medicare, the problem gets even worse.

Our approach in this chapter is to tell you what we think. We think the best way to help you is to tell you what you ought to buy and then tell you how to buy it. This avoids describing all sorts of policies that really aren't worth the money, then telling you not to buy those. Of course, the choice is yours, but we think our approach makes sense.

Our *first* assumption is that you will not have a large amount of personal resources and that your earnings potential is limited. This means that the most important thing an insurance policy can do for you is to *protect the assets you have and keep you out of debt*. The *second* thing we assume is that you want to devote as small a portion of your income, beyond your health insurance premiums, to health care as you possibly can. There are more pleasant uses for the money. This means that you want to minimize your potential out-of-pocket expense. Our *third* assumption is that, like most older people, you are a little bit frightened of the cost of health care and want to buy some peace of mind as well as some insurance.

Traditional Insurance Policies

These come in two main types, either of which could be sold as a Medicare supplemental policy:

- **Service benefit policies** generally pay all the costs of a "service," such as hospitalization, surgery, outpatient care, and the like. Because of the way these policies relate to Medicare, they usually pay all of the difference between the amounts charged and what Medicare pays, leaving you with no out-of-pocket costs for the use of Medicare benefits. Generally, however, they cover nothing that Medicare does not cover. Your Medicare coverage and your insurance coverage run out together. As we've noted, this is not a real concern since most Medicare beneficiaries do not exhaust their hospital or skilled nursing facility benefits. Your real costs are likely to be on the outpatient side. These policies cover the 20 percent copayment. If the insurer uses its own fee schedule, however, they may not cover the difference between 100 percent of the Medicare approved rate and what the doctor actually charged.

- **Indemnity benefit policies** provide a fixed amount per day or per service. Usually the policy states the amounts as something like "$532 per day or actual charges, whichever is lower." A policy that has high maximum payments relative to actual costs may *look* like it "covers everything," but the language of the policy, not one or two experiences with it, should be looked into.

- **"Medigap"** or **Medicare supplemental** policies are specially designed policies coordinated with Medicare and are not intended as your primary health insurance. They pay the traditional hospital and major medical expense package of benefits, less what Medicare pays. There may be several options. The lowest of the low will work almost like a limited indemnity benefit policy. The highest of the high may cover so much that it will seem like a health maintenance organization. The big difference will not be in what is covered but in how much of the charge for it is covered.

- **Employer retiree health insurance** or health insurance for Medicare beneficiaries who work after 65 usually pays for all or most of a defined set of services, so they look like service benefit plans with low out-of-pocket costs to those enrolled. Since Medicare has become the *secondary* payer for plans covering employees over 65, they have gotten somewhat less generous. One of the possibilities offered by these plans may be a health maintenance organization option. (Ask for the pamphlet, "Medicare and Employer Health Plans" at your Social Security Office. If they're out, ask them to reorder HCFA publication 02150.) Be aware that there are problems associated with rejecting your employer's health plan if you are over 65 and continue working. In that case, the employer cannot offer you a plan that is the equivalent of a Medigap policy. It can only pay for the services that Medicare does not cover at all.

HCFA certifies insurance policies as meeting minimum standards for Medicare supplemental insurance *if* the company issuing the policy requests it. Companies are not supposed to claim that their policies have been approved by HCFA unless they have such approval in writing. It is entirely possible that some companies claim that their policies have been certified when they have not. Medicare requires all supplemental insurance companies to meet the minimum standards developed by the National Association of Insurance Commissioners. We suggest you check with the Insurance Commissioner (or equivalent official) in your state to check the exact status of any policy that claims to be certified.

You'll recall that our criteria for Medicare supplemental insurance were as follows:

- To protect your assets and keep you out of debt
- To reduce your out-of-pocket expenses as much as possible
- To give you peace of mind

We can use them to screen the types of Medicare supplemental insurance available.

The first thing that's clear is that service benefit plans are unlikely to meet your needs. They have all of the defects of Medicare itself, minus the copayments and deductibles. They provide no protection on the outpatient side, which is where you need it more and more. This leaves indemnity plans, Medigap plans, and employer plans.

Of these three, we believe *you should keep any employer plan that you have.* It may require a small contribution, but these plans were modeled after employee plans in more generous days, and companies haven't gotten around to cutting them substantially yet. With rare exceptions, they are as good as high-option Medigap policies, and possibly better. Further, a number of court cases have severely limited the right of companies to reduce benefits once you have retired, and, as we write this in mid-1988, Congress has just modified the federal bankruptcy laws so that employers' obligations to retiree medical and life insurance plans can no longer be discharged in bankruptcy proceedings. The company *must* pay. (But, obviously, it cannot do so if it genuinely has no assets left.) With your employer plan, you should, of course, make sure that you are enrolled in Part A of Medicare when you turn 65. You should also purchase Part B, doctor insurance. Why? First, if you don't purchase it during your **individual enrollment period,** you will have to wait until the next **general enrollment period** and will pay an additional 10 percent premium for every year you wait. Second, enrolling keeps the cost to your employer down and helps to preserve the benefits of your plan. Third, because premiums for Part B cover only 50 percent of the cost, enrolling gives your employer's plan a de facto injection of federal money. (For these reasons, many companies require their retirees and over-65 employees to enroll in Part B.)

If you don't have employer-provided retiree health insurance or it is a wholly unsatisfactory plan, we recommend that you purchase indemnity insurance. This is the point where we have to tell you what *not* to do:

- *Do not* purchase limited-purpose insurance, such as cancer insurance, accident insurance, and so on. Benefits in these policies are limited to certain diagnoses, they are generally full of other limitations, and many are simply fraudulent, designed never to pay off.

- *Do not* buy a policy that excludes preexisting conditions, if at all possible. If you do, make sure that the exclusion is limited to six months at most. Federal law prevents any company from calling any policy that excludes preexisting conditions for more than six months a "Medicare supplement." The fact that this is against the law doesn't mean that it won't be done, of course. What you're sick with now is what you're most likely to be sick with in the future. Buying a policy that excludes it is like buying no insurance at all.

- *Do not* buy policies that duplicate ones that you already have. Congressional hearings revealed that *25 percent* of the funds spent on Medigap insurance are spent on duplicate coverage. Most policies have **coordination of benefits** provisions that ensure that only the amount charged by the provider is paid. You get no benefit from duplicate coverage, only the insurance companies do.

- *Do not,* we hate to have to say, buy a policy just because it is endorsed by a famous figure. The endorser's chief reason for endorsing the policy is the money he or she gets for doing it. Policies that are advertised this way are not necessarily bad. Neither are they necessarily good.

- *Do not* buy policies advertised with television spots and magazine ads that claim you'll face bankruptcy if you don't buy them. This is not necessarily true of insurance in general and is certainly not true of any one policy.

- *Do not* buy policies by mail if at all possible. Buy a policy through the mail *only* if you are sure that it is the best. Before you buy, call or write the company and see if there is an office or agent near you. If so, deal with that office directly.

- *Do not* buy policies that have dollar limits on total annual payments, or payments over your lifetime, unless those limits are *reasonably* high. Consider an annual limit of $5,000, which at least one Medigap policy has. This is *less than one shot of tissue plasminogen activator (TPA)*. It is *less than one-fourth of a bypass operation*. It is *less than one-tenth of a heart transplant*. It is probably *less than the combined helicopter and emergency room charges for a trauma center*. The ideal Medigap policy has no annual limits and a lifetime limit of at least $500,000.

- *Do not* purchase nonrenewable policies, ones that have unduly restrictive renewal clauses.

- *Do not* replace existing coverage without careful consideration of the advantages and disadvantages of both policies.

- *Do not* buy a policy just because it claims to pay for reductions in Medicare payments due to the Gramm-Rudman-Hollings balanced budget law. The Medicare law relieves beneficiaries of responsibility for paying for the reductions in payments to providers. You'll be paying for something Medicare already provides if you fall for this one.

Some do's:

- *Do* make sure that the company that sells the policy is licensed in your state.

- *Do* check the rating of the company in *Best's Insurance Reports — Life/Health*, which is available in most public libraries. This will give you an objective rating of the merits of the company and its policies.

- *Do* make sure that you know *exactly* what your premium will be and *exactly* what it covers. Many features that companies quite honestly say they offer are available only as riders or amendments to the basic policy, and cost extra. The fact that a company offers a feature does not necessarily mean that it is included in your premium. Get a complete schedule of benefits, and ask the salesperson to mark the benefits your premium covers.

- *Do* pay by check, made out to the company, not the salesperson. This gives you proof that you paid, in the form of a canceled check, and keeps the salesperson from pocketing your payment.

- *Do* take advantage of any "free look" provisions mandated by the laws of your state. These allow you to buy a policy and cancel it with no obligation within a certain period if you decide that it is not what you want.

- *Do* ask the salesperson or agent for information on the average out-of-pocket expenses for holders of the policy. This will tell you how much protection you really are buying.

- *Do* look very carefully at the coverage offered for doctors' fees over and above the Medicare approved price. A policy that covers only your 20 percent copayment is better than nothing but leaves you exposed to bills that are two to three times the size of what Medicare pays, or more. Remember that the out-of-pocket limit applies only to Medicare approved fees.

- *Do* choose a policy that has a **stop-loss provision,** if you can get it. Even if there isn't one in the policy you are considering, the agent may be able to add it in the form of a **rider,** for which there will be an additional (usually small) fee.

- *Do* look for a policy that covers the prescription drug charges that Medicare doesn't pay, such as the $600 deductible and the 50 percent (in 1991) copayment. Prescription drug coverage is relatively expensive. Studies on older people have shown that they spend either a relatively small amount on prescription drugs or a lot. A policy that does not protect against the small expenditures, but protects against the large ones via a stop-loss provision, makes sense.

- *Do* call your state insurance department and make sure that the policy is approved by them before you buy. (Approval to sell a policy in a state does not mean that it is a good one, simply that it violates none of the laws and conditions on insurance in that state.) A list of state insurance departments is provided in appendix C.

- *Do* ask about typical out-of-pocket expenses. Remember that you are trying to reduce the proportion of your income that you spend on health care.

- *Do* make sure the policy you select is automatically adjusted to cover increases in Medicare's copayments and deductibles.

You can use the form on page 126 to check your policy against our recommendations.

The Merits of Health Maintenance Organizations

We discussed health maintenance organizations (HMOs) a good deal in chapters 2 and 5. Those chapters give you some of the flavor of HMOs. The big advantage of an HMO, given our assumptions about what you want, is that all but a trivial portion of care is prepaid. There are no worries about having the cash to go into the hospital. There are no service-specific charges, so there is no need to negotiate with the doctor about taking **assignment**. There are far fewer, or no, forms to fill out. One payment covers everything.

Depending on the costs of medical care in your area and the particular HMO and options you pick, the individual HMO premium may range from nothing to around $100 per month.

An HMO premium may seem high. But remember, you are likely to spend 15 percent or more of your income on medical care. The HMO premium, in contrast to traditional Medigap coverage, picks up many out-of-pocket expenses that you would otherwise have to pay. More important is the peace of mind achieved by knowing that this is the *only* cost, except for nominal copayments. The proper comparison of two insurance plans is always this: *Compare premiums plus out-of-pocket costs for one plan to premiums plus out-of-pocket costs for the other.*

You should get exact figures from the HMOs that you consider enrolling in. They should be able to provide you with average out-of-pocket costs for their Medicare members. Keep in mind that HMO benefit packages differ to some degree. Medicare requires the low-option plan in Medicare approved HMOs to be at least equal to Medicare benefits, *without* the Medicare copayments and deductibles. Compare these to 15 percent of your annual income. Depending on your income, the HMO may save you anywhere from nothing (a

MEDICARE SUPPLEMENTAL
INSURANCE COMPARISON WORKSHEET

Use the information provided by the insurance companies to complete this worksheet.

Company Name	Policy 1	Policy 2	Policy 3	Policy 4
Policy/Plan Name				
Premium: May be affected by age and sex Monthly/Quarterly	$	$	$	$
Semi-Annually/Annually	$	$	$	$

Does the Supplemental Policy cover the Deductibles and Copayments listed below?	If so, place a Checkmark in the appropriate column for each policy.			
Medicare Part A: Hospital Insurance Yearly deductible $560				
Skilled Nursing Facility Care 1st to 8th day copayment: 1989 $22.00 1990* $				
*Beginning in 1990 should cover at least 20% of the average daily charge in a SNF				
Blood: Deductible equal to first three pints of blood				
Medicare Part B: Medical Insurance Initial deductible $75 20% copayment				
Out-of-pocket limit: 1990 $1,370 1991 $1,530 1992 $1,700 1993 $1,900				
Prescription drugs: Deductible and copayment 1991 $600 50% copayment 1992 $652 40% copayment 1993 $710 20% copayment				
Mammography screening: Any expense not covered by Medicare beginning in 1990				
IV Drug Therapy (In home): Deductibles and copayments 1990 $550 50% copayment 1991 $600 50% copayment 1992 $652 40% copayment 1993 $710 20% copayment				

break-even situation, but with added peace of mind) to a lot. Use the forms on pages 128–130 to compare several HMOs.

Because the one big issue with HMOs is freedom of choice of doctors and hospitals, a number of alternatives that look like HMOs in some respects have emerged in recent years. **Preferred provider organizations (PPOs)** have closed panels of doctors like HMOs, but not quite: for an extra fee, you can go to the doctor or hospital of your choice; the PPO just covers less of the cost to you if you stray from the preferred providers. The extra cost can be trivial, or it can be so high that the PPO is, in effect, an HMO for all but the affluent. Generally, their benefits are not as generous as those of HMOs, but they are a little better than traditional fee-for-service plans (example: Blue Cross and Blue Shield). PPOs are just one variety of **competitive medical plans (CMPs)** with which HCFA has been experimenting. Basically, CMPs are prepaid plans that do not have to meet the very stringent (and costly) federal requirements for Medicare HMOs. They receive a set amount, based on the average cost of treating a Medicare beneficiary in the counties they serve, adjusted for local wage and price differences. For this they are supposed to offer medical care. Depending on the cost of care in the area and the options available within the CMP, they can be as generous as an HMO but should not offer less than the standard Medicare benefits. There may be a lot of advantage, or no advantage, for you in belonging to a CMP.

A major *disadvantage* of HMOs, for those who travel a good deal, is their reluctance to cover health care other than severe emergencies outside of their service area. If your HMO is in North Dakota and you are vacationing in Florida, you can expect that it will cover an emergency room visit for something serious, but not a trip to a local doctor for a cold. Many HMOs provide a toll-free number to call for preapproval of treatment. If you are committed to your HMO and want to travel, you should take note of the many storefront medical treatment offices that are opening around the country. (One wag called them "doc-in-the-boxes.") You can use them for treatment of illnesses that are not serious as you travel.

Joining an HMO is *not* forever. You have the right to drop out, and you will be covered by Medicare just as before. You can give one a try with no fear.

You may decide that the HMOs or other alternative care plans in your area are too expensive. There may be no HMO accepting Medicare patients (or no HMO) in your area. You may decide that, no matter how great the savings and the peace-of-mind factor, HMOs are

MEDICARE HMO WORKSHEET

HMO Name	Plan 1	Plan 2	Plan 3
Additional Premium May be affected by age and sex			
Monthly	$	$	$
Quarterly	$	$	$
Semi-Annually	$	$	$
Annually	$	$	$

Does the HMO cover these deductibles and copayments?	If "yes," place a checkmark in the appropriate column.		
Medicare Part A: Hospital Insurance			
Yearly deductible $560			
Skilled Nursing Facility Care 1st to 8th day copayment:			
1989 $22.00			
1990* $			
*Beginning in 1990 should cover at least 20% of the average daily charge in a SNF			
Blood: Deductible equal to first three pints of blood			

Medicare Part B: Medical Insurance
   Initial deductible $75
   20% copayment			

Out-of-pocket limit: 1990 $1,370			
1991 $1,530			
1992 $1,700			
1993 $1,900			
Prescription drugs: Deductible and copayment			
1991 $600 50% copayment			
1992 $652 40% copayment			
1993 $710 20% copayment			
Mammography screening: Any expense not covered by Medicare beginning in 1990			
IV Drug Therapy (In home): Deductibles and copayments			
1990 $550 50% copayment			
1991 $600 50% copayment			
1992 $652 40% copayment			
1993 $710 20% copayment			

MEDICARE HMO WORKSHEET, CONT'D

Section I: Organization/Facilities	Plan 1	Plan 2	Plan 3
Travel time to primary care site			
Advance time to make appointments			
Telephone access to primary care doctor			
Emergency care procedure			
Out-of-area care procedure			
Cleanliness of facility			
Modern in appearance			
Staff behavior toward patients			
Patient waiting time			
Health promotion classes (list the type available if any)			
Member grievance process			
Years in business			
Federally qualified			
Other factors:			
Section II: Primary Care Physician			
Physician's name			
Specialty board certified			
Years in practice/Years in HMO/PPO			
Partners/Back-up coverage			
Use of physicians' assistants, nurse practitioners, etc.			
Prevention oriented			
Average time spent with patients			
Prescribes generic drugs			
Uses extraordinary life-saving measures			
Admits to hospital			
Communicates well with patients			
Subscribes to PMS Code of Practice			
Other:			

Section III: Back-up System	Plan 1	Plan 2	Plan 3
Additional hospitals in plan			
Travel time to each			
Second opinion surgical program			
Referrals to non-HMO/PPO specialists			
Quality assurance program			
Procedure for changing primary care doctor			

just not for you. You want to refer yourself to specialists, keep your own family doctor, whatever. In that case, you will be looking at

Filing Claims for Supplemental Insurance

One of the things you have to face with traditional insurance, and occasionally with health maintenance organizations, is filing a claim. Being insured by Medicare and a Medigap policy means that you have to file twice for everything, except when for hospital bills and doctors who take assignment. In these cases, the bill you get will be for what Medicare *didn't* pay. With other types of providers, you will probably have to file a claim with Medicare. Some Medigap insurers will ask you to file a claim with Medicare, wait until you get your **Explanation of Medicare Benefits (EOMB)** from Medicare, and then file with the carrier for the remainder. (See the sample form on pages 132–133.)

One of the things insurance was supposed to protect against is high out-of-pocket expenses. Being put in a situation where you may be under pressure to pay before you get the claim check is no fun, and it's almost guaranteed if you have a doctor who doesn't take assignment. The key to making sure that your insurer's money and Medicare's money is used, rather than yours, is *filing claims fast*.

Medicare carriers are under pressure to pay doctors and hospitals quickly, because the HCFA is under pressure from them. Most carriers can turn checks fairly fast. They may also have profiles on your doctor, know what your doctor's charges are, whether or not he or she takes assignment, and so on.

How to file a Medicare claim is explained in appendix D. The important point to remember about Medigap insurance is that it does not duplicate Medicare coverage, so you should answer the question about other insurance (see HCFA claim form 1490S on pages 134–135) with "no." Answer "yes" only if you have coverage that duplicates Medicare and does not supplement it.

Your Medigap insurer's claim form will tell you if you are required to submit a copy of the EOMB with a claim. It's convenient just to send the EOMB, but we recommend that you *never* do this. First, the EOMB is official correspondence between an agency acting for the U.S. government and you. Second, you will need it to make sure that your insurer has paid the difference between the provider's charge and the Medicare payment. Third, you won't be able to keep your claims log straight without it. Fourth, if you are still working, you'll need it to keep your medical expense deduction right if you itemize.

A typical supplemental insurance claim form asks for a lot of standard information: your name, your policy number, your Social Secu-

YOUR EXPLANATION OF MEDICARE BENEFITS

Read this notice carefully and keep it for your records.
This is not a bill.

HEALTH CARE FINANCING ADMINISTRATION

Iphigenia Smith
4321 Edgar Allen Poe Drive
San Diego, CA 99110

Dec. 31, 1987
Need help? Contact:
TRANSAMERICA OCCIDENTAL
  LIFE INSURANCE
1149 South Broadway
Box 54905 Terminal Annex
Los Angeles, CA 90054
Phone: 213 Area: 748-2311
  Other Areas: 1-800-252-9020

This tells you if Assignment was taken and the dollar amount billed.

Assignment was taken on your claim for $45.00 from MIDWAY MEDICAL CLNC. (See item 4 on back.)

This indicates the service and date provided.

		Billed	Approved
1 Office Service	Dec 05, 1987	$45.00	$40.00

Approved amount limited by item 5c on back.

This indicates amount Billed and Approved.

Total approved amount	$40.00
Medicare payment (80% of the approved amount minus 2.324%)	$31.26

This indicates the Approved amount and Medicare's 80 percent.

MIDWAY MEDICAL CLNC agreed to charge no more for the above approved services than the amount approved by Medicare. We are paying a total of $31.26 to MIDWAY MEDICAL CLNC.

This is what Medicare pays.

You are responsible to the physician / supplier for the difference of $8.00 between the approved amount and the Medicare payment. If you have other insurance, it may help with the part Medicare did not pay.

This explains what You pay.

A new law has reduced your Medicare payment by 2.324% for services from November 21, 1987 to March 31, 1988. You are not responsible for the 2.324% reduction on this assigned claim.

This explains any change in billing and what — if any — affect on you.

(You have met the deductible for 1987)

This indicates whether or not you have met the $75 deductible.

132

IMPORTANT: If you do not agree with the amounts approved you may ask for a review. To do this you must *write* to us before *Jun 31, 1988.* (See item 1 on the back.)

This gives you the time frame to file any appeal.

DO YOU HAVE A QUESTION ABOUT THIS NOTICE? If you believe Medicare paid for a service you did not receive, or there is an error, contact us immediately. Always give us the:

Medicare Claim No. 987 65 4321A   Claim Control No. 7350 316 290

Use these numbers when making any inquiry on your claim.

PATIENT'S REQUEST FOR MEDICAL PAYMENT

IMPORTANT—SEE OTHER SIDE FOR INSTRUCTIONS

PLEASE TYPE OR PRINT INFORMATION

MEDICAL INSURANCE BENEFITS SOCIAL SECURITY ACT

NOTICE: Anyone who misrepresents or falsifies essential information requested by this form may upon conviction be subject to fine and imprisonment under Federal Law. No Part B Medicare benefits may be paid unless this form is received as required by existing law and regulations (20 CFR 422.510).

1 Name of Beneficiary from Health Insurance Card
(Last)   (First)   (Middle)

SEND COMPLETED FORM TO:

The Part B Carrier for your state will be listed in this space.

2 Claim Number from Health Insurance Card

Patient's Sex
- ☐ Male
- ☐ Female

3 Patient's Mailing Address (City, State, Zip Code)
Check here if this is a new address ⟶ ☐

_____
(Street or P.O. Box — Include Apartment Number)

_____
(City)   (State)   (Zip)

3b Telephone Number
(Include Area Code)

(___ ___ ___)

___ ___ ___ - ___ ___ ___ ___

4 Describe the Illness or Injury for which Patient Received Treatment

4b Was condition related to:
A. Patient's employment
- ☐ Yes   ☐ No

B. Accident
- ☐ Auto   ☐ Other

4c Was patient being treated with chronic dialysis or kidney transplant?
- ☐ Yes   ☐ No

5
a. Are you employed and covered under an employee health plan? ☐ Yes ☐ No

b. Is your spouse employed and are you covered under your spouse's employee health plan? ☐ Yes ☐ No

c. If you have any medical coverage other than Medicare, such as private insurance, employment related insurance, State Agency (Medicaid), or the VA, complete:
Name and Address of other insurance, State Agency (Medicaid), or VA office

Policy or Medical Assistance No.

Policyholders Name:

NOTE: If you DO NOT want payment information on this claim released, put an (X) here ⟶ ☐

6 I AUTHORIZE ANY HOLDER OF MEDICAL OR OTHER INFORMATION ABOUT ME TO RELEASE TO THE SOCIAL SECURITY ADMINISTRATION AND HEALTH CARE FINANCING ADMINISTRATION OR ITS INTERMEDIARIES OR CARRIERS ANY INFORMATION NEEDED FOR THIS OR A RELATED MEDICARE CLAIM. I PERMIT A COPY OF THIS AUTHORIZATION TO BE USED IN PLACE OF THE ORIGINAL, AND REQUEST PAYMENT OF MEDICAL INSURANCE BENEFITS TO ME.

Signature of Patient (If patient is unable to sign, see Block 6 on reverse)

6b Date signed

IMPORTANT
ATTACH ITEMIZED BILLS FROM YOUR DOCTOR(S) OR SUPPLIER(S) TO THE BACK OF THIS FORM

Form HCFA-1490S (SC) (2-87)

DEPARTMENT OF HEALTH AND HUMAN SERVICES—HEALTH CARE FINANCING ADMINISTRATION

HOW TO FILL OUT THIS MEDICARE FORM

Medicare will pay you directly when you complete this form and attach an itemized bill from your doctor or supplier. Your bill does not have to be paid before you submit this claim for payment, but you MUST attach an itemized bill in order for Medicare to process this claim.

FOLLOW THESE INSTRUCTIONS CAREFULLY:

A. Completion of this form.

Block 1.   Print your name shown on your Medicare Card. (Last Name, First Name, Middle Name)

Block 2.   Print your Health Insurance Claim Number including the letter at the end **exactly** as it is shown on your Medicare card. Check the appropriate box for the patient's sex.

Block 3.   Furnish your mailing address and include your telephone number in Block 3b.

Block 4.   Describe the illness or injury for which you received treatment. Check the appropriate box in Blocks 4b and 4c.

Block 5a.   Complete this Block if you are age 65 or older and enrolled in a health insurance plan where you are currently working.

Block 5b.   Complete this Block if you are age 65 or older and enrolled in a health insurance plan where your spouse is currently working.

Block 5c.   Complete this Block if you have any medical coverage other than Medicare. Be sure to provide the Policy or Medical Assistance Number. You may check the box provided if you do not wish payment information from this claim released to your other insurer.

Block 6.   Be sure to sign your name. If you cannot write your name, make an (X) mark. Then have a witness sign his or her name and address in Block 6 too.

If you are completing this form for another Medicare patient you should write (By) and sign your name and address in Block 6. You also should show your relationship to the patient and briefly explain why the patient cannot sign.

Block 6b.   Print the date you completed this form.

B. Each itemized bill MUST show all of the following information:

- Date of each service

- Place of each service   —Doctor's Office   —Independent Laboratory
  - —Outpatient Hospital   —Nursing Home
  - —Patient's Home   —Inpatient Hospital

- Description of each surgical or medical service or supply furnished.

- Charge for EACH service.

- Doctor's or supplier's name and address. Many times a bill will show the names of several doctors or suppliers. IT IS VERY IMPORTANT THE ONE WHO TREATED YOU BE IDENTIFIED. Simply circle his/her name on the bill.

- It is helpful if the diagnosis is shown on the physician's bill. If not, be sure you have completed Block 4 of this form.

- Mark out any services on the bill(s) you are attaching for which you have already filed a Medicare claim.

- If the patient is deceased please contact your Social Security office for instructions on how to file a claim.

- Attach an Explanation of Medicare Benefits notice from the other insurer if you are also requesting Medicare payment.

COLLECTION AND USE OF MEDICARE INFORMATION

We are authorized by the Health Care Financing Administration to ask you for information needed in the administration of the Medicare program. Authority to collect information is in section 205 (a), 1872 and 1875 of the Social Security Act, as amended.

The information we obtain to complete your Medicare claim is used to identify you and to determine your eligibility. It is also used to decide if the services and supplies you received are covered by Medicare and to insure that proper payment is made.

The information may also be given to other providers of services, carriers, intermediaries, medical review boards, and other organizations as necessary to administer the Medicare program. For example, it may be necessary to disclose information about the Medicare benefits you have used to a hospital or doctor.

With one exception, which is discussed below, there are no penalties under social security law for refusing to supply information. However, failure to furnish information regarding the medical services rendered or the amount charged would prevent payment of the claim. Failure to furnish any other information, such as name or claim number, would delay payment of the claim.

It is mandatory that you tell us if you are being treated for a work related injury so we can determine whether worker's compensation will pay for the treatment. Section 1877 (a) (3) of the Social Security Act provides criminal penalties for withholding this information.

✿ U.S. GOVERNMENT PRINTING OFFICE: 1987-706-734

rity number, the number from your Medicare insurance card, whether or not you have Part B (doctor insurance), your address, your telephone number, and so on. You should make a note in your claims log (appendix B) that you have filed a claim *before* you mail it. Don't rely on memory.

If you do not get the amount you believe the policy should pay, or the insurer rejects the claim, see chapter 8, which is a troubleshooting kit for all sorts of situations. The one thing you should know before you go into a full-scale effort is that insurers often reject claims *because they're duplicates*. Your claims log will help you avoid being thrown by this. We believe that insurers would be well advised simply to notify you that the claim is a duplicate, and that processing of the original is still going on, rather than telling you it has been rejected, but that day has not arrived yet.

In this chapter you will learn: Why it's important to negotiate with your doctor ▪ When to negotiate with your doctor ▪ How assignment can save you money ▪ How the maximum allowable actual charge can save you money ▪ What is meant by fully informing a patient ▪ How to get the right diagnosis ▪ When to get a second opinion

5. Negotiating with Your Doctor

The images that comes to mind when people think of negotiating are usually confrontational: strikes and diplomatic encounters. They also think that the term implies that something has gone wrong, and the negotiating is being done to set it right. People also think in terms of winners and losers. The word — at least as defined by good ol' *Webster's* — doesn't have the connotations of confrontation, things going awry, and wins and losses. "Negotiations" can simply mean "the carrying on of business" or "dealing with some matter that requires ability for its successful handling."

It's fair to say that there is a confrontation of sorts going on between many members of the medical profession and American society, that it's happening because things have gone wrong, and that there will be winners and losers. But that doesn't have to be the case in your dealings with doctors. We make no secret of the fact that if it does come down to a win/loss situation, we prefer the consumer, the patient — you — to be the winner. But often the discussions that we suggest in this chapter can be carried out so that you *and* the doctor win.

Of course, a win-win situation depends on what each party views as a successful outcome. Let's use accepting **assignment** as an example. If you use a doctor who does not currently accept assignment, and you persuade him to accept it in your case (the best outcome) or at least for the treatment of the moment (better than nothing), he is giving up the right to charge you more than 20 percent of the Medicare approved price. He is also agreeing to let his billing service, rather than you, handle most of the paperwork. He may consider this a loss; that is fine. On the other hand, he may have kept you as a patient, rather than having you start going to someone else. In that case, it's a win. A win for both of you. How he looks at it is up to him. In any case, negotiating shouldn't be an exercise in doctor-bashing. Think of it, rather, as helping your doctor to help you as much as he can, and educating him about the medical marketplace. Negotiating is getting the best service for the best price.

It has been said that "the man (or woman) who asks for nothing is quite likely to get it." To negotiate successfully, you have to know what you're trying to get. We specify some goals for you in this chapter. You should aim for this:

- Paying no more than the Medicare approved charge for the services you receive
- Getting the best possible treatment to produce what you consider the best overall outcome
- Staying in control of your treatment — being able to make and enforce the choices that you think best for you and avoiding unnecessary risk and expense — at all times, even if you are unable to communicate your wishes

For each of these issues, we give you the background you need to deal with the issue, some suggestions for dealing with the general situation, and some examples (or scenarios) of successful negotiations.

Why It's Hard to Negotiate with Doctors

Nurses (among others) have a longstanding joke that the initials "M.D." stand for "mostly divine." With divine beings, one does not negotiate. One prays. It is therefore not surprising that the idea of negotiating with your doctor is foreign to most people.

It should not be foreign. It should be standard practice. There are a number of reasons why it isn't. At a time when doctors were among the few educated people in society — when only about 4 percent of the population had a college education and most adults had not finished high school — it was unrealistic to expect that the patient could understand matters well enough to negotiate treatment without a crash course in biology. Rather than provide it, doctors relied on intimidation, furthered by their extremely rare level of learning and high social position to get patients to cooperate. This has always been the style of physicians in largely unlettered societies. In the late nineteenth century, the style of medicine practiced today was struggling to establish itself as the only "scientific" kind of medicine, and to end legislative control of medicine and establish control by the profession. This effort reinforced the tendency to treat the patient as a child — a sick child, at that.

Another reason has its roots in the history of American medicine. In the nineteenth century, the group of medical practitioners who had the M.D. degree — only one of the kinds of degrees, or certificates of study, issued to the various types of medical practitioners — made a move to take over all of medical practice through the legislatures. This was done at a time when those with the M.D. degree, who practiced a kind of medicine that is called "allopathic," had no greater claim to a scientific foundation for their practices that any of the other schools did. (Those other schools, for example, practiced osteopathic, chiropractic, naturopathic, and homeopathic brands of medicine. They still survive.)

Part of the strategy for taking over the whole medical field was a conscious, long-range effort to place holders of the M.D. degree (as opposed to other kinds of doctors such as osteopaths) on a pedestal. The strategy required a "mythology of medicine" — a presentation of M.D.-style medicine as far more scientific, far more founded in careful, controlled experiments, than it really was (or, for that matter, far more scientific than it is today). Doctors are still trained in the mythology. The game still goes on. A federal court recently concluded that the **American Medical Association** had deliberately engaged in an attempt to restrain the practices of chiropractors.

In fact, medicine still has much in common with engineering. The engineer solves problems by trying out solutions, based on general knowledge of a problem, until something works. If she's good, it works on the first try. If not, she keeps trying. Medicine still has little in common with the hard sciences, such as physics, where the classic experiments work all of the time.

Finally, doctors consciously and unconsciously cultivate an aloofness, an above-the fray attitude and a hypercompetent appearance. To some extent, this is a matter of emotional survival. But this attitude is acknowledged by many to get in the way of sympathizing with patients' personal concerns about illness, growing old, and death.

With these factors still dominant in medical training and practice, it's up to the patient — you — to educate doctors to treat you as you wish to be treated.

Why It's Important

Medicare beneficiaries — whether over 65 or disabled — need to negotiate more than most people. There are several reasons for this:

- Most Americans experience their first serious illnesses only when they are about 50 or older. Yuppies may have heart attacks in their 30s, but serious illness, for most people, comes with age.

- Because of this, the most expensive illnesses come when people have reduced incomes, are not fully employed, and are dependent on Medicare for health coverage.

- Medicare pays most of the hospital expenses of the elderly, but the proportion of nonhospital expenses covered is falling rapidly. This is happening at a time when care is increasingly being shifted out of the hospital into other settings. Medicare was designed largely as hospital insurance and has not caught up with the reality of current medical practice.

- Almost no form of supplemental insurance covers everything that the elderly need.

- The cost of treatment, the physical and psychological burdens of treatment, and the effect on relatives are all determined mostly by the doctor.

- The doctor, in large measure, determines how and when people die.

If you want to have *any* influence on the cost of your treatment, how much (or little) you benefit from it, and how and when you go, you have to negotiate with doctors. There's no other option.

There are three more reasons to take this business of negotiating seriously. First, doctors in many areas are hungry for patients right now, and getting hungrier. The United States is heading toward a ratio of 2 doctors per 1,000 population, while there is good evidence that 1.2–1.4 per 1,000 is what is really needed. From the patient's side, the doctor glut shows up in increased exposure to treatments designed to augment the doctor's income rather than the patient's health. From the doctor's side, it means a scramble for a static pool of patients. It means that the loss of a single patient is more serious, and more effort needs to be made to keep patients happy. There are still regions of the country whcre one or two doctors monopolize a specialty, but they are growing fewer.

Second, the new breed of doctors — the most recent graduates of medical school — are much more inclined to involve patients in treatment decisions than are their older colleagues. Part of the reason for this is dissatisfaction with the traditional style of practice. Another reason is the knowledge that fully informing patients (or doing what they *think* is fully informing patients) protects them to some degree from malpractice suits — they can blame a poor outcome partly on the patient's dumb choice. You can take advantage of their sincere desire to inform you to get better care at a better price.

Third, when one enters a large hospital with lots of departments and lots of specialties — particularly a teaching hospital — several doctors are likely to be involved in the patient's care. The admitting physician may shrink into the background as surgeons, radiologists, nuclear medicine specialists, internists, cardiologists, pulmonary medicine specialists, intensivists, and a corps of residents and doctors gets into the act. Often, no one person is clearly in charge. Some doctors and hospitals realize the danger (to patients and to their malpractice insurer) in this situation and are trying to do something about it, but those efforts are in their infancy. It may well be that if you want anyone to be in charge, it will have to be you. Thus it is essential that you and someone you trust be prepared to negotiate your care.

The First Big Issue: Prices

We said that throughout this book we give you bits of the history of the Medicare program and just enough technical detail to make you an empowered consumer, but not enough to overwhelm you. The first big issue is prices. Talking about prices in Medicare requires, first and foremost, that we talk about **assignment.** Assignment is defined as the transfer of benefits of a policy to another party; for example, telling your insurance company to send the check directly to your doctor or hospital, rather than to you.

Assignment in Medicare means this: a doctor who "takes assignment" on all or part of your treatment accepts what Medicare pays, less the deductibles and your 20 percent copayment, and agrees to do most of the paperwork. You only have to deal with the paperwork that relates to your insurance company (if you have supplemental insurance for Medicare).

Assignment is one of those topics that has a long, complicated history and deserves a bit of background information. When a doctor agrees to take assignment, she agrees to accept the payment that the Medicare carrier has decided is appropriate for the service she rendered. This does *not* mean that she has agreed to accept it as payment in full. She is supposed to charge you 20 percent of the Medicare price; Medicare pays the other 80 percent. The Medicare check goes to her. You have to deal only with your portion of the bill and with your insurance company. If you have insurance that covers the 20 percent that Medicare doesn't pay (called the copayment), you may pay nothing. If your supplemental insurance has a copayment provision, you may have to pay something even after your insurance company has paid. This varies from policy to policy.

Until recently, doctors could pick and choose whether or not to take assignment on a service-by-service basis. Now they are either participating doctors — which means that they take assignment on all services they render — or nonparticipating, which means that they can still pick and choose among patients and services, taking assignment on some but not on others.

Doctors and Their Prices: History Past and Present

The Code of Hammurabi, a compilation of Babylonian law that dates to about 1750 B.C. — almost forty centuries ago — sets limits on how much doctors may charge. (It also prescribes strict punishments for bad results of treatment.) Some 140 years before the American Revolution, the colony of Virginia set maximum allowable prices for doctors' services. As you can imagine, control of doctors' fees has been a big issue with the medical profession from the time it first recognized itself as such.

Doctors in the United States argued strongly with everyone who has tried to limit fees in some way. When health insurance became generally available because of employer funding after World War II, health insurers faced a dilemma. They had to get doctors to accept enough payment from them to convince the insured that expenses really were covered. They had to make the amount small enough that policies were affordable. The result was the **usual, customary, and reasonable (UCR)** reimbursement system, which is explained in chapter 2.

Why Assignment and Participation Are Important Issues for You

The importance of assignment and participation can best be explained by examples. Suppose you have a cardiac catheterization. (This is a procedure in which a small tube is inserted into the arteries of the heart, or into the heart itself, for diagnosis and sometimes treatment. Dye can be injected to show the arteries and detect blockages, arteries can be dilated with a balloon, drugs can be injected to abort heart attacks.) The doctor charges $3,000. He is free to pull this number out of his hat; there are no set prices. It may be much more, or much less, than his colleagues charge. Most studies show that at least a 2-to-1 ratio can be found in a given community — that is, the highest-charging doctor will charge at least twice as much as the lowest-charging. (Remember, however, that price has nothing to do with quality. High prices do not necessarily mean better care.)

If he is a participating doctor, he has agreed to accept assignment — which, again, means accepting the Medicare approved payment as payment in full — for all services he renders to Medicare beneficiaries. (Again, this does not mean you pay nothing; Medicare pays 80 percent, and you (or your insurance company) pay 20 percent.) Does this mean that Medicare will pay 80 percent of $3,000? No. It means that Medicare will pay 80 percent of the "reasonable" charge, the "customary" charge, or the actual charge, whichever is least. The amount of which Medicare pays 80 percent is called the "approved charge."

The approved charge for a physician service is the *lowest* of the following:

- The amount you were actually charged for the service
- The midpoint of all the charges that your doctor made for this service during the period from July 1, two years ago, to June 30, last year (called the "customary charge")
- An amount large enough to cover 75 percent of the bills submitted for this service by all the doctors in the relevant locality (called the "prevailing charge")

The approved charge is determined by the Medicare carrier, under instructions from Medicare. It applies to doctors in the area the carrier serves. Let's say that the prevailing charge is $2,000. Medicare will pay the doctor 80 percent of that — $1,600 — and you or your insurance company will pay the remaining 20 percent — $400. Your doctor will file the claim, the check will go to him, and he will bill you for the remaining $400. You will pay it or file a claim with your insurance company. If you have not met your $75 annual deductible, it will be subtracted from the amount that Medicare pays. You and your insurance company will pay it, depending on your policy. Both situations are illustrated in the following chart:

Example 1: Effect of Assignment on Doctor Bills	
Actual charge:	$3,000
Medicare approved charge:	$2,000
Medicare pays: 80% of $2,000 =	$1,600
You pay: $2,000 − $1,600 =	$ 400
If $75 Medicare Part B deductible not met:	
Medicare approved charge:	$2,000
Less: Part B deductible:	$ 75

Medicare pays: 80% of $2,000 (= $1,600),
   less $75 = $1,525
You pay: $ 475
If you have reached the out-of-pocket limit for Part B
claims ($1,370 in 1990, $1,530 in 1991, $1,700 in
1992, and $1,900 in 1993), you pay: Nothing

By becoming a **Medicare-participating physician,** your doctor has
agreed to eat the other $1,000. It's no great loss. He knew that he
wasn't going to get it anyway. But when the reasonable and customary
charges of doctors are figured, he will enter the equation with a $3,000
charge, not a $2,000 one. He is likely to get a little higher payment
from Medicare the next year as a result. *The system contains a built-
in incentive for him and his colleagues to drive prices up.*

But what happens if you go to a nonparticipating doctor? The biggest change is that you will pay the difference between the *total
amount* the doctor charged and 80 percent of what Medicare pays.
Let's look at an example, using the same numbers as before: You go
to a doctor for a heart catheterization, for which he will charge
$3,000. The Medicare allowance in this case is $2,000. Medicare will
pay the doctor 80 percent of that, or $1,600. You, or your insurance
company, will be responsible for the difference between $3,000 and
$1,600, or $1,400. By using a nonparticipating doctor, you will have
to pay over *three times as much* as you would have paid for the same
services from the participating doctor. And you will have to file the
claim with Medicare, the check will be paid to you, you will have to
pay the doctor, and you will have to file a claim with your insurance
company for the difference. And, regardless of how much you have
spent on doctor bills during the year, the out-of-pocket limit *does not
apply.* It is limited to *Medicare approved* charges only.

Here's the arithmetic again:

Example 2: Effect of Lack of Assignment on Doctor Bills	
Actual charge:	$3,000
Medicare approved charge:	$2,000
Medicare pays: 80% of $2000 =	$1,600
You pay: $3,000 − $1,600 =	$1,400

If $75 Medicare Part B deductible not met:

Medicare approved charge:	$2,000
Part B deductible:	$ 75
Medicare pays: 80% of $2,000, less $75 =	$1,525
You pay:	$1,475

If you have reached the out-of-pocket limit for Part B claims ($1,370 in 1990, $1,530 in 1991, $1,700 in 1992, and $1,900 in 1993), you still pay: $1,475

Example 3: Comparison of Effects of Taking and Not Taking Assignment

	Doctor takes assignment	Doctor does not take assignment
Actual charge:	$3,000	$3,000
Medicare approved charge:	$2,000	$2,000
Medicare pays:	$1,600	$1,600
You pay:	$ 400	$1,400
If $75 Medicare Part B deductible not met:		
Medicare approved charge:	$2,000	$2,000
Less: Part B deductible:	$ 75	$ 75
Medicare pays:	$1,525	$1,525
You pay:	$ 475	$1,475

If you have reached the out-of-pocket limit for Part B claims ($1,370 in 1990, $1,530 in 1991, $1,700 in 1992, and $1,900 in 1993):

Medicare approved charge; $2,000		$2,000
Medicare pays:	$1,525	$1,525
You pay:	$ 0	$1,475

The only saving grace provided with regard to services by nonparticipating doctors is the **maximum allowable actual charge (MAAC)** established by Medicare. If the doctor's charges to you exceed the MAAC, neither you nor your insurance company have to pay the difference between the MAAC and what the doctor charged. Let's say the MAAC for a cardiac catheterization is $2,500. In that case, Medicare will pay $1,600 — 80 percent of the reasonable cost. You (or your insurance company) will pay the difference between the MAAC of $2,500 and the $1,600 payment from Medicare, or $964. The doctor has to eat the other $500. And his higher price does not enter into the calculation of the prevailing charges for the next year, because it has been replaced by the MAAC. The next chart shows an example of the effect of a MAAC.

Example 4: Comparison of Effects of Taking and Not Taking Assignment When Maximum Allowable Actual Charge Is Involved		
	Doctor takes assignment	Doctor does not take assignment
Maximum allowable actual charge for service:	$2,500	$2,500
Actual charge:	$3,000	$3,000
Medicare approved charge:	$2,000	$2,000
Medicare pays:	$1,600	$1,600
MAAC:	$2,500	$2,500
You pay:	$ 400	$ 900
If $75 Medicare Part B deductible not met:		
Medicare approved charge:	$2,000	$2,000
MAAC:	$2,500	$2,500
Less: Part B deductible:	$ 75	$ 75
Medicare pays:	$1,525	$1,525
You pay:	$ 475	$ 975
If you have reached the out-of-pocket limit for Part B claims ($1,370 in 1990, $1,530 in 1991, $1,700 in 1992, and $1,900 in 1993):		
Medicare approved charge; $2,000	$2,000	$2,000
Medicare pays:	$1,525	$1,525
You pay:	$ 0	$ 975

It should be obvious that persuading your doctor to take assignment on all your bills — or going to a doctor who accepts assignment — can save you large sums of money. Since most people over 65 are not particularly wealthy, the potential savings really count. You should not feel that you are cheating your doctor by asking him to accept assignment. The charge that Medicare has determined as "reasonable," in most cases, takes what other doctors charge into account. Remember, too, that the relationship of real costs to charges in all of American medicine is not tight. It is unlikely that whatever Medicare pays is below what it cost your doctor to provide the service, plus a reasonable profit. Your doctor may *feel* that the Medicare payment is too low. Unless he presents you with hard evidence that Medicare is not covering his real costs, don't worry. Point out to him that other doctors who accept assignment seem to do well.

Some New Incentives for Doctors to Accept Assignment

The States: Medical licenses are still granted by states, not by the federal government, even though proposals for a national medical license are growing more frequent. (The reasons for these demands range from evidence that many states handle the licensing of doctors in a haphazard way to the desire to have uniform disciplining of incompetent practitioners).

Because the states have the licensing power, they can attach requirements to the license. The Commonwealth of Massachusetts has passed a law requiring that all doctors accept assignment for Medicare and accept Medicaid patients, as conditions of licensure. Doctors who do not agree cannot get a license to practice in Massachusetts. The law has survived through several levels of review by appeals courts. To date the program has been very successful, and physicians' claims that doctors would leave the state have proven false. In fact, the number of doctors in Massachusetts has increased.

The Federal Government: The federal government has not yet attempted to require that doctors accept assignment as a condition to being in the Medicare program. Instead, from 1980 through 1988, the Reagan administration attempted to use free-market incentives to encourage greater physician participation. Some of the incentives actually do have a chance of encouraging more doctors to participate.

Some of the incentives are of direct benefit to you:

- A *Directory of Participating Doctors in Your Area* is available to you free of charge. You should receive a notice of the availability of this directory annually, and you can obtain one at any time by writing to the Medicare carrier for your state. Copies are available for review at Social Security offices. Medicare-participating doctors also can display emblems or certificates that show they accept assignment on all Medicare claims. The directory shows the specialties of the doctors as well. (A list of Medicare carriers is contained in appendix A.

- If your hospital refers you to a doctor for outpatient care, the hospital must *inform you if the doctor is a nonparticipating doctor and identify at least one participating doctor from whom you can obtain the same services*, "if practicable."

- If a nonparticipating physician is preparing to perform **elective** surgery on you and will not take assignment, and if the charge for surgery will exceed $500, *you must be provided with written notice of the estimated actual charge, the estimated approved charge, and the estimated expense to you* (or your insurance plan). This will give you time to seek the same services from a participating doctor or to negotiate with your doctor to provide the services on assignment.

There are a few additional incentives for doctors. Each **Explanation of Medicare Benefits** (the paper that the Medicare carrier sends to tell you what it paid for [see a copy in appendix E]) that contains unassigned charges will include a message reminding you that you would have fared better if you had obtained the services from a participating doctor. In addition, claims that do not require investigation by the Medicare carrier to resolve a discrepancy are paid for participating doctors about a week earlier than those for nonparticipating doctors. If a doctor has cash flow problems, this can make a big difference and be a real incentive to become a participating doctor.

Negotiating with Your Doctor About Fees

The most effective way to negotiate fees with your doctor is with your feet: attempt to find a doctor who is a Medicare participant. Doctors need customers these days, and the need will grow. It will be very easy, as time goes by, to find a participating doctor — even if you don't live in Massachusetts.

But there may be reasons for not using a participating doctor:

- You may not be able to find one.
- You may have been getting genuinely good service from your family doctor, who for whatever reason does not participate.
- A specialist your family doctor refers you to may be the only one in town, or a good one, and may not participate.

Whether or not the doctor participates, you have a reason to negotiate fees. You especially have a reason if the doctor doesn't participate, because in that situation the amount that you wind up paying out of pocket — or that has to be covered by your insurance — may be three to four times the amount that Medicare considers to be the reasonable *total* charge for such services. In other words, it is just good business to bargain.

There are other reasons for negotiating. Many doctors' prices are pulled out of thin air. They are not set by any market forces the way the prices for other services are. For most services, prices are publicly available and advertised. With doctors, it doesn't work that way, if only because the prices aren't published. The Medicare system of "prevailing charges" — inherited from Blue Cross and Blue Shield, which were set up by hospitals and doctors — is as good a price-fixing mechanism as any ever invented, and the doctors aren't vulnerable to an antitrust suit, either. As long as people tolerate this by not negotiating fees, prices will remain secret, and everyone will have to pay far more than necessary for medical care.

Finally, the strongest reason to negotiate fees is that, for your doctor, medicine is (whatever else he thinks it is) a business. It is subject to far less regulation than other businesses that involve far smaller portions of the American economy and have far smaller potential for harm.

The Second Big Issue: Treatment

Now let's discuss negotiating with your doctor about treatment. The basic questions you should ask and discuss with your doctor are these:

- Does she recognize her obligation to inform you fully?
- What are her criteria for the success or failure of a treatment?
- How sure is she of your diagnosis? How did she establish it? What alternatives did she consider?
- If she has recommended surgery, is there a medical treatment option? If she has recommended a medical treatment, is there a surgical option? How long should you stay with the medical option before looking at surgery?
- If she has recommended surgery, where can you get a second opinion? What are the various surgical options?
- If she has recommended medical treatment, what are the various medical options?
- Is she willing to accept your prior instructions concerning your treatment in the event that you become unable to do so?

- If (when) she calls in specialists, how will you and she maintain control of the team treating you?
- What steps will be taken to control potentially harmful diagnostic tests?

The Doctor's Obligation to Inform You Fully

The number of situations in which it is legally permissible for a doctor *not* to inform you fully about your condition and the treatment options available has shrunk dramatically over the last two decades. It is safe to say that in most states the only situations in which a full explanation of your situation can legally be withheld from you are those in which your mental competence is in doubt. Standards for finding you incompetent are becoming stricter. However, this does *not* mean that you will, in fact, be fully informed.

Ideally, your doctor should sign the **People's Medical Society (PMS) Code of Practice**, which is included in this book as appendix F. This is the most detailed attempt we know of to define what informed consent *ought* to mean from the patient's point of view. Unfortunately, if the number who have agreed to sign the code is any indication, most doctors don't agree with the PMS view of informed consent; you have to be on your guard. This does not mean refusing to trust your doctor. It does mean recognizing that she may have not one but several blinders on. Below we show the PMS Code of Practice in the form of questions you should ask your doctor:

- Does he post a printed schedule of fees for office visits, procedures, testing, and surgery?
- Does he provide itemized bills?
- Is he available for nonemergency telephone consultation during certain hours each week?
- Does he schedule appointments to allow the time necessary to see you, with minimal waiting time? Will he promptly return phone calls and report test results to you?
- Will he allow and encourage you to bring a friend or relative into the examining room with you?
- Will he facilitate getting your medical and hospital records to you and provide you with copies of your test results?
- Will he let you know your prognosis, including whether or not your condition is terminal or will cause disability or pain?
- Will he explain why further diagnostic activity or treatment is necessary?
- Will he discuss diagnostic, treatment, and medication options for

your particular problem with you (including the option of no treatment) and describe in understandable terms the risk of each alternative, the possibility of pain, the effect on your functioning, the number of visits each alternative would entail, and the cost of each?

- Will he discuss his qualifications to perform the proposed diagnostic measures or treatments?
- Will he let you know of organizations, support groups, and medical and lay publications that will assist you in understanding, monitoring, and treating your problem?
- Will he agree not to proceed until you are satisfied that you understand the risks and benefits of each alternative and has your agreement on a particular course of action?

If you ask the doctor these questions, you'll be pretty well informed about your treatment and the doctor's style of practice. But to get a serious response, you still have to work around some obstacles that impede communication.

First, a general prejudice exists in our society against the aged (and the disabled). There is a general prejudice against people who appear less than middle-class in social status. Nothing in the education of a doctor necessarily removes either of these prejudices. As a Medicare beneficiary, you are (automatically) either aged or disabled. As a recipient of Social Security, you may be poor. (The average Social Security payment in the United States in 1986 was $5,856 for an individual, $9,996 for a couple).

Second, doctors are told that they must arrange treatment according to your best interests, but that means *the doctor's* view of your best interest. Nothing in the training of doctors prepares them to be more sympathetic to your view of your own best interests than to their own. They are raised in the tradition of "doctor knows best." If you want them to treat you according to your view of your best interest, you have to tell them. Loudly. Clearly. Especially loudly.

Third, doctors in general and American doctors in particular don't like to treat chronic conditions. (Chronic conditions are those that are marked by long duration and frequent recurrence and are hard or impossible to cure once and for all.) Doctors want a clear victory over disease, and they want it quickly.

Fourth, you may have difficulty in seeing, hearing, or speaking. This will make communicating with you more difficult. On top of your chronic conditions, this will make you even more frustrating to the doctor, and you more frustrated with him.

Fifth, you may have dementia — the general label for a condition in which your brain is not working as well as it did at one time. It may be mild to severe, acute or chronic. It may or may not be caused by, or made worse by, drugs the doctor has prescribed for you. The problem is that once there is any sign of it, you are likely to be treated as though you had no brains (and no free will) at all. The doctor will see his job as curing you in spite of yourself. All your protests, reasonable or not, will be discounted. There is also a medical prejudice in the belief that anyone who is not a perfectly functioning adult either has a diminished pain response or doesn't mind pain. (It is only now being recognized that very small children *do* need anesthetics for surgery.) If you're uncomfortable or in pain, you will be less likely to make yourself heard, and so . . .

It's up to you to make sure that you are informed enough to give consent to whatever the doctor has in mind for you. Trust in him is not enough. Liking him is not enough. Both are good, but they don't add up to *knowing* what he plans for your treatment, what alternatives are available, and what might go wrong with each. *You can't count on him to overcome all the prejudices about the elderly and the disabled in our society.*

You'll note that the PMS Code of Practice requires the doctor to allow someone else to be with you when you are examined. Having a friend or relative assist you in dealing with the doctor will help with the fourth and fifth points we've just made. But more important, having someone with you will keep the doctor on his toes. That means you get better care. In fact, if you feel that you are functioning at less than full capacity, or if there is some sign that the doctor believes so, we recommend that you insist on having someone with you. (Some of us may never attain what the medical profession considers "full capacity.")

With all the hurdles that have to be jumped to get to the point where you feel fully informed, some criteria are needed. We believe you can feel fully informed if (and *only* if)

- You understand what is wrong with you, what the doctor thought was wrong with you before he arrived at the current diagnosis, and how he arrived at the current diagnosis.
- You understand the medical and surgical treatments available, and the risks and benefits of each; the doctor should have given you some objective measure of the risks.

Let's look at an example. For a while, you've been feeling run down and have had a vague, dull pain in your abdomen. Lately, it has become much sharper, and you are having diarrhea. Going to the bathroom relieves the pain, but only for a short time. You've been taking some medicine you bought off the shelf at the drugstore, but lately it isn't working. You have started to lose weight and to have soaking sweats at night. You've been putting off going to the doctor because you're afraid he'll find cancer. But you now feel so bad that you want something done. Wisely, you decide to go to the doctor.

He examines you and discovers that you are bleeding slowly from somewhere in your digestive tract. He draws blood for tests and asks the laboratory (which is fortunately in the same building as his office) to get the results back to him "stat" (medicalese for "right now!"). You sit in the waiting room for about an hour, with time out for a few trips to the bathroom. The nurse calls you back to the examining room. The doctor says, "You definitely have a bleeding problem somewhere inside. You're anemic, which could account for the tiredness. I was worried that you might have a tumor in the colon, but the blood tests show signs of something called inflammatory bowel disease."

He continues, "I want to do a colonoscopy on you. It's a simple procedure I can do here in the office. We place a small tube with a light and a lens into your colon through the rectum. I can take biopsies to confirm my guess, and also look for tumors. If you have polyps, which could cause the bleeding, I can remove any I see. We'll sedate you lightly. All you'll have is a few cramps, and you won't remember much."

You ask what he suspects — a tumor, inflammatory bowel disease, or something else. He tells you that you might have a tumor, or inflamed bowel, or both, or possibly a parasite causing diarrhea. You ask why he can't use X rays and tell him that you don't like the sound of the colonoscopy.

"I could take a large bowel series," the doctor replies, "which involves an enema of barium. It's nearly as uncomfortable as the colonoscopy and doesn't differentiate between some of the conditions I think you might have. We might still wind up with a colonoscopy after the X rays if we find polyps. I want to examine a stool specimen for parasites, but I'm pretty sure you don't have them. The other symptoms don't fit." You ask if there are any other tests that might be used. The doctor says no. It's X rays or the colonoscopy. You ask about the risks.

The doctor says, "It's possible that I will accidentally perforate your bowel; that happens about once for every 450 colonoscopies done in the United States. My record is better. I've done two thousand of these and only perforated somebody's bowel twice. If this happens, I will have to put you in the hospital. It's almost certain that surgery will be needed. Survival for major perforations of the bowel without surgery is poor."

You ask what will happen with each of the conditions the doctor suspects. He tells you that with a benign tumor, you'll continue to be miserable; with a cancerous one, you might die. A parasitic infection might clear up, or leave you growing weaker and weaker. It could be treated with drugs, but these would have no effect if there were no parasites. An attack of inflammatory bowel disease could subside on its own, or it could ultimately lead to serious surgery to remove a large part of the intestines. There are fairly good drugs to treat it.

You reluctantly agree to the colonoscopy, which is a bit more unpleasant than the doctor made it sound, but not as bad as you feared. The biopsy shows that you have a mild case of inflammatory bowel disease. The doctor prescribes medicine for the cramps and diarrhea and tells you that he is putting you on steroids.

"Like a weightlifter?" you ask in some puzzlement. The doctor tells you no, there is another kind of steroid. You ask about side effects. He tells you that there are some serious ones, but they are only associated with long-term use. He suspects that you will be off them in a month or two. You ask about short-term side effects. He tells you that these include weight gain, a puffy face, and lowered resistance to infection. You ask if there are any others. The doctor tells you that there is something called "steroid psychosis" and that he usually puts patients who are on high doses in the hospital. He tells you that the dose he proposes for you is not high enough to worry about.

You go home, take the drug, and almost immediately feel better. The diarrhea stops, the cramps go away, you stop soaking the sheets with sweat at night, and you feel even better. In fact, you feel wonderful. Then you clearly feel your heart missing beats. You call the doctor in a panic. He tells you to come to the office right away. He orders an electrocardiogram, which shows nothing seriously out of order except missed beats, and more blood tests, again "stat."

"Steroids can cause increased potassium loss in the urine," the doctor tells you. " Potassium is an element in the blood that helps control heartbeat and muscle contraction. Yours is very low. Apparently your body reacts more strongly to that effect than most. I'll prescribe a potassium supplement for you."

You point out, with a bit of embarrassment, that the doctor mentioned nothing about heart problems when he prescribed the drug. You also ask if feeling abnormally good is another side effect. The doctor admits that these are side effects he didn't tell you about because he did not think them likely in your case. He tells you that he will reduce the dosage of steroid in a few days, and he devotes a lot of time to warning you about stomach irritation from the potassium supplement.

The point of the story is this: you'll have to *work* to get this much; your doctor should be able to give it to you. If he doesn't know, make him look it up. With in-office computer services for doctors now readily available, he can get the answer within seconds. Making him look up the answer will contribute to his continuing professional education, raise the general level of medical practice in the United States, and possibly save your life.

Let's continue with our list of criteria for being a more informed consumer. We believe you can feel fully informed if (and only if)

- You have a clear understanding of the doctor's criteria for the success or failure of a treatment — whether or not he expects a complete recovery, and if he does not, what improvement he hopes for. (More on this later.)

- You know the best that can be expected from the treatment you are receiving for a person of your age, sex, and general condition. Sometimes cures aren't possible, but it may be possible to make you much more comfortable. Doctors call treating a condition that can't be cured in order to make the patient more comfortable and better able to function "palliation." If you *both* understand what he's after, you will control your treatment much more effectively.

- You understand who will be in charge (you) if you are referred to a specialist and you've had a chance to make your own choice.

- If surgery is recommended, you have received a second opinion from someone who is not professionally or financially associated with the doctor who recommended the surgery.

- The doctor has disclosed any financial benefit he will receive from recommending a treatment or prescribing a drug. (The AMA code of ethics requires this, and state laws should.)

- You have made arrangements to ensure that your wishes are carried out if you are unable to remain in charge of your treatment.

- If you brought a friend to the visit with the doctor, does your friend feel comfortable on the above points.

Let's look at a hypothetical example. You have had arthritis for several years but have been taking aspirin and exercising as prescribed. You have been doing well in general, and you have been free of pain and stiffness most of the time. Now, suddenly, your right knee is almost too painful to move. You increase the dosage of aspirin as your doctor instructed you, but that doesn't seem to help. You call him, and he tells you to come to the office the next day. He looks at the knee, which is hot, red, and swollen.

He takes some blood for a test, suggests that you rest the knee as much as possible and splint it at night, and gives you a prescription for a nonsteroidal antiinflammatory drug (these drugs are like aspirin but much more powerful). The test results come back and show that you have rheumatoid arthritis on top of the osteoarthritis that was already damaging the knee. (Both forms of arthritis can damage joints. Rheumatoid arthritis is generally much more severe.) Various drugs for both forms of arthritis are tried without success. You develop stomach bleeding with one of the antiinflammatory drugs and have to be put on steroids for a short while. This produces a good deal of relief, but your doctor does not want to use steroids for any length of time. Finally, he recommends replacement of the knee with an artificial one. You ask why.

"You've effectively lost use of the knee," he says. "If we could get it quieted down for a while, we could work on some physical therapy and try to preserve enough function to let you at least walk. But we just can't do it. I think surgery is the only alternative." He gives you the name of an orthopedic surgeon, Dr. Konrad Kowboi, who has done numerous knee replacements.

You go to see the surgeon. He examines the knee and says he agrees that surgery is needed. He can do it on Wednesday, and he starts to ask his nurse to reserve a room for you at the hospital. You ask him to wait a minute. Doesn't he want to look at your X rays? Your medical record?

"No," he replies, "I trust Howard Fassnacht [your doctor] implicitly. If he says you need surgery, I'm ready to do it." You say that replacing a knee sounds like an awfully drastic step. What's involved?

"We just cut the old knee out, and put the new one in." You ask if you will be able to walk, to climb stairs, to ride your bike as you used to like to do.

"Sure. I'll make sure that you'll have no limitations." You are worried by the surgeon's offhand manner and tell him that you want a second opinion. He scowls. "My schedule fills up pretty fast, and that knee is deteriorating further every second. I might not be able to get you in when you absolutely have to have it." You stand firm and tell him that you will call him when you get a second opinion. You call the Medicare second opinion hotline (1-800-638-6833 [1-800-492-6603 in Maryland]) and get the names of some doctors who will give second opinions. One of them is Vanessa Virtuevessel, an orthopedic surgeon in a group practice with three other surgeons at a local clinic. You call for a second opinion appointment. The nurse tells you that she will mail you a form to sign so that Dr. Fassnacht can release your records and X rays. When you go to the clinic, you discover that Dr. Virtuevessel has your chart spread out on her desk and X rays up on the light box. Even you can see that the knee doesn't look good. As she examines you, you explain that you were uncomfortable with the surgeon's breezy approach and too-deft answers.

Dr. Virtuevessel says, "I'm sorry that Dr. Kowboi made you feel uneasy. He's a bit like that sometimes. We surgeons sometimes cut first and ask questions later. But I think both Dr. Fassnacht and Dr. Kowboi are right. You've had reasonable trials of all the drugs you can tolerate. Your rheumatoid factor (a measure of how severe the disease is) is quite high. I think we ought to replace the knee."

You are immediately calmed by Dr. Virtuevessel's manner. You ask if she can do the surgery. She replies that as the source of the second opinion, she can't ethically do it. You ask her to recommend someone else. She tells you that any of the other two orthopedic surgeons in the group can handle knee replacements.

"You should understand," she adds, "that we're a partnership, and I will receive some of the surgery fee in the form of profits at the end of the year. We also rent space to a physical therapist. If you use him, I will receive some of the rent. If this makes you uncomfortable, I can recommend someone outside our group." You're impressed with her honesty and tell her that someone from the group will be fine — if they're good.

"Both of them are board-certified. We have their résumés on file with the nurse, if you want to see them." You ask if there are any statistics on their results. Dr. Virtuevessel makes a face. "The state just made us start keeping numbers on that. The nurse has the file." You ask about the usefulness of the new knee. Dr. Virtuevessel says that with good healing, you will eventually be able to walk and climb stairs and ride the bike, but you will have to set the seat high to avoid too much bending of the artificial knee.

You look at the statistics on her two partners. You notice that, even though both have good results, Dr. Norman Noscrub has had many more patients with postoperative infections than the other, Dr. Stanley Sterildrape. You decide on Dr. Sterildrape.

You ask Dr. Fassnacht to be in charge of your overall care in the hospital. You have filed a living will and want to make sure that your wishes are carried out if anything goes wrong. Since Dr. Fassnacht has agreed to your wishes, you want him in control of the team of doctors treating you. The hospital records him as the "physician in charge" on your case. Everything goes well, and after a few months of rehabilitation, you are back on the bike.

This is an idealized picture to some degree, but it represents what *should* happen when the patient and the patient's chosen doctor are in control, and nothing happens without their approval. If you don't feel that your situation meets these criteria, do not allow the doctor to pass go. Negotiate and, if you can't win, seek another doctor.

The Doctor's Criteria for Success and Failure (and Yours)

This may seem to be a strange subject to raise. Don't doctors know when a treatment has succeeded or failed? Generally, yes. Aren't the criteria — what to look for — to determine success or failure set by the medical profession? Not at all.

We've all seen at least one television movie in which the life (or appearance, or sanity) of a patient was saved because one doctor kept on pushing after all his colleagues had given up. There is much truth in this fiction. Doctors are people, and they differ. Some of them will try any new thing that they read about in the medical journal that arrived yesterday afternoon. Others will not adopt new treatments until they feel that the treatment is completely proven and most other doctors have adopted them.

Some pore over the medical journals like pirates in search of buried treasure. Others have read nothing in years, choose their continuing education courses by the quality of the resort at which they are held, and sleep through the classes. Some prescribe with abandon, believing that "there's a pill for everything." Others are so afraid of the negative side effects of drugs in the elderly that they neglect drugs that could be useful. Surgeons think internists are unduly cerebral, and cautious to a fault. Internists think surgeons live by the motto "If it moves, cut it." One cardiologist may prescribe stopping smoking, losing weight, a walking program, and nitroglycerin tablets. Another may prescribe the same, plus a triple bypass.

Some strive to treat the whole person, and are satisfied with a patient who has avoided the risks of surgery and is handling his condition well on medical therapy. Others see no irony in the claim that "the operation was a success, but the patient died."

This wide variety of approaches is not necessarily bad (it gives you the option of shopping around), and it does not mean that doctors know nothing. It simply indicates that medicine is, as Lewis Thomas, M.D. wrote, "the youngest science." Various experts have estimated that it was not until somewhere between 1920 and 1950 that one had an equal chance of being helped or harmed by an encounter with a doctor. Before that, one was more likely to be harmed.

Medicine has also evolved (some would disagree about the choice of verb) into a bewildering variety of specialties and subspecialties. Most assume that if a patient has been referred to them (or has called for an appointment), choosing them was obviously the right thing to do, and they will plow ahead until it becomes obvious that they are not helping. "If you go to Midas, you get a muffler," is the way one doctor has put it.

Doctors respond to peer pressure (as do all people) and tend to practice like their colleagues. The gang at the hospital across town may have a completely different approach.

The upshot is that you have to find out what it is the doctor is trying to do for you, and tell him whether or not that is what you want. We can't stress one point strongly enough: *Nothing in a doctor's training equips him to make the choice for you. Nothing in his training makes him better able to make the choice than you can.* Doctors don't share their standards of success and failure with patients because they have never realized that you have your own standards. They are a parent, you are a child. The prejudices we described above get in the way, too. It's up to you to find out two things:

- What outcome does the doctor expect and accept?
- What are the alternatives?

A patient may feel that what the doctor has recommended — say, medical treatment and use of a portable oxygen tank — is a fine outcome, and preferable to the 20 percent risk of death, and the 15 percent risk of a worsened condition, attached to surgery. But the *doctor* may well have recommended this because success, for him, is keeping the patient out of the operating room. Another patient may decide that anything is preferable to being attached to an oxygen tank for the rest of his life, and will accept the doctor's recommendation for surgery. The *doctor* may have recommended this because, for him, success is avoiding dependence on oxygen. The reasons the doctor recommends a treatment may have nothing to do with the way *you* look at it.

People tend to think that because a doctor recommends something, he must know how to balance medical considerations with considerations of the "quality of life," based on some more or less objective set of values shared with the patient. Nothing could be further from the truth.

A doctor's education is usually exclusively in medicine or the sciences that make up the foundation for medicine, unless his undergraduate professors or the medical school have decided to help him be a more broadly educated human being somewhere along the line. The doctor may have no acquaintance with the humanities, with philosophy, with values, with literature, art, music, or history. The typical doctor is probably less well equipped to deal with issues of value and choice than the typical English major. The upshot: find out what your doctor is thinking, and why — then make your own choices.

How Sure of the Diagnosis Is the Doctor? How Did He Get to It?

Some diagnoses are obvious. Many are not. The diagnosis recorded at hospital admission is wrong about 40 percent of the time.[2] A portion of this admission diagnosis error rate reflects the current state of medicine and not necessarily a failing on the part of the doctor. (Even the suspicion of some diagnoses, such as a heart attack or a ruptured appendix, is a good reason to send someone to the hospital; tests done in the hospital may establish some other diagnosis as correct, but the decision to hospitalize, based on the knowledge the doctor had at the time, was correct.) Another portion is simply error, sometimes fatal error.

Is Overtesting or Undertesting the Problem?

Autopsy results show that there is always a certain percentage of cases in which a diagnosis of an incurable, fatal disease is made when the correct diagnosis is a disease that is not fatal if treated. Since the diagnosis led to no treatment or only palliative treatment, the patients in these cases died unnecessarily. The few studies that have been done on this issue show that *the percentage of these types of cases has probably been rising over the last three decades.* It reached 10 percent of cases in a study done in the early 1980s. To put it in the most forceful terms possible: misdiagnosis accounts for 10 percent of all deaths in which the patient died in the hospital. At least as measured by this

---

[2] Alan Brewster, M.D., personal oral communication. Other studies have shown diagnosis error rates of 10 percent to 81 percent, depending on study methods. See, for example, the studies cited in Charles B. Inlander, Lowell Levin, and Ed Weiner, *Medicine on Trial* (New York: Prentice-Hall, 1988), pp. 67–80.

kind of fatal mistake, the problem of misdiagnosis is getting worse, not better.[3]

What can you do to protect yourself and ensure that you get the best (and right) treatment? You need to get your doctor to share her diagnostic thinking with you. What else did she think you might have? What is in favor of the diagnosis she chose? How sure is she? What test results — if any — tipped the scales in favor of one diagnosis over another? How does the diagnosis affect the treatment? What else can she do to make the diagnosis more certain?

You can help deal with the problem of misdiagnosis by keeping several points in mind: first, your symptoms may be real, and troubling to you, but they do not necessarily indicate something that can be, or should be, medically treated. The labor that accompanies the birth of a child is painful, but pregnancy is not a disease. Many people have a tendency to "somatize" — to express problems in their lives as physical symptoms. The symptom can be reduced by drugs, but will it not go away until the problem is solved. An understanding friend may be better equipped to help than a doctor. Sometimes even talking to a pet may be of more value than everything in the pharmacy. It's ultimately up to each individual to know the difference. The doctor can only help, by communicating what the tests show.

The second point is this: doctors talk about the "sensitivity" and the "specificity" of tests. "Sensitivity" refers to the ability of the test to detect *something*, regardless of what it is. "Specificity" refers to how accurately the test distinguishes between the various somethings that might be there. The ideal test is 100 percent sensitive — it detects something every time something is present — and specific to only one something. Every test in existence falls short of this ideal. Many, in addition to being less than 100 percent sensitive — that is, they miss something that is really there — give "false positives," — indicating that something is wrong when it isn't. Most are less than specific — they narrow the possibilities to a few things, assuming something is really there, but they don't tell which one. Example: elevated amounts of enzymes produced by the liver can indicate that one has liver damage, or that one is taking one of the many drugs that harmlessly elevate the level of these enzymes.

Since perfect tests don't exist, doctors have to use the ones they have.

[3] H. H. R. Friederici and M. Sebastian, *Archives of Pathology Laboratory Medicine*, (June 1984): 521, cited in Inlander et al., *Medicine on Trial*, p. 72.

Almost all tests have some risk associated with them. So the dilemma arises: "For $200 worth of tests, and a small amount of risk, I am 97 percent sure of what this patient has. For $2,000 more, and more risk, I can be 99 percent sure. Is it worth it?"

Worth it for whom? You? The doctor? Her malpractice insurer? Many doctors say that they do more testing than they feel is wise simply to protect themselves from malpractice suits. Taken at face value, this means that *doctors think they are doing too many tests now. If they considered only their patients' welfare, they would do fewer.*

This suggests that the problem you face, as a patient, is not under-testing that may miss a diagnosis — even though the results from the autopsy studies we mentioned are disturbing. The danger you face is *overtesting.* Pennsylvania Blue Cross and Blue Shield apparently agree; they have decided to pay for some tests only in special situations.

What can you do to protect yourself?

- At each step of the process, ask your doctor why she is doing each test and what information she expects to gain from it.
- Ask her about the risks associated with it.
- Ask her how sure she is of the diagnosis now, and ask her to express it *in percentage terms.* If she says she is more than 50 percent sure, ask how sure she expects to be as a result of the test. If she indicates less than 85 percent certainty, ask *how* the test will narrow the diagnostic range.
- Most important, ask her why she can't make the diagnosis from your history alone.

Don't let her proceed until you're satisfied.

Surgery and the Medical Alternatives; Medicine and the Surgical Alternatives

Surgery is serious business. But so is medicine. Drs. Paul Gertman and Knight Steele did a study of **iatrogenesis** — doctor-induced illness — on a medical service (a division of a hospital that primarily offers one branch of medicine, such as internal medicine, cardiac care, or surgery) at the Boston University Hospital. They found that more than one-third of the patients had some doctor-caused illness, the severity ranging from mild to fatal. Nine percent had doctor-caused illnesses that were either disfiguring or life threatening. Two percent died. Gertman and Steele used very strict criteria for iatrogenesis and noted that their results probably underestimated the actual occurrence.

So medical treatment and surgery are both risky. Avoiding the danger is not a simple matter of staying out of the operating room. In negotiating the risks and benefits of both surgery and medical treatment, you need to figure out your doctor's reasoning, just as you had to do with the matter of diagnosis. Again, there are no right and wrong answers here that the doctor learned in medical school. Balancing the risks and benefits is ultimately your decision.

First you need to find out what your doctor thinks a good outcome is. You may be surprised at how little she will be satisfied with. (Example: Parkinson's disease, a disorder in which uncontrollable trembling and twitching of the hands and loss of coordination develops, is primarily a disease of those over 60. It can often be controlled with drugs, but these have significant side effects. With constant monitoring, and surgical therapy if necessary, most patients can achieve a high degree of control of symptoms. But they won't if the doctor considers reduction of hand tremors as the best possible outcome and does not work at balancing the drugs used, or consider surgery.)

After you've squared expectations with the doctor, you need to find out how beneficial, and how risky, the various medical and surgical alternatives are likely to be. This is your decision, not the doctor's. His job is to give you the facts. Even so, it's important to recognize that, overall, surgery is generally riskier than medical treatment. There is another virtue to the conservative approach that many internists take: it is usually, although not always, possible to proceed with surgery after a trial of medical therapy. The reverse may not be possible — the offending organ may have been removed.

You should understand the one big exception to this advice is **cancer**. For some **tumors**, medical therapy may be the best approach, but in general, it is best to remove suspected **malignancies** surgically as soon as possible. The primary reason is that cancers can **metastasize**, or spread throughout the body. Cancers that have metastasized are much harder to treat. The secondary reason is that tumors grow, and what can be a small operation that leaves an inconspicuous scar for a small tumor may turn into a major, disfiguring one if it is allowed to grow. Even here, the approaches taken by various experts may differ. What you need to know are the risks and benefits of each.

Let's say that you need surgery. The first thing you should do is find out all you can about the type of operation that will probably be used in your case. The books in appendix G, which are usually available in public libraries, will help.

The second thing you should do is obtain a second opinion for nonurgent, or **elective**, procedures. You should get this second opinion from someone other than the surgeon who will do the surgery and who is not connected financially with the doctor who recommended it. This is something you should ask about, even though the doctor should disclose any financial connection he has with the one who recommended surgery. Medicare has a second opinion hotline you can call to find doctors who will render a second opinion: 1-800-638-6833 (1-800-492-6603 in Maryland). You should obtain from the second physician the same sort of information you received (or tried to get) from the first: risks and benefits of the various courses of treatment.

You should seek a third opinion if the second opinion does not concur with the first. Find out why there is disagreement. Most often, there will be disagreement because the medical profession hasn't agreed on a right (or wrong) approach. But there may be doubt about the diagnosis. (Example: An internist feels a lump in your breast and suggests that you see a surgeon for a needle biopsy, an in-office procedure in which a fine, hollow needle is used to remove a tiny bit of tissue for examination. The surgeon can't feel the lump and suggests that you have a mammogram. The mammogram, as is usually the case with older women, shows all sorts of changes, none of them particularly benign and none of them clearly suggestive of cancer. The surgeon refers you back to the internist, who can feel no lump this time. Nothing has been established, you're worried, and both doctors are concerned and embarrassed. A third opinion, perhaps from an oncologist [a specialist in the treatment of cancer] could help.)

Suppose you decide on surgery. The job is still not finished. You should insist on seeing the **anesthesiologist** or **anesthetist** who will give the anesthesia. You should ask what he will do if the first approach, for some reason, does not work. (Example: The anesthetist decides on spinal anesthesia but can't get the needle into the spinal canal, so a general anesthetic is used instead.)

You should ask about preoperative sedation (a shot or pill to relax you before you go to surgery) and plans for repeating it if you do not get to the operating room on time. (Example: You are scheduled for removal of a portion of an enlarged prostate gland via a cystoscope [a hollow tube that can be inserted into the bladder through the penis, and through which an instrument can be used to remove diseased prostate and bladder tissue.] You have been very worried about this ever since the urologist [a surgeon specializing in operations on the kidneys, bladder, and urinary tract] described the procedure to you. You're told that you will be heavily sedated for this, and possibly out completely if you respond to the drug that way. You're given a shot and you spend a pleasant, dreamy hour lying on the gurney. An emergency case bollixes the operating room schedule and you are taken in two hours late — more awake than you've ever been in your life.)

The anesthesiologist or anesthetist will usually be happy to write an order for repeating the preop sedation *if* you remind him.

You should, of course, make him aware of any drug allergies that you may have. Sometimes an allergy to one drug means potential problems with a whole class of drugs.

The preoperative consent form that you will be asked to sign may have a clause in it allowing the surgeon to perform any procedure he deems necessary, after he gets "inside." Signing an operative consent this broad completely defeats all the careful effort that you have devoted to making sure that you stay in control of your treatment. Your surgeon has a pretty good idea of what he will find when he starts; if you discuss limiting the operative consent to those things *when you agree to surgery* (not when the consent form is handed to you in the hospital), he may be willing to eliminate the overbroad clause.

To sum up:

- Make sure you know what outcome from the surgery is expected and what can go wrong.
- Ask for the possible results in numerical terms — 85 percent chance of a good result, 15 percent chance of a bad one, and the like. Don't accept general reassurances like "everything will be fine."
- Don't sign a blanket operative consent.
- Insist on seeing the anesthesiologist. Let him know about allergies, make arrangements for repeating preoperative sedation, and make sure you understand what arrangements have been made for alternative anesthesia.

Specialists

Today more doctors are specialists rather than generalists. The all-purpose doctor of yore is today a minority. There are at least two reasons for this: first, the specialties are far more lucrative than internal medicine, general practice, and family practice. Second, because the general fields are so broad, and an internist's training in particular overlaps those of other specialties, **residencies** in these fields are very demanding. (A residency is a period of time, usually three to five years, spent in training at a hospital before a doctor obtains certification from one of the numerous national medical boards that she is adequately trained in her field.) So is practice, once the doctor is into it. The fact is that one has much more control over one's time if one is an eye surgeon, limited to one type of treatment for one organ, than if one is an internist, whose purview is any nonsurgical treatment of anything.

As we noted earlier, the **fee-for-service system** is heavily biased in favor of procedures, discrete and well-defined things that a doctor can do, usually of a surgical nature. Cognitive skills, such as making the diagnosis that may avoid an unnecessary operation costing tens of thousands, are far less well rewarded. So the United States has too many surgeons and not enough generalists. The medical students go where the livin' is easiest.

You face different situations when you are referred to a specialist as an outpatient, and when you are hospitalized.

Outpatient Referrals: Some abuses of referrals have taken place under Medicare (and other insurance systems). The most common is called "Ping-Ponging," when a specialist and a generalist refer a patient back and forth between them, getting a fee at each visit while the patient flies across town like a Ping-Pong ball across the table. Generally, referral to a specialist on an outpatient basis should be for a *limited* term, and for either diagnostic testing treatment the generalist is not qualified to give or doesn't have the equipment for, or a consultation.

You can save yourself needless repeat testing, exposure to multiple X rays, and the like if you make sure that a copy of your medical record and test results (including X-ray films) is either mailed to the specialist in advance or given to you to take with you to the appointment. This is simple common sense, but it rarely happens. The specialist may have no more to go on than what was said in the initial phone call from your doctor. Insist that your records and test results get to the specialist no later than you do.

The simple answer is for you to obtain a *current* copy of your medical record. This is yet another case where patients have to do something the doctors should be doing in order to make sure it gets done at all. You have a definite right to your medical record in only a few states, and even then there are restrictions. We suggest that you find a consumer-oriented doctor who will request the records and then give you a copy. It's the simplest, cheapest, and fastest way.

If you are referred more than once to the same specialist, or to another specialist for what seems to be the same reason, stop your doctor and ask why the referrals are going on. Don't accept another one unless you are satisfied with the reasons. If your doctor is referring you because she genuinely does not feel competent to perform the service the specialist is providing, fine; a doctor who knows her limits is a wonderful thing. But if these are not the reasons, each referral is costing you unnecessarily, even if all the doctors involved take assignment. Again, you should be the judge and decide for yourself whether or not to see the specialist you're referred to.

Specialists in the Hospital: Your situation in the hospital is different. There are services and departments within hospitals, such as medicine, surgery, intensive care, trauma, geriatrics, and so on. Let's say that your doctor admits you for medical treatment of a problem. You are admitted under her care to the medical service, the part of the hospital that handles general problems that don't fall under some specialty, such as obstetrics or psychiatry. If it is a teaching hospital, a corps of **residents**, senior medical students, and nurses in training will descend upon you. Many of them will be charged with some aspect of your care and will be reading your chart to carry out orders or writing more orders in your chart for others to carry out. If you don't have a personal physician in the area and have been admitted under the care of the house staff, you are fair game for all of the residents and all of the **attending physicians** on the service.

Additional testing reveals that you need surgery. You are transferred to the surgical service. Let's say that you have medical problems that are complicated enough to require continuing care by an internist, even as preparations for surgery go on. You will now have the residents and senior students of the surgical service on the case as well. Any attending physician who is called in as a consultant and becomes interested in your case ("good teaching material") will stay on it, and bill for the visits that satisfy her curiosity, unless she is told to stay away by whoever's in charge (who may be hard to identify). The medical myth working here is that since every doctor works to the highest standard, and the hospital oversees them all, you are safe even if no one is obviously in charge, and the pharmacy computer is the only defense against incompatible and contradictory treatments.

Some hospitals have recognized that the situation we have described is fraught with risk. They are designating a "physician in charge" of each case who is supposed to coordinate everything done by everybody. If you, or someone who has your **power of attorney** (a legal document giving him or her the power to act for you in certain situations) in the event you are too ill to exercise control, are not in charge, *no one* may be.

A key reason to make sure that one person is in charge is that to reach agreement on assignment with each of the doctors involved in your case may leave you with a bill of catastrophic proportions. Remember the example from earlier in the chapter, in which you paid $400 in one case, and $1,400 in the other? Multiply this by ten doctors, and you could wind up owing $14,000 in doctor bills, which in most cases is *completely avoidable* by seeking out doctors who will take assignment. Someone has to be in charge of this. It is hard for you to do it from a hospital bed. A friend or relative with the power of attorney is a good idea.

Dying

Death and dying have always been major human preoccupations; many psychologists have noted that people (at least in developed Western countries, in the late twentieth century) spend the first half of our lives trying to deal with our adolescence and the last half trying to come to terms with death.

One of the more dubious achievements of late-twentieth-century medicine has been the development of the ability to delay death almost inevitably. It can be delayed long after a person has entered a **permanent vegetative state** and will never exercise any of the faculties that make him or her human again. Even after the **brain stem** has lost the ability to control breathing, even after the heart has lost the ability to beat on its own, "life" of a sort can be continued with **respirators** and **pacemakers**. The **artificial heart**, which may someday be used to keep potential organ donors "alive" indefinitely, can be called in if these fail. Some people resist all the technology and die anyway; one cynical physician has expressed it as "You die, but you die with your **electrolytes** in balance."

Doctors, who are often so ready to inject their value judgments into treatment decisions with no formal training to do so, have shrunk from it here. They have forced most decisions in this area into the courts, and the case law that is developing is quite clear: you *always* have a right to refuse treatment — of any sort — if you are mentally competent and have not fallen into the clutches of a hospital. This principle, at least, is well established: the competent individual can refuse to *begin* treatment. The cases that have garnered so much attention recently have been about stopping treatments already begun.

The evolving case law suggests that even "treatments" such as supplying food or water, which one or more of your doctors may regard as merely humane measures designed to comfort you, are not part of medical practice per se. If you are not mentally competent, the recent cases suggest, the wishes you expressed while alive must be respected. (Of course, expressing those wishes in a formal way via a **living will** or **durable power of attorney** can avoid a host of problems.

Quality of Life: Is It Worth the Living?

Deciding how you want to be treated at the end of your life requires some imagination and rather fearless self-analysis. First, recognize that experience of illness and the medical world, for most people, is rather limited. One should not judge one's ability to accept pain on the basis of a visit to the dentist, with Novocain and nitrous oxide. Pain has heights that most people will never scale. (Ask anyone who has passed a kidney stone.) Relief for pain is limited to what the doctor feels he can prescribe without killing you. Whatever that dose is, the nurses will give less, because they are afraid of addiction, even if you have two weeks to live. An *extremely* painful condition is unlikely to be given adequate relief in a hospital. (A hospice is another matter. See chapter 7, page 221.)

Even if you are not in real pain, you may be acutely uncomfortable. A **nasogastric tube** that moves constantly and irritates the throat with each swallow, a dry mouth and cracked lips from being denied any more fluid than ice chips, a catheter that creates the sensation of having to urinate desperately even while it drains urine, and **intravenous lines** that prevent you from using your hands or bending your arms, plus the sensation of whatever incision you've had, even if there's no pain until you move, are triple-distilled misery. Add the pain of cancer and nausea from chemotherapy to the mix, and one has a "quality of life" that many would argue is not worth living unless there is the hope of a cure.

Your Rights Right Now

A 28-year-old **quadriplegic** woman suffering from severe cerebral palsy and arthritis sufficiently painful to require morphine, Elizabeth Bouvia, was in almost this same situation (substitute the pain of severe arthritis for the cancer), and she petitioned a California court to let her die. She was being kept alive by feedings through a **nasogastric tube**. She asked to have the tube removed, which would eventually lead to death by starvation. The hospital and her doctors refused. The California Second Circuit Court of Appeals ruled that, as an article in the *New England Journal of Medicine* paraphrased it, "a patient need not be comatose or terminally ill to refuse medical treatment, even when the treatment may be life-saving and even when its absence may lead to an earlier death. The court added that the right to refuse medical treatment was virtually absolute and the patient's motives were not a matter for debate or decision by others" (*New England Journal of Medicine* 318 [1988]: 288).

The *Bouvia* case is important because it is the only one to date in which a conscious, coherent individual requested the withdrawal of medical treatment solely on quality of life grounds and was upheld in court. Other cases having to do with artificial feeding and **hydration** are important because they are rapidly establishing a judicial/medical consensus that, as the same article put it,

> *The focus of discussion should be the patient's wishes, not the type of treatment or the patient's **prognosis**. Artificial feeding can be viewed on a level with other medical interventions — **cardio-pulmonary resuscitation**, mechanical ventilation, **dialysis,** and antibiotic therapy. It should not be considered a part of "ordinary care" or the routine provision of nursing care and comfort. Competent patients have the right to refuse this treatment after assessing for themselves the benefits and burdens. This right is not limited to comatose or terminally ill patients. For incompetent patients, feeding, like other treatments, can be stopped in accordance with the patient's previously expressed wishes.* (New England Journal of Medicine *318 [1988]: 288)*

This consensus is, however, an *emerging* one, not firmly fixed in law, and will probably be subject to much attempted cutting and trimming. For the moment, however, what these cases establish — after much needless suffering and expense on the part of the persons and families involved — is that courts in several states are inclined to view patients' own assessments of their quality of life as the deciding factor in refusing or stopping treatment. The Supreme Court's refusal to review one of these cases, *Brophy v. New England Sinai Hospital*, indicates that it would be inclined to agree. The *New England Journal of Medicine* paraphrased the court's decision this way:

> *The state had no duty to preserve life when the patient would feel that the means of doing so demeaned his or her humanity. Only Brophy could make decisions about the quality of his life — not physicians or third parties, including the court. . . . Even though he was not terminally ill, he had the right to refuse life-sustaining treatments, including artificial feeding . . . the discontinuation of Brophy's feeding would not represent suicide or direct killing, the court ruled, nor would it subject him to a painful death by starvation. Instead, it would merely allow the underlying disease to*

*take its natural course. (*New England Journal of Medicine *318* [*1988*]: *287)*

Again, what applies to artificial feeding applies even more strongly to respirators and artificial hearts. *You have a constitutional right to refuse any medical treatment.*

Having the right does not mean that others will honor it. It is probably safe to assume that, in the current state of the law, you or your family will have to bear at least some legal expenses, and needless anguish, if you do not take definite steps to make sure that your doctor knows your wishes and is willing to honor them.

You can do this in several ways. Thirty-nine states allow **living wills** as of mid-1987. (Sample living wills for states that have, and do not have, living will laws, and material on establishing a **durable power of attorney** in the various states, can be found in appendix H).

Given the current state of the law, we believe that you should both establish a living will and execute a durable power of attorney, giving control of decisions about your health care to a trusted friend or relative in the event you are no longer able to make them. The living will allows you to specify exactly what you mean, and doing both covers all bases. Phrases such as "no heroic measures" and "no artificial life support" are too vague to be enforceable on your doctors and the hospital and will in all likelihood land the matter back in court, which is what you want to avoid. The material in appendix H will help you tailor your living will to reflect your wishes.

There is one area where you, the doctor, and the hospital will wind up talking the same language without much effort: "no code" orders. This means "Do not attempt cardiopulmonary resuscitation" — if your heart stops, let it stay stopped. You can specify to your doctor that you do or do not want a no-code order written. Perhaps the most relevant (and well-hidden) fact here is that only about 4 percent of patients who have cardiopulmonary resuscitation are discharged from the hospital alive. In that sense, contrary to what we see on television, it's a procedure that has a 96 percent failure rate.

In this chapter you will learn: How review agencies can get you into or keep you out of the hospital ▪ How to contact the Peer Review Organization in your area ▪ How to make an ally of your doctor ▪ How to request reconsiderations and appeals ▪ When to file a request for an expedited review ▪ How to request a hearing before an Administrative Law Judge

---

6. Medicare and Hospitals

The purpose of this chapter is to explain how to make sure you get what you are entitled to under Medicare from hospitals. Chapter 2 explained the diagnosis-related groups (DRG) system, which is the way Medicare currently makes payments to hospitals. Chapter 5 explained how to negotiate with your doctor and the hospital about your treatment. This chapter is a legalistic one, designed to show you how to make sure Medicare pays for the care you need.

PROs and URCs

There is a lot of variation between regions of the country in the rate at which people of all ages are admitted to hospitals and in what they are admitted for. Research has shown that this has little to do with the demographics of the populations being served — with how old people are, how sick they are, and so on. It has much more to do with the practice patterns of the doctors in a community. It is also affected to some extent by the availability of hospital beds. For this and other related reasons, Medicare and the various providers of health insurance have been concerned to make sure that people stay out of the hospital if they don't really need to be there. They are also concerned with getting people out as soon as they are ready to go, either home or to a **skilled nursing facility (SNF)**.

The most recent study done on this subject, conducted by the RAND Corporation and reported in April 1988, showed that Medicare spends over $2 billion every year on unnecessary hospital care.

The mechanisms that Medicare uses to deal with this problem have accumulated over the years, the **Joint Commission on the Accreditation of Healthcare Organizations (JCAHO)** has added others, and the DRG system brought the **peer review organizations (PROs)** with it. These are layered on top of one another. For the first time in Medicare's history, the Peer Review Organizations are involved in deciding whether or not you can get into the hospital, as well as when you have to leave. And, of course, your doctor has a lot to do with whether or not you go into the hospital. We'll discuss the roles of each of these in turn.

Your Doctor   The medical profession is losing its control over American health care. Experts differ over whether this is a good or bad thing and about the extent of the loss. Most agree that it has happened because the medical profession is seen by many opinion leaders as having broken the "social contract" with society that gave it that control in exchange for selfless dedication to people's health. At the same time, technology has made it possible to render in the doctor's office or an **ambulatory surgery** center much care that formerly could be given only in a hospital. This has meant that there are new income opportunities for doctors. For example, they can operate on you in an ambulatory surgery center in which they have part ownership and receive fees for the use of the facilities that formerly would have gone to the hospital. Your doctor is being pulled in many different directions.

Generally, a doctor who wants to keep you out of the hospital is a good thing. What is important for you is that you understand what your options are and why the doctor is proposing to treat you outside the hospital.

According to the **American Medical Association's (AMA's)** code of ethics, the doctor is obliged to inform you if he is referring you to a facility that he partly owns or from which he derives a profit. This does not apply, of course, to treatment in his own office but to referral to an **ambulatory surgery** center, outpatient **radiotherapy** center, or **outpatient rehabilitation center.**

If he is performing surgery in his office or in an ambulatory surgery center, be sure to ask what you need to do to prepare for the operation and what you can do for pain relief afterward. One of the biggest complaints that patients have about ambulatory surgery concerns pain relief afterward. (The **procedure** itself is often more pleasant than it would be in the hospital.) You will usually be advised not to eat any-thing for several hours before the procedure and to have someone to drive you home afterward if you will be given **sedation** or a **general anesthetic** of some sort. The most important thing to discuss is any reason why you think you should be treated in the hospital; make sure you understand his reasons and agree with them. You are always free to seek another doctor, even in a **health maintenance organization (HMO)** or **competitive medical plan (CMP).**

In some cases, the peer review organization decides that a patient's surgery must be performed outside the hospital. We'll tell you what to do about that a little later.

The latest source of pressure affecting your doctor is the hospital's response to the DRG system. Remember that the hospital gets to keep any profit it makes on a case and must "eat" any loss. This has led to pressure on doctors from hospitals, to admit as many patients as pos-sible and then, to get them out of the hospital as soon as possible. The results of these pressures is that Medicare patients are being discharged "quicker and sicker." There are a number of reasons to think that this is a good trend and that it might actually protect patients from the potential harm resulting from long hospitals stays. It does represent a change from past practice and an additional pressure on your doctor.

Peer Review Organizations

Medicare's latest attempt to control the costs and monitor the quality of health care for Medicare beneficiaries are the **peer review organi-zations (PROs).** PROs are groups of doctors who have contracts with Medicare to review various aspects of treatment Medicare pays for. Usually, one PRO covers an entire state or a large portion of it. The idea is that the medical profession will remain self-policing, since the reviewers are doctors; at the same time, Medicare can obligate them to focus on what it considers to be problem areas through contracts. The PROs are supposed to work toward targets, such as "Unnecessary hospital admissions should be reduced by 35 percent over the next two years." The key term for Medicare is "35 percent"; the key word for the doctors is "unnecessary." How the two perspectives work together determines what the PRO in a particular area is concentrating on at any given time. The areas currently under review around the nation include the following:

- Reviews of proposed hospital admissions for various procedures
- Reviews of lengthy hospital or skilled nursing facility stays
- Reviews of discharges, readmissions, and deaths

■ Reviews of charts after discharge, to measure the appropriateness of admissions and the quality of care given

The **Health Care Financing Administration (HCFA)**, which runs Medicare, is basically free to add review functions to PRO contracts whenever it sees a need to review some aspect of the quality of care paid for by HCFA programs, including Medicare. Depending on your diagnosis, the previous performance of your doctor and hospital, and the operations or procedures that are proposed for you, the PRO may be reviewing your care before, during, or after your treatment. We'll explain what to do in each situation.

The Hospital Utilization Review Committee

One of the requirements for hospitals to be accredited is to have a committee of doctors that looks at utilization of services, called (generically) **utilization review committees (URCs)**. (Some hospitals give them slightly different names.) According to JCAHO rules, these committees are supposed to operate in the same manner regardless of who is paying for your care. To make matters even more confusing, the PRO can elect to delegate some or all of its review responsibilities for individual cases to the URC of a hospital, if it believes that the URC is performing well. So you may get a notice regarding your care, before or after you enter the hospital, from the URC, from the PRO, or from the UCR-acting-as-PRO. (The stationery the notice is on will be different.)

There are good reasons to have hospital URCs looking at care in addition to PROs. They are much better structured to deal with problems of individual doctors than the PROs, are closer to the scene, and can act more quickly. (Whether this makes a bit of difference depends on the internal politics of the hospital and how freely the URC is allowed to operate. In some institutions, it's a paper tiger.)

Medicare Intermediaries and Carriers

Medicare's **intermediaries** and **carriers** have review responsibilities, too, basically related to oddities that show up during their processing of claims. These functions overlap those of the PROs and the URCs to some extent.

Your Retiree or Employee Insurance Plan

Several years ago Congress made Medicare the *secondary* payer for Medicare beneficiaries who are still working and have health insurance through their employer or who have employer-provided retiree health insurance. This change made employers sit up and take notice of retiree health costs. Many have established preadmission and postadmission review procedures or hired firms to review the cost and quality of care they pay for. These may affect your hospital stay.

Getting In: The First Hurdle

The various review bodies making decisions about whether or not you can go to the hospital at all are the following:

- Your doctor
- A reviewer for your employee or retiree health plan
- The hospital's utilization review committee
- The carrier or intermediary
- The peer review organization

In reading the rest of this section, it is important to remember that *only your doctor or the hospital utilization review committee, acting in accordance with medical staff bylaws, can deny your admission to the hospital.* The only thing the others can decide is whether they will pay for the hospital stay or the procedure. *You are always free to seek admission to the hospital if you think you need it.*

Your Doctor

If your doctor decides that you do not need hospital care, you can discuss it with him or find another doctor. There are no avenues of appeal that result in someone's giving your doctor an order to admit you against his will. You probably would not want to be treated by a doctor who is being forced to do something against his better judgment anyway. You can, of course, ask for a second opinion, and the doctor rendering it may be able to convince your doctor that you do need hospitalization. But remember — for most conditions, you're safer outside the hospital than in.

Your Retirement or Employee Health Plan Reviewer

If your employee or retiree health plan reviewer decides that the plan will not pay for hospital care, Medicare will still pay for what the employer plan does not cover as long as the services you need are Medicare-covered and medically necessary. *The employee or retiree health plan review has no effect on Medicare's decisions.* If this situation arises, we suggest that you contact your employer and your doctor. Your employee or retiree health plan will have some procedures for appeals, and you should pursue this channel first if your situation is not an emergency. The first rejection may have come from a computer, a nurse reviewer, a doctor, or a combination of all three. In cases that are appealed, most of the review entities make use of expert physician consultants to decide cases, in order to protect themselves from liability. A rejection of an appeal from one of these services generally is solid evidence that you do not need hospitalization. You should ask your doctor about the medical necessity for the treatment he proposes.

If your appeal is denied, you or your doctor should contact the Medicare **intermediary** or **carrier** and ask if there is a problem with the admission, given your (current or former) employer's refusal to pay. Generally, you will be told that Medicare will cover the treatment and that the carrier and your employer will fight it out later. This is a tricky area that is not exactly the responsibility of any one of Medicare's review agents right now. You should document all your contacts with your employer and the reviewer in writing. A suggested appeal letter is shown below.

Sample Appeal Letter for Rejection of Admission Request by an Employee or Retiree Health Plan Reviewer

Your name
Your street address
Your city, state and ZIP code

The date [Important!]
Office to which appeals are addressed
Street address
City, state, and ZIP code
ATTN: Proper person, if any

REFERENCE: Your employer/retiree medical plan number
             Your medicare number

Dear Madam or Sir:

I have been advised that you have rejected my doctor's plans to hospitalize me for (name of condition, or operation, or both).

My physician, Dr. _____, feels strongly that I should be treated in the fashion he has suggested. I am attaching a letter from him, plus additional medical evidence (if any), in support of my request for a reconsideration of your decision.

I look forward to hearing from you.

Sincerely yours,
Your signature

Your doctor will usually handle such appeals for you, but you can strengthen the case for review and add pressure to the reviewers by acting on your own.

The Hospital's Utilization Review Committee

It is unlikely, but not impossible, that you will be informed that your admission to the hospital will not be accepted by the hospital's URC. There are really only two instances: In the first, the PRO has delegated review of proposed admissions and procedures to the hospital's URC. In the second, the URC will be reviewing your doctor's cases for admission because of some problems he has had with unnecessary admissions in the past, or — more rarely still — if the hospital's URC is reviewing all nonemergency admissions because of problems in the past or a PRO mandate. Hospitals are so hungry for bed-filling patients now that any hospital-initiated preadmission review is unlikely.

Two different situations need to be carefully distinguished here: if the hospital's URC is acting on its own, you essentially have no appeal. Your doctor's right to admit you is limited by the hospital's bylaws and the conditions of his membership in the medical staff. Generally these do not allow him to admit cases the URC says should not be admitted.

If the URC is acting as the agent of the PRO, things are different. *You have a right to appeal the PRO's decision.* We'll cover how in an upcoming section on PROs.

Carriers and Intermediaries

Carriers, you'll recall, handle Medicare doctor insurance (Part B) for Medicare. Intermediaries handle Part A, for hospital insurance. Under the new Medicare catastrophic coverage law, the carriers have the job of tracking all your medical claims to make sure you do not have to pay excess charges once you have hit the Part B out-of-pocket limit ($1,370 in 1990, $1,530 in 1991, $1,700 in 1992, and $1,900 in 1993). Medicare will no doubt develop regulations that allow you to appeal a finding by the carrier that you have not met the out-of-pocket limit when, in fact, you have, and to receive a refund of any excess payments you may have made.

The Peer Review Organization

As explained earlier, the PROs have been set up to measure, preserve, and, one hopes, improve the quality of care under Medicare. They can do anything within their contracts in this field that the Medicare law permits. The law permits them to deny you admission under the following circumstances:

- There is a problem with unnecessary admissions in your area and Medicare has contracted with them for a preadmission review service.
- You are scheduled to have one of the procedures for which second opinions, preadmission review, or outpatient surgery is required, and one or more conditions have not been met.

They can do nothing, in regard to Medicare patients, that their contracts do not call for.

If you are denied admission by a PRO preadmission review or by a decision that your operation must be done in an outpatient facility, you can request a reconsideration. The instructions at the end of this chapter explain how.

Staying In: The Second Hurdle

People have the idea that they are supposed to stay in the hospital until they are completely well. The simple fact is that Medicare never intended this, and it isn't a good idea anyway. Medicare intended to pay for hospitalization only as long as it is **medically necessary**; that is, as long as the hospital is the only place you could receive the needed care. Most hospital patients are able to be discharged to a **skilled nursing facility (SNF)**, to **home health care,** or to their homes, after relatively short stays. Medicare will not pay for the nonmedical care of people who have limited ability to care for themselves, unless their conditions can be expected to improve with further medical treatment.

Only about 5 percent of older citizens are in a SNF or under custodial care in a nursing home at any one time. This figure reflects two facts: first, most older citizens are at least healthy enough to care for themselves, and second, most don't have the money for nursing homes, which can cost around $22,000 per year. Nursing homes are, in many cases, not the ideal solution for care of the chronically ill.

Not needing hospital care does not mean that you are completely well. It is likely that you will go home from the hospital needing some further recuperation. As we discussed in chapter 5, it is important to find out how well you can be and to make realistic plans within those limits. Being told that you are ready to be discharged should not be a crisis if you have discussed your situation with your doctor or have asked relatives to make provisions for your postdischarge care.

The Effect of the Diagnosis-Related Groups System

As stated earlier, the only limit on your hospital stay is its **medical necessity.** You *cannot* be discharged for any of the following reasons:

- Because your care has cost more than the money amount of your DRG
- Because you have been in the hospital more days than the number of days assigned to your DRG

- Because your hospital has not requested **outlier** payments
- Because your hospital has not received outlier payments

Only medical necessity should govern your length of stay. When you go into the hospital, you are supposed to receive a notice telling you that you cannot be discharged "because your DRG has run out." A copy is shown on pages 181–183.

The same logic and the same procedures that we discussed above under *getting in* apply to *staying in*. We'll discuss the few differences for each of the following:

- Your doctor
- A reviewer for your employee or retiree health plan
- The hospital's utilization review committee
- The carrier or intermediary
- The peer review organization

Your Doctor

Discuss discharge plans with your doctor before you go into the hospital or as soon as possible after admission in an **emergency** or **urgent** situation. You should ask what course your care is likely to take, what might go wrong, what limitations on your ability to care for yourself you can expect after your hospitalization, and what plans you should be making for discharge. Asking these questions *now* puts you in control of the process to some extent.

Your Employee or Retiree Health Plan Reviewer

Just as is the case with admission, a decision by your employer or retiree health plan reviewer that hospital care is not needed has no effect on Medicare, as long as the care you need is covered by Medicare and is medically necessary. A finding by your employer health plan reviewer should alert you to the possibility that the PRO or the hospital's URC may find that your continued stay in the hospital is not medically necessary. Again, you should discuss the situation with your doctor and make plans for discharge if he does not seriously disagree with the reviewer.

The Hospital's Utilization Review Committee

The hospital's URC review of your case has no effect on Medicare *unless* the PRO has delegated review of continued hospital stays to it. If you receive a notice that your continued stay in the hospital is no longer needed, you have the right to request a reconsideration and to appeal if the reconsideration is not favorable. The last part of this chapter explains how.

AN IMPORTANT MESSAGE FROM MEDICARE

YOUR RIGHTS WHILE YOU ARE A MEDICARE HOSPITAL PATIENT

- You have the right to receive all the hospital care that is necessary for the proper diagnosis and treatment of your illness or injury. According to Federal law, **your discharge date must be determined solely by your medical needs,** not by "DRGs" or Medicare payments.

- You have the right to be fully informed about decisions affecting your Medicare coverage and payment for your hospital stay and for any post-hospital services.

- You have the right to request a review by a Peer Review Organization of any written Notice of Noncoverage that you receive from the hospital stating that Medicare will no longer pay for your hospital care. Peer Review Organizations (PROs) are groups of doctors who are paid by the Federal Government to review medical necessity, appropriateness and quality of hospital treatment furnished to Medicare patients. The phone number and address of the PRO for your area are:

_____

_____

_____

TALK TO YOUR DOCTOR ABOUT YOUR STAY IN THE HOSPITAL

You and your doctor know more about your condition and your health needs than anyone else. Decisions about your medical treatment should be made between you and your doctor. **If you have any questions about your medical treatment, your need for continued hospital care, your discharge, or your need for possible post-hospital care, don't hesitate to ask your doctor.** The hospital's patient representative or social worker will also help you with your questions and concerns about hospital services.

IF YOU THINK YOU ARE BEING ASKED TO LEAVE THE HOSPITAL TOO SOON

- Ask a hospital representative for a written notice of explanation immediately, if you have not already received one. This notice is called a "Notice of Noncoverage." You must have this Notice of Noncoverage if you wish to exercise your right to request a review by the PRO.

- The Notice of Noncoverage will state either that your doctor or the PRO agrees with the hospital's decision that Medicare will no longer pay for your hospital care.

  + If the hospital and your doctor agree, the PRO does not review your case before a Notice of Noncoverage is issued. But the PRO will respond to your request for a review of your Notice of Noncoverage and seek your opinion. You cannot be made to pay for your hospital care until the PRO makes its decision, if you request the review by noon of the first work day after you receive the Notice of Noncoverage.

+ If the hospital and your doctor disagree, the hospital may request the PRO to review your case. If it does make such a request, the hospital is required to send you a notice to that effect. In this situation the PRO must agree with the hospital or the hospital cannot issue a Notice of Noncoverage. You may request that the PRO reconsider your case after you receive a Notice of Noncoverage but since the PRO has already reviewed your case once, you may have to pay for **at least one day of hospital care** before the PRO completes this reconsideration.

IF YOU **DO NOT** REQUEST A REVIEW, **THE HOSPITAL MAY BILL YOU** FOR ALL THE COSTS OF YOUR STAY BEGINNING WITH THE THIRD DAY AFTER YOU RECEIVE THE NOTICE OF NONCOVERAGE. THE HOSPITAL, HOWEVER, CANNOT CHARGE YOU FOR CARE UNLESS IT PROVIDES YOU WITH A NOTICE OF NONCOVERAGE.

HOW TO REQUEST A REVIEW OF THE NOTICE OF NONCOVERAGE

• If the Notice of Noncoverage states that your **physician agrees** with the hospital's decision:
  + You must make your request for review to the PRO by **noon of the first work day** after you receive the Notice of Noncoverage by contacting the PRO by phone or in writing.
  + The PRO must ask for your views about your case before making its decision. The PRO will inform you by phone and in writing of its decision on the review.
  + If the PRO agrees with the Notice of Noncoverage, you may be billed for all costs of your stay beginning at noon of the day **after** you receive the PRO's decision.
  + Thus, you will **not** be responsible for the cost of hospital care before you receive the PRO's decision.

• If the Notice of Noncoverage states that the PRO agrees with the hospital's decision:
  + You should make your request for reconsideration to the PRO **immediately** upon receipt of the Notice of Noncoverage by contacting the PRO by phone or in writing.
  + The PRO can take up to three working days from receipt of your request to complete the review. The PRO will inform you in writing of its decision on the review.
  + Since the PRO has already reviewed your case once, prior to the issuance of the Notice of Noncoverage, the hospital is permitted to begin billing you for the cost of your stay beginning with the third calendar day after you receive your Notice of Noncoverage **even if the PRO has not completed its review.**
  + Thus, if the PRO continues to agree with the Notice of Noncoverage, **you may have to pay for at least one day of hospital care.**

NOTE: The process described above is called "immediate review." If you miss the deadline for this immediate review while you are in the hospital, you may still request a review of Medicare's decision to no longer pay for your care at any point during your hospital stay or after you have left the hospital. The Notice of Noncoverage will tell you how to request this review.

POST-HOSPITAL CARE

When your doctor determines that you no longer need all the specialized services provided in a hospital, but you still require medical care, he or she may discharge you to a skilled nursing facility or home care. The discharge planner at the hospital will help arrange for the services you may need after your discharge. Medicare and supplemental insurance policies have limited coverage for skilled nursing facility care and home health care. Therefore, you should find out which services will or will not be covered and how payment will be made. Consult with your doctor, hospital discharge planner, patient representative and your family in making preparations for care after you leave the hospital. **Don't hesitate to ask questions.**

ACKNOWLEDGEMENT OF RECEIPT — My signature only acknowledges my receipt of this Message from (name of hospital) on (date) and does not waive any of my rights to request a review or make me liable for any payment.

_____

Signature of beneficiary or
person acting on behalf of beneficiary.

The Peer Review Organization

One of the jobs of the PRO is to review cases that have extended hospital stays. This review can be triggered in a number of ways. See the end of this chapter for instructions on how to appeal a decision not to pay for more time in the hospital.

The PRO's decision affects Medicare's payment for your hospital stay in the following way: you can stay in the hospital until the third day following the date you received the notice that your continued stay was no longer necessary. If you do not request a reconsideration, Medicare will cease payment on the third day following the notice. If you do request reconsideration and get a favorable ruling at any stage of the process, Medicare will pay for time spent in the hospital up until you are discharged or die. If you lose the appeal, you or your insurer must pay for these days.

There is an oddity in the law on this that you should be aware of. If you request an *expedited* reconsideration of the PRO's decision, it *may* come before the two days to which you would otherwise be entitled have passed. Some Medicare experts believe that this is not the result Congress intended. The moral of the story is that you should not request an expedited reconsideration unless you are unable to make reasonable plans for posthospital care in the event you lose.

Making Sure Your Care Is Adequate

Making sure that you receive adequate care in the hospital is a subject that is beyond the scope of this book. There is, in fact, a book devoted exclusively to this subject: *Take This Book to the Hospital With You*, by Charles B. Inlander and Ed Weiner. We suggest that you read it. It contains valuable advice for any hospital stay, whether or not Medicare pays for it.

There is a temptation for hospitals to provide less than adequate care to Medicare beneficiaries. First, they are afraid that your care will cost more than the DRG for your condition(s) will pay. Second, they are afraid that they will not be able to maximize the profit they could make on the DRG. Right now, economic reality for hospitals is that they can make the most money by admitting you unnecessarily and then giving as little care as possible. This is the situation the PROs were set up to police. There are **perverse incentives** in any payment system, and the DRG system is better, from a number of angles, than the pay-for-each-day system that preceded it.

The key point to remember is that your status as a Medicare patient should make no difference. Hospitals make about 50 percent of their revenues from Medicare patients. The hospital needs you as much as you need it.

All this assumes, of course, that you know what good care is. This is something about which lay opinions have been disregarded in the past. The Hospital Patient's Bill of Rights (see appendix I) gives you an indication of what the hospital industry thinks you should think good care is. This document has no legal standing. We think that the PMS Code of Practice, located in appendix F, is better. Both should serve to give you some idea of an ideal you should expect your hospital care to live up to. We've discussed how to negotiate for the kind of hospital care you want in chapter 5.

Controlling the Doctors

All the controversy about hospitals and Medicare makes us forget that it is ultimately the doctors who control the hospital, at least as far as medical care is concerned. There is a good deal of self-doubt in the profession about the way things are done now. You can see a wide sampling in *Medicine on Trial*, by Charles B. Inlander, Lowell Levin, and Ed Weiner. The material covered in that book is beyond the scope of this one.

We do want to mention one thing to watch out for, something that doctors regret but feel they can't control: the clinical "cascade." What happens is this: You go in for a relatively simple treatment, and you have a bad reaction to the dye used in a test, or something else goes not exactly according to your doctor's original plan. She asks a specialist to look at you. The specialist treats you for the bad reaction to the dye, but thinks he spots something else, so he orders some tests. They show a possible abnormality, you're in the hospital, so it might as well be checked out now, and . . .

All too soon you are the recipient of as much medical attention as the hospital can muster, being treated for reactions to treatments that were given because you had reactions to other treatments, with your admitting doctor somewhere in the background, peering over the shoulders of the specialists and house staff who have you surrounded.

The only one who can stop this is *you*, sad to say. You should question every treatment, and insist on knowing, at every moment, which doctor is primarily responsible for your care. You should negotiate for assignment with every doctor who treats you. If you need to ask whether or not you will be billed for a service, do so. Refuse it if the doctor will not take assignment, and ask whoever is in charge of your case to find someone who will.

If you are too ill to deal with this, we suggest that you give someone you trust, and who is willing to steer your care, a **durable power of attorney.** This was discussed at considerable length in chapter 5. A durable power of attorney will enable him or her to handle these matters for you.

Remember:

- You have a right to the same quality medical care as anyone else the hospital serves.
- You have the right to refuse services you do not want.
- You have the right to leave the hospital, even against medical advice.

Reconsiderations and Appeals

This section covers how to obtain reconsideration of the following:

- Decisions about hospital care by the peer review organizations
- Decisions about payment for hospital care
- Decisions about payment of doctor's bills

Peer Review Organization Decisions

The PRO is involved in determining the following:

- Whether or not Medicare will pay for your hospital admission
- Whether or not Medicare will pay for your continued stay in the hospital
- Whether or not Medicare will pay for your admission to a skilled nursing facility
- Whether or not Medicare will pay for your continued stay in a skilled nursing facility
- Whether or not Medicare will pay for an outpatient procedure to be done in the hospital
- Whether or not Medicare will require a second opinion before paying for surgery

Key Points:
- In all your dealings with the peer review organizations, there is one issue only: the *medical necessity* of your being cared for at all, or the *medical necessity* of your being cared for *in the way your doctor wants to do it.* All other issues are extraneous. Stay focused on this point.

- There is a great deal of uncertainty in medicine. It is unlikely that what your doctor wants to do is totally unreasonable. You and he should emphasize *why* it is acceptable as good medical care.

- Keep copies of everything you send to the PRO. It is advisable to send materials *certified mail, return receipt requested.* This gives you proof of the date you mailed material and the date on which the PRO (or other recipient of your papers, such as your Social Security district office) received it.

- If you are dealing with a decision that your continued stay is no longer medically necessary, make sure you understand when Medicare will no longer pay for your hospital stay.

- A PRO review of care that you have already had *never* requires you to pay for it. You cannot retroactively be required to pay for care you've already received, unless you can reasonably be expected to have known that it wasn't covered. (See chapter 2 for more information on this.)

Procedure

The procedure that follows is *generic.* It applies to all actions by the PROs. Only the evidence submitted would differ.

Notices: Your denial is called a Notice of Noncoverage, and it will explain why something is being denied.

If you receive such a notice *while you are in the hospital,* it's important to understand that there are two tracks possible. If you are asking the *PRO* to review the hospital's decision, you are not responsible for services received before you get the notice of the PRO's decision. If you are asking the PRO to rethink its own decision, the hospital may start billing you beginning with the third calendar day after you received the Notice of Noncoverage. If the PRO does not reverse its position and you decide not to stay in the hospital, you may have to pay for the third day. If you decide to stay, you are responsible for the further cost of your care.

How to Appeal (Request a Reconsideration) of a Peer Review Organization Decision: You can appeal the decision of the PRO by filing a request for reconsideration with the PRO itself, at the address for the PRO shown on the notice you received; at any **Social Security office**; or at a Railroad Retirement Board office, if you are a railroad retirement beneficiary.

Your doctor and the hospital also have the right to file an appeal. They do *not* have the right to an "expedited reconsideration" that you have.

Time to File the Request for Reconsideration: You must file your request for reconsideration within sixty days of the date you receive the notice of denial. Unless you can prove otherwise, the notice is deemed to have been received by you five days after the date on it. (Example: The notice is dated January 5. You are deemed to have received it on January 10, unless you can prove you received it later. Your sixty-day period for appeal started on January 10. The last day you can file an appeal is March 10, the sixtieth day after the deemed receipt of the notice.) Some more examples of how the dates run are provided below.

Time Periods for Filing Requests for Reconsideration		
NOTICE OF NONCOVERAGE MAILED	DEEMED RECEIVED	LAST DAY TO FILE REQUEST
January 2	January 7	March 7
March 15	March 20	April 17
November 27	December 1	January 29 (of next year)

"Good Cause" for Late Filing: Generally, you will be allowed to file late if there is what the PRO considers to be "good cause" for it. The regulations are very broad, and it is hard to see what exactly might count. The regulations give examples such as serious illness, a death in the family, failure to receive information you had requested before the sixty-day limit, a misunderstanding of what the PRO notice told you, and so on.

Obtaining Information: Both you and your doctor have a right to see the information on which the PRO based its decision. You should ask for this when you file your request for reconsideration. You may add to the information anything you or your doctor want to add.

Expedited Reconsideration and Time Limits: You can request that the PRO make an expedited review or reconsideration of the denial. How fast "expedited" has to be depends on the circumstances:

- Within three working days if you are still a patient in the hospital (this doesn't really apply here, of course, since you're trying to get in)
- Within three days if the initial determination was a denial of hospital admission and you are still in the hospital

- Within ten working days if you are in a skilled nursing facility
- Within thirty working days in all other situations, and in every situation where someone other than you files the appeal. Having expedited redetermination available is a very important reason for *you* to file the appeal and have the doctor or hospital submit information as part of an appeal.

What to Include: You should file your claim using HCFA Form 2649, which is shown on page 190. Other forms for other situations are also shown:

- HCFA HA501.1 — Request for a Hearing on Part A Claims. This form is used to request a hearing if you are not satisfied with the results of your request for reconsideration.
- HCFA 1964 — Request for Reconsideration on Part B Claims. This is used initially to request a reconsideration of a denial for services under Part B, doctor insurance. It is analogous to the 2649.
- HCFA 1965 — Request for Hearing on Part B Claims. Like the HA501.1, this is used to request a hearing if you are not satisfied with the results of your request for reconsideration.

You never have to use these forms, but using them will help you record all the information you need. You can supplement them with a letter if you wish.

You can request an appeal with just a letter, but using the form will ensure that you include everything that is needed. You should ask your doctor to provide medical documentation. It is important for both you and your doctor to focus on the issue at hand, and not editorialize. The general issue you will be dealing with in PRO denials of admission is the *medical necessity* for you to be hospitalized at all, to have a procedure done in the hospital, or to have it done at all. Keep the focus on these issues. They will boil down to appropriate medical judgment. Your doctor will probably want to submit information regarding your condition, plus evidence from the medical literature indicating that what the PRO wants done is unwise.

Notices and Appeals: When the PRO provides you with its reconsidered decision, it must do so *in writing* and inform you of the following:

- The decision
- The reasons for it

DEPARTMENT OF HEALTH, EDUCATION, AND WELFARE
HEALTH CARE FINANCING ADMINISTRATION

Form Approved.
OMB No. 066-R-0067

REQUEST FOR RECONSIDERATION OF PART A HEALTH INSURANCE BENEFITS

INSTRUCTIONS: *Please type or print firmly.* Leave the block empty if you cannot answer it. Take or mail the WHOLE form to your Social Security office which will be glad to help you. Please read the statement on the reverse side of page 2.

1. BENEFICIARY'S NAME	2. HEALTH INSURANCE CLAIM NUMBER

3. REPRESENTATIVE'S NAME, IF APPLICABLE

(□ RELATIVE □ ATTORNEY □ OTHER PERSON) □ PROVIDER FILING

4. PLEASE ATTACH A COPY OF THE NOTICE(S) YOU RECEIVED ABOUT YOUR CLAIM TO THIS FORM.

5. THIS CLAIM IS FOR

□ INPATIENT HOSPITAL □ SKILLED NURSING FACILITY (SNF) □ HEALTH MAINTENANCE ORGANIZATION (HMO)
□ EMERGENCY HOSPITAL □ HOME HEALTH AGENCY (HHA)

6. NAME AND ADDRESS OF PROVIDER *(Hospital, SNF, HHA, HMO)*	CITY AND STATE	PROVIDER NUMBER
7. NAME OF INTERMEDIARY	CITY AND STATE	INTERMEDIARY NUMBER

8. DATE OF ADMISSION OR START OF SERVICES	9. DATE(S) OF THE NOTICE(S) YOU RECEIVED

10. I DO NOT AGREE WITH THE DETERMINATION ON MY CLAIM. PLEASE RECONSIDER MY CLAIM BECAUSE

11. YOU MUST OBTAIN ANY EVIDENCE *(For example, a letter from a doctor)* YOU WISH TO SUBMIT.

□ I HAVE ATTACHED THE FOLLOWING EVIDENCE:

□ I WILL SEND THIS EVIDENCE WITHIN 10 DAYS:

□ I HAVE NO ADDITIONAL EVIDENCE OR OTHER INFORMATION TO SUBMIT WITH MY CLAIM.

12. IS THIS REQUEST FILED WITHIN 60 DAYS OF THE DATE OF YOUR NOTICE?

□ YES □ NO

IF YOU CHECKED "NO" ATTACH AN EXPLANATION OF THE REASON FOR THE DELAY TO THIS FORM.

13. ONLY ONE SIGNATURE IS NEEDED. THIS FORM IS SIGNED BY:

□ BENEFICIARY □ REPRESENTATIVE □ PROVIDER REP.

SIGN HERE ▶

14. STREET ADDRESS

CITY, STATE, ZIP CODE

TELEPHONE	DATE

15. If this request is signed by mark (X), TWO WITNESSES who know the person requesting reconsideration must sign in the space provided on the reverse side of this page of the form.

DO NOT FILL IN BELOW THIS LINE — FOR SOCIAL SECURITY USE — THANK YOU

16. ROUTING

□ INTERMEDIARY

□ HCFA, RO-MEDICARE

□ BSS, ODR

18. SSA OR INTERMEDIARY DATE STAMP

17. ADDITIONAL INFORMATION

FORM **HCFA-2649** (8-79 FORMERLY SSA-2649)
DESTROY PRIOR EDITIONS

INTERMEDIARY

Page 1 of 4

REQUEST FOR HEARING
<u>PART A</u> HEALTH INSURANCE BENEFITS

Take or mail original and all copies to your local Social Security office.

CLAIMANT'S NAME

WAGE EARNER'S NAME (Leave blank if same as above)

HI CLAIM NUMBER

NAME AND ADDRESS OF INTERMEDIARY

CLAIM FOR
- ☐ Hospital Services
- ☐ Extended Care Facility Services
- ☐ Home Health Agency Services
- ☐ Emergency Services

PERIOD IN QUESTION
FROM: TO:

NAME AND ADDRESS OF PROVIDER

I disagree with the determination made on the above claim and request a hearing before a hearing examiner of the Bureau of Hearings and Appeals. My reasons for disagreement are: (additional pages may be added if necessary.)

Check one of the following:

☐ I have additional evidence to submit. (Attach such evidence to this form or forward to the Social Security Office within 10 days.)

☐ I have <u>no</u> additional evidence to submit.

Check <u>ONLY ONE</u> of the statements below.

☐ I wish to appear in person before the hearing examiner.

☐ I waive my right to appear and give evidence, and hereby request a decision on the evidence before the hearing examiner.

Signed by: (Either the claimant or representative should sign-Enter addresses for both. If claimant's representative is not an attorney, complete Form SSA-1696)

SIGNATURE OR NAME OF CLAIMANT'S REPRESENTATIVE
☐ ATTORNEY ☐ NON-ATTORNEY

CLAIMANT'S SIGNATURE

ADDRESS

ADDRESS

CITY, STATE, AND ZIP CODE

CITY, STATE, AND ZIP CODE

TELEPHONE NUMBER

DATE:

TELEPHONE NUMBER

Claimant should not fill in below this line

Is this request filed within 6 months of the reconsideration determination?   ☐ Yes   ☐ No
If "No" is checked: (1) attach claimant's explanation for delay, (2) attach any pertinent letter, material, or information in the Social Security Office.

ACKNOWLEDGMENT OF REQUEST FOR HEARING

Your request for a hearing was filed on_____at _____
The hearing examiner will notify you of the time and place of the hearing at least 10 days prior to the date which will be set for the hearing.

| Hearing Examiner Copy | TO:
☐ Hearing Examiner _____ (Location) | For the Social Security Administration |
| Claim File Copy | TO:
☐ BHI, Reconsideration Branch

☐ BHI, Regional Office _____
(Only emergency services in other than Federal Hospitals) | By:_____
(Signature)   (Title)

_____
(Street Address)

_____
(City)   (State)   (ZIP Code) |

Interpreter Needed_____   Servicing District Office Code_____
(Language)

Form HA 501.1
(2-72)

HEARING EXAMINER

DEPARTMENT OF HEALTH AND HUMAN SERVICES
HEALTH CARE FINANCING ADMINISTRATION

Form Approved
OMB No. 0938-0033

REQUEST FOR REVIEW OF PART B MEDICARE CLAIM
Medical Insurance Benefits - Social Security Act

NOTICE—Anyone who misrepresents or falsifies essential information requested by this form may upon conviction be subject to fine and imprisonment under Federal Law.

Carrier's Name and Address

The name and address of the
Carrier for your state will
be listed in this space.

1 Name of Patient

2 Health Insurance Claim Number

3 I do not agree with the determination you made on my claim as described on my Explanation of Medicare

Benefits dated:

4 MY REASONS ARE: *(Attach a copy of the Explanation of Medicare Benefits, or describe the service, date of service, and physician's name—NOTE.—If the date on the Notice of Benefits mentioned in item 3 is more than six months ago, include your reason for not making this request earlier.)*

5 ☐ I have additional evidence to submit. *(Attach such evidence to this form)*

☐ I do not have additional evidence.

COMPLETE ALL OF THE INFORMATION REQUESTED. SIGN AND RETURN THE FIRST COPY AND ANY ATTACHMENTS TO THE CARRIER NAMED ABOVE. IF YOU NEED HELP, TAKE THIS AND YOUR NOTICE FROM THE CARRIER TO A SOCIAL SECURITY OFFICE, OR TO THE CARRIER. KEEP THE DUPLICATE COPY OF THIS FORM FOR YOUR RECORDS.

6

SIGNATURE OF **EITHER** THE CLAIMANT **OR** HIS REPRESENTATIVE

Representative	Claimant
➡	➡
Address	Address
City, State, and ZIP Code	City, State, and ZIP Code
Telephone Number	Date	Telephone Number	Date

Form **HCFA-1964** (1-78) (Formerly SSA-1964)   **CARRIER'S COPY**   (over)

DEPARTMENT OF HEALTH AND HUMAN SERVICES
HEALTH CARE FINANCING ADMINISTRATION

Form Approved
OMB No. 0938-0034

REQUEST FOR HEARING - PART B MEDICARE CLAIM
Medical Insurance Benefits - Social Security Act

NOTICE—Anyone who misrepresents or falsifies essential information requested by this form may upon conviction be subject to fine and imprisonment under Federal Law.

Carrier's Name and Address	**1** Name of Patient
The name and address of the Carrier for your state will be listed in this space.	**2** Health Insurance Claim Number

3 I disagree with the review determination on my claim, and request a hearing before a hearing officer of the insurance carrier named above.

MY REASONS ARE: *(Attach a copy of the Review Notice. NOTE.—If the review decision was made more than 6 months ago include your reason for not making this request earlier)*

4 Check one of the Following:

☐ I have additional evidence to submit. *(Attach such evidence to this form or forward it to the carrier within 10 days.)*

☐ I do not have additional evidence.

Check <u>Only One</u> of the Statements Below:

☐ I wish to appear in person before the Hearing Officer.

☐ I do not wish to appear and hereby request a decision on the evidence before the Hearing Officer.

5 EITHER THE CLAIMANT OR REPRESENTATIVE SHOULD SIGN IN THE APPROPRIATE SPACE BELOW:

Signature or Name of Claimant's Representative ➡	Claimant's Signature ➡
Address	Address
City, State, and ZIP Code	City, State, and ZIP Code
Telephone Number	Date	Telephone Number	Date

(Claimant should not write below this line)

ACKNOWLEDGMENT OF REQUEST FOR HEARING

Your request for a hearing was received on _____. You will be notified of the time and place of the hearing at least 10 days before the date of the hearing.

Signed	Date

Form **HCFA-1965** (8-79) (Formerly SSA-1965)

CARRIERS COPY

- A statement of the effect the decision has on what Medicare will pay for or has paid for
- A statement of your appeal rights, with complete instructions for filing the appeal

When you receive a notice of a reconsidered decision that is not in your favor, consider whether you want to request a hearing. A hearing is more formal than a reconsideration, and it entitles you to appear before an **administrative law judge** (**ALJ**). If you do request a hearing, it is wise to have a lawyer involved. Hearings can involve subpoenaing witnesses and other legal steps. It is less formal than a court case, but far more formal than a request for reconsideration. Medicare is emphasizing doing all business possible, including hearings, over the phone. Although a hearing can be conducted over the phone, you should carefully consider appearing in person. It is sometimes easier to make your case in person, depending on the circumstances.

Only you, not your doctor or the hospital, have this right. The rules for filing an appeal are exactly the same as for filing for reconsideration with the PRO — sixty days, counted from five days after the date of the notice, and all that. You should file your appeal on HCFA HA-501-US, unless the information you received with the PRO's Notice of Reconsideration tells you to do something else.

The first thing the ALJ will attempt to determine is whether or not the controversy involves at least $200 (with the price of health care these days, it almost surely will). If the ALJ determines that the amount is less than $200, he will notify you and any other concerned parties that he has determined this and that they have fifteen days to show why he is wrong. If no evidence is submitted within fifteen days, the request for a hearing is dismissed. (You will not have to worry about this if you don't receive such a notice.)

You will be notified by the ALJ of the date of the hearing at least ten days before it is filed.

If the ALJ's decision is unfavorable, you can appeal to the Social Security Appeals Council. Your attorney can tell you how to do this. The Appeals Council does not take all the appeals addressed to it. If $2,000 or more is at issue, you can appeal an Appeals Council decision, or the ALJ's decision if the Appeals Council refused a hearing, to the federal courts. This must be done within sixty days of the date of the Appeals Council decision on your case, or its decision not to hear it.

Requesting Reconsiderations on Payment

The procedures in this section apply to denial of payment for all services, other than doctors' services, after you have left the hospital. They also apply to notices regarding hospital care that you receive from the Medicare intermediary while you are in the hospital.

Notices: Your notice of denial will come either in the form of an **Explanation of Medicare Benefits (EOMB)** or in the form of a letter. In any case, it must be in writing. It will explain the reason that something is being denied. A typical EOMB is shown on pages 132–133.

How to Appeal (Request a Reconsideration) of a Payment Denial or Intermediary Determination that Care Is Not Medically Necessary: You can appeal the PRO decision by filing a request for reconsideration with the intermediary itself, at the address shown on the EOMB, at any Social Security office, or at a Railroad Retirement Board office, if you are a railroad retirement beneficiary, or at any office of the **Health Care Financing Administration.**

Your doctor and the hospital have the right to file an appeal only if you do not plan to do so and you certify this in writing on a form they will provide. They do *not* have the right to an "expedited reconsideration" that you have.

Time to File the Request for Reconsideration: You must file your request for reconsideration within sixty days of the date you receive the notice of denial. Unless you can prove otherwise, the notice is deemed to have been received by you five days after the date on it. (Example: The notice is dated January 5. You are deemed to have received it on January 10, unless you can prove you received it later. Your sixty-day period for appeal started on January 10. The last day you can file an appeal is March 10, the sixtieth day after the deemed receipt of the notice.)

Request for Extension of Time to File: If you need more than sixty days to file your appeal, you can request more time at any Social Security office, Medicare office, or the Railroad Retirement Board. You cannot file an extension request with an intermediary. You will be notified in writing of the time granted you.

"Good Cause" for Granting a Time Extension: Generally, you will be allowed to file late if there is what the PRO considers to be "good cause" for it. The regulations are very broad, and it is hard to see what

exactly might count. The regulations give examples such as serious illness, a death in the family, failure to receive information you had requested before the sixty-day limit, a misunderstanding of what the PRO notice told you, and so on.

Obtaining Information: Both you and your doctor have a right to see the information on which the PRO based its decision. You should ask for this when you file your request for reconsideration. You may add to the information anything you or your doctor want to add.

Expedited Reconsideration: There is a procedure for expedited appeals under Part A (hospital insurance), but it may be used only if both the person appealing and the secretary of Health and Human Services (HHS) agree that the only issue is a constitutional one. This is a rare situation.

What to Include: You should file your claim using HCFA Form 2649. You can request an appeal with just a letter, but using the form will ensure that you include everything that is needed. You should ask your doctor to provide medical documentation. It is important for both you and your doctor to focus on the issue at hand, and not editorialize. The general issues you will be dealing with are as follows:

- The medical necessity of the service
- Whether or not Medicare covers it
- Whether or not you are entitled to it
- Whether or not the amount paid is what ought to have been paid

Medical necessity issues will boil down to appropriate medical judgment. Your doctor will probably want to submit information regarding your condition, plus evidence from the medical literature that indicates that the decision is unwise.

Time Limits: The regulations provide no time limit for a decision on a Part A request for reconsideration.

Notices and Appeals: When you are provided with the reconsidered decision, it will include, in writing, the following:

- The decision
- The reasons for it

- A statement of the effect the decision has on what Medicare will pay for, or has paid for
- A statement of your appeal rights, with complete instructions for filing the appeal

When you receive a notice of a reconsidered decision that is not in your favor, consider whether you want to request a hearing. A hearing is more formal than a reconsideration, and entitles you to appear before an ALJ. If you do request a hearing, it is wise to have a lawyer involved. Hearings can involve subpoenaing witnesses and other legal steps. It is less formal than a court case, but far more formal than a request for reconsideration.

Only you, not your doctor or the hospital, have this right. The rules for filing an appeal are exactly the same as for filing for reconsideration — sixty days, counted from five days after the date of the notice, and all that. You should file your appeal on HCFA HA-501-US, unless the information you received with the Notice of Reconsideration tells you to do something else.

You may request a hearing only if the amount in controversy is $100 or more.

You should also note that your request for a hearing will be deemed received *five days* after the date on it, unless you can show that it was received earlier. If you are within five days of the sixty-day limit, send it *certified mail, return receipt requested,* so you will have proof of the date it was actually received.

The first thing the ALJ will attempt to determine is whether or not the controversy involves at least $200 (with the price of health care these days, it almost surely will). If the ALJ determines that the amount is less than $200, he will notify you and any other concerned parties that he has determined this and that they have fifteen days to show why he is wrong. If no evidence is submitted within fifteen days, the request for a hearing is dismissed. (You will not have to worry about this if you don't receive such a notice.)

You will be notified by the ALJ of the date of the hearing at least ten days before it is filed.

If the ALJ's decision is unfavorable, you can appeal to the Social Security Appeals Council. Your attorney can tell you how to do this. The Appeals Council does not take all the appeals addressed to it. If $1,000 or more is at issue, you can appeal an Appeals Council decision, or the ALJ's decision if the Appeals Council refused a hearing, to the federal courts. This must be done within sixty days of the date of the Appeals Council decision on your case, or its decision not to hear it.

If you receive a favorable determination, Medicare will pay its usual amounts for the services rendered. If you do not receive a favorable determination, you pay.

In this chapter you will learn: What Medicare covers under skilled nursing care ▪ How Medicaid can help pay for nursing home care ▪ What to look for when selecting long-term care insurance ▪ How to evaluate a nursing home ▪ What home health care services are covered

7. Nursing Homes, Home Health Care, and Medicare

The nursing home business is a $40-billion-per-year industry. Of the nation's 31.3 million citizens aged sixty-five and above, 2.3 million (7.4 percent) live in nursing homes. The average cost of a year's stay is $22,000. The average stay, 465 days, costs $28,000. The average charge is around $60 per day. The Brookings Institution, a Washington think tank, estimates that by the year 2018, almost 8 percent of the elderly will live in nursing homes, at an annual cost of $55,000.

We explained in chapter 3 that Medicare does not, as many people think, pay for nursing homes. It does pay for **skilled nursing facilities** (**SNF**) care, but only for 150 days per calendar year. What follows is a brief summary of the explanation of coverage in chapter 3.

Care in a SNF is less intense than that you received in a hospital, but more intense than that provided in **intermediate care facilities** (**ICFs**) or custodial care. ("Custodial care" is defined as the provision of room, board, and personal services, generally on a long-term basis, without additional medical services such as those provided by SNFs and ICFs. Some facilities provide all three levels of care — skilled, intermediate, and custodial — in the same building or in different buildings on the same grounds.)

Many of the services listed under hospitals are covered under SNFs.

The exceptions are services that SNFs do not normally provide, such as operating rooms. Medicare permits small hospitals (ninety-nine beds or less) that have empty beds to run a SNF within their walls, using beds that have been designated as "swing beds." Swing beds are used as SNF beds or as hospital beds, depending on which are needed.

You are entitled to 150 days of SNF care during each calendar year. For the first eight days, a coinsurance equal to one-fifth of the national average daily charge for SNF care must be paid (the amount is $22.00 for 1989) The next 142 days are paid in full. From the 151st day forward, you pay for all SNF care.

Medical necessity is *the* key issue in payment for SNF services. The SNF regulations go to great lengths to define what is and is not SNF care. The key is that care complex enough to require the services of a nurse or skilled rehabilitation personnel is covered; care that you could do yourself is not. But complications may require SNF-level care, even for situations that would normally not be covered. Basically, SNF care is rehabilitation; if your condition cannot be expected to improve as a result of SNF care *and* you do not need observation by skilled personnel, your care will not be covered. Obviously, what your doctor writes in the chart makes a big difference in what gets covered. If you are worried about coverage of SNF services, discuss this with your doctor.

Do You Really Need a Nursing Home?

Nursing homes cost about $22,000 per year. Medicaid, another state/ federal program that provides health care, does pay for nursing homes, but the price may be the loss of substantial amounts of assets and income. The old law virtually guaranteed that the spouse who stayed at home would have to impoverish him- or herself to pay for the care of the spouse in the nursing home. The new Medicare catastrophic coverage provisions greatly reduce the burden but can still lead to a substantial loss of assets. Beginning January 1, 1989,

- In any month in which a married person is in a nursing home, no income of the at-home spouse is to be considered available to the spouse in the nursing home.

- Income is considered the property of the person to whom it is paid. Income paid to both spouses is attributed 50 percent to each.

- The home, household goods, and personal effects of both spouses are not counted in considering Medicaid eligibility.

- All assets other than these will be counted and divided in two. If the at-home spouse has less than $12,000, the spouse in the nursing home may transfer assets to him or her to make up to $12,000 available to the at-home spouse. (States may, at their option, raise this figure to any amount less than $60,000. The $12,000 amount will be indexed to inflation.

- The assets that remain in the name of the spouse in the nursing home are considered available to pay for his or her nursing home care. All assets in excess of $60,000 are attributed to the spouse in the nursing home and are considered available to pay for nursing home care.

- States must allow nursing home residents to retain certain sums for medical expenses not covered by Medicare or Medicaid before contributing to the expense of their nursing home care. The states may place "reasonable limits" on the amounts spent.

Beginning September 30, 1989,

- The states must allow the at-home spouse sufficient income from the other spouse to bring total household income of the at-home spouse to at least 122 percent of the federal poverty level for a two-person household. In 1989, this will be $789 per month. On July 1, 1991, it will be raised to 133 percent of the poverty level, and to 150 percent on July 1, 1992. States will not be required to allow more than $1,500 per month, except by court order or change in regulations.

These changes greatly ease the situation of the spouse who remains at home, but if assets and income are substantial, one may be forced to use most of them to pay for a nursing home before becoming eligible for Medicaid. Even after one is eligible, the income of the spouse who remains at home is limited.

Some companies are beginning to offer nursing home insurance, but it is, at present, expensive and somewhat restricted in what it will pay for.

Before discussing how to choose a nursing home, we want to raise a question that is rarely asked: *Do you really need a nursing home?*

It is true, of course, that some older people are crippled by arthritis, have Alzheimer's disease, or have another form of senile dementia that makes it impossible for them to live without constant supervision; others have another problem that requires constant, round-the-clock custodial care. These people are only about 5 percent of the elderly. (There are, of course, others who are cared for by a spouse or other relative.) The majority of the over-65 population seems to do quite well without nursing home care.

In our experience, many older people think they need nursing home care because they are no longer able to do one or a few of the things they did when they were young. If you are no longer able to drive, this does not mean you need a nursing home — it means you need transportation. If you are unable to cook, this does not mean you need a nursing home — it means you need someone to prepare meals for you. Most of the elderly face difficulties that are no more severe than those faced by younger handicapped people who are able to live independently.

Part of the reason many older people think they need a nursing home if they are no longer able to do everything they used to do is that they share society's prejudice against the aged. A problem that is a handicap heroically overcome in a 35-year-old is an infirmity that demands that a 65-year-old be tucked away in a nursing home — or so people think. We discussed some of these prejudices as they affect your dealings with your doctor in chapter 5. We suggest you read that section "The Doctor's Obligation to Inform You Fully" again. Are you, perhaps, prejudiced against the elderly yourself?

The Health Status Checklist on page 203 will help you assess the level of care that you (or an aged relative) need. In using it, think very carefully about the person's level of functioning. If you're not sure, put a question mark. On items with a question mark, you may want to seek some professional advice in evaluating the person's capabilities.

Caring for a bedridden, elderly person can be a full-time job. The caregiver must be on the lookout for the development of pressure sores (decubitus ulcers), incontinence, dehydration, malnutrition, development of contractures from too little limb movement, and the unusual drug reactions that are common in the elderly.

For those who are not bedridden, adult day care, home health care, homemaker services, sharing a home with other elderly people, Meals on Wheels, shopping services, and adult foster care may be alternatives that will avoid a nursing home stay. For the availability of these services, you can check with your local agency on aging, the medical social services office of the hospital (if the person is in the hospital awaiting discharge), and departments of social services. Many are listed in the telephone book under the names we've used above, for example, "shopping services."

Health Status Checklist*

Read each statement *very carefully* before deciding if it applies to the person in question, then place a check mark in front of those that describe the person's condition. Think in terms of *"Does this person have difficulty with"*:

_____ 1. *Bathing* — Requires assistance from another person

_____ 2. *Continence* — Difficulty in controlling either the bladder or bowels

_____ 3. *Dressing* — Either requires assistance or does not dress at all

_____ 4. *Eating* — Requires assistance, either from a person or via tube or intravenously

_____ 5. *Mobility* — Either requires the assistance of a person to walk or is confined to chair/bed

_____ 6. *Using toilet room* — Either requires assistance from another person or does not use one at all

_____ 7. *Speech* — Either completely lost or is so severely impaired that it can be understood only with difficulty (person cannot carry on a normal conversation)

_____ 8. *Hearing* — Either completely lost or so impaired that only a few words a person says or loud noises can be heard

_____ 9. *Vision* — Either blindness or so severely impaired that television cannot be seen eight to twelve feet away (features of a familiar person can be recognized within two to three feet)

_____ 10. *Mental status* — Cannot understand (or remember) simple instructions, requires constant supervision or restraints for his or her own safety

*Suggested by the Department of Health and Human Services, Long-term Care Survey.

Paying for Custodial Care in a Nursing Home

As we have seen, Medicare does not cover care in a nursing home that is custodial, or nonmedical in nature. Two alternatives may help you pay for custodial care if you really need it: Medicaid and private nursing home insurance.

Medicaid

The Medicaid program provides medical care for the poor. It was tacked onto the Medicare bill at the last possible second, and its passage by Congress, together with Medicare, amazed its advocates. The program still shows the features of its hasty design.

Medicaid is intended for the very poor who have nowhere else to turn, but not all of the very poor are covered. It is a state-run program that receives federal funds. States make many of the rules, and the trend in recent years has been to make Medicaid requirements more stringent. Congress recently liberalized them for persons who need nursing home care. Beginning January 1, 1989,

- In any month in which a married person is in a nursing home, no income of the at-home spouse is to be considered available to the spouse in the nursing home.

- Income is considered the property of the person to whom it is paid. Income paid to both spouses is attributed 50 percent to each.

- The home, household goods, and personal effects of both spouses are not counted in considering Medicaid eligibility.

- All assets other than these will be counted and divided in two. If the at-home spouse has less than $12,000, the spouse in the nursing home may transfer assets to him or her to make up to $12,000 available to the at-home spouse. (States may, at their option, raise this figure to any amount less than $60,000. The $12,000 amount will be indexed to inflation.)

- The assets that remain in the name of the spouse in the nursing home are considered available to pay for his or her nursing home care. All assets in excess of $60,000 are attributed to the spouse in the nursing home and are considered available to pay for nursing home care.

- States must allow nursing home residents to retain certain sums for medical expenses not covered by Medicare or Medicaid before contributing to the expense of their nursing home care. The states may place "reasonable limits" on the amounts spent.

Beginning September 30, 1989,

- The states must allow the at-home spouse sufficient income of the other spouse to bring total household income of the at-home spouse to at least 122 percent of the federal poverty level for a two-person household. In 1989, this will be $789 per month. On July 1, 1991, it will be raised to 133 percent of the poverty level, and to 150 percent on July 1, 1992. States will not be required to allow more than $1,500 per month, except by court order or change in regulations.

The current regulations require that the assets and income of *your* spouse and your parents be considered in determining your eligibility for Medicaid, with few exceptions. This is a very important point: your spouse and parents do not *actually* have to give anything toward the cost of your care, but your *eligibility* is determined as though they do. The exact requirements, as well as the amount of assets and income you may retain and still be eligible, vary from state to state, because of the latitude allowed by the federal government in setting some of the income and asset limits. Check the list of Medicaid state offices in appendix N to find out where to call to determine the exact eligibility requirements for your state.

You are automatically eligible for Medicaid if you are eligible for, or receiving, **Supplemental Security Income (SSI)** payments for aged, blind, and disabled, but you must apply at a state welfare office. If you meet the requirements for SSI, there is little chance that you would have to give up additional income or assets to qualify for Medicaid.

If your income, less certain deductions and medical bills, is within certain (low) limits, you may be eligible for Medicaid as medically needy. You must "spend down" to pay medical bills to the point at which you are eligible; after that, Medicaid pays for all of them as long as you are eligible.

Medicaid services in some states are more restrictive than Medicare services. If the service you are receiving is covered under Medicare and not Medicaid, Medicaid will not pay the Medicare copayments and deductibles applicable to that service. Otherwise, it will, although there may be additional limits. To find out if you are eligible for Medicaid, apply at any state welfare office. The welfare office is required to take your application and make a formal determination of eligibility even if you are told informally that you are not eligible.

When you apply, you should bring proof of age, financial status, and any disability you may have. The proof of financial status should include bank statements for checking and savings accounts, rent or mortgage payment receipts, loan papers for your car or the title to it, any documents relating to stock or bond ownership, and check stubs for any regular payments you receive. You should also have the amount of your Social Security check, if yon receive Social Security payments. You should always have your Social Security number. Bring your medical bills, or copies of them, for the last year.

When you call the welfare office for your appointment, ask what is needed. This will save you a delay in getting your eligibility determined and perhaps avoid another trip.

You can transfer your assets to someone other than your spouse or parents (for example, to a child) in order to become eligible for Medicaid, but you must have done so *more than two years* before you become eligible for Medicaid. The exception to this is the division-of-assets provision of the new Medicare catastrophic coverage law. Under it, the spouse who is entering the nursing home can transfer assets up to $12,000 (or higher, if a state elects, with a limit of $60,000) to the spouse who is staying at home. Outside this provision, if you want to transfer your assets in order to become eligible for nursing home coverage under Medicaid, *you should do so only with the services of a lawyer who understands the Medicaid program*. This is both to protect you and to ensure that you actually will be found eligible for Medicaid based on the action you took. There is no point in transferring assets only to find that you are still not eligible.

This translates into what we've said before: *You should explore all other alternatives before deciding to enter a nursing home.*

Private Insurance for Nursing Home Care

In early 1987 there were only two companies offering nursing home insurance. Today there are now more than seventy. Now for the bad news: *many of them exclude so much that you may be paying more than $100 per month for unusable coverage.*

The May 1988 issue of *Consumer Reports*, a highly respected magazine that rates various products and accepts no advertising, cut through a great deal of confusion by offering a set of features that should be found in a good policy. These are as follows:

- The policy should provide a daily nursing-home benefit of at least *$80.*
- The waiting period before benefits begin should be no more than *twenty days.*
- The maximum benefit period should be at least *four years* for one stay. If no time period is given, the dollar ceiling per benefit period should be at least 1,460 (365 days times 4) times the daily benefit.

- The maximum benefit period for all stays should be *unlimited*.
- It should pay full benefits for **skilled nursing facilities (SNF), intermediate care facilities (ICFs),** and custodial care.
- If there is a rule requiring that you be in a hospital before entering the nursing home, *coverage should begin within thirty days after a hospital stay of three days or more.*
- It should pay *home care benefits*.
- These should be paid *without* requiring a prior nursing home or hospital stay.
- It should have *waiver of premium,* which means that you need not pay premiums while you are in a hospital or nursing home. (You may have to pay extra for waiver of premium, but it should be available at least as an option.)
- It should be *guaranteed renewable for life.*
- The policy should specifically state that *Alzheimer's disease is covered.*
- The premium should stay *level for life.*
- The *Best's rating* of the company should be *A* or *A+*. (Best's is a service that, among other things, assesses the financial health of insurance companies.)

Consumer Reports did not recommend a premium, which varies with the age of the policyholder. The magazine recommends that if the insurance salesperson does not provide adequate answers, ask for a specimen policy. If he or she will not provide one, write the company, ask for one, and give the salesperson's name and address. If they will not send one, look for another company.

Some other points to watch out for:

- The policy may say that the premium is level for life but actually permit increases if the company applies for one covering all the insured, or all the insured in one state. Ask about this.

- Find out if the company can decide whether or not you qualify for payments (usually on the basis of medical necessity). If so, what are your appeal rights?

- Find out how many nursing homes in your state the policy will pay for. Some policies pay only for selected homes.

- Find out whether or not a need for nursing home care caused by a pre-existing condition is covered. It almost surely will not be covered in full. The question is, how bad are the restrictions? A waiting period during which Medicare will pay for the nursing home (remember, **skilled nursing facility** only), after which the policy picks it up, is not bad. A two-year exclusion is too much; nursing home stays last an average of 465 days, or 1.3 years.

Finally, resign yourself to the fact that no policy currently offered has adequate inflation coverage. No policy *Consumer Reports* reviewed had an unlimited daily benefit. The Brookings Institution has estimated that private insurance will cover only 7–12 percent of nursing home expenses in the year 2018, and that, at best, no more than half of the elderly will buy nursing home coverage.

Consumer Reports advises that no one under 60 buy a nursing home policy unless it offers some definite way to cover cost increases due to inflation. For those over 60, policies should be bought only by those who have more than modest assets. The rest of us should rely on Medicaid for nursing home coverage.

Selecting a Nursing Home

You can begin the process of selecting a nursing home by eliminating those you know you don't want to use. Don't consider nursing homes that are as follows:

- Too far away to allow visiting by relatives and friends
- Too expensive
- Not properly certified or licensed
- Not offering the medical or other services needed
- Unsuitable for some other reason, such as being owned by a religious denomination with which you do not want to associate

You can find out whether or not a home is properly certified or licensed by contacting the state agencies regulating nursing homes that are listed in appendix K at the back of this book.

Pages 209–214 contain a checklist for use in reviewing up to four nursing homes at one time. We suggest that you copy it (on a photocopying machine) for use on a clipboard as you review homes in your area.

When you examine the checklist closely, you will note that some of the questions are starred. These questions can be answered only by your own observations.

Remember that you don't necessarily have to answer every single question on this checklist. You should try very hard to answer the ones that are important to you. If you forget to ask something important during your visit, you can always call later and try to get the answer.

However, if you find that you didn't observe something important, the only way to get the answer is to schedule another visit. The best thing to do is to look over the checklist carefully before you end each interview you have during your visit, to make sure you have asked and answered all the relevant starred questions. Then look over the rest of the questions before you end your tour, to make sure that you have seen everything you need to see to answer them. *We suggest that you don't rely on memory. Circle the answer to each question as you observe/ask it.*

NURSING HOME CHECKLIST

THE BUILDING AND GROUNDS	NURSING HOMES			
	A:	B:	C:	D:
Outside				
1. Is the building neat and well maintained?	Y N	Y N	Y N	Y N
2. Does it appear fireproof? (Wood-framed buildings can be dangerous.)	Y N	Y N	Y N	Y N
3. Are the sidewalks clean and well maintained?	Y N	Y N	Y N	Y N
4. Do the sidewalks have wheelchair ramps?	Y N	Y N	Y N	Y N
5. Does the entrance have handrails and wheelchair ramps?	Y N	Y N	Y N	Y N
6. Is the home located within easy walking distance of public transportation?	Y N	Y N	Y N	Y N
7. Are the grounds spacious?	Y N	Y N	Y N	Y N
8. Are they well maintained?	Y N	Y N	Y N	Y N
9. Is there an area where patients can sit?	Y N	Y N	Y N	Y N
10. Do they sit outside (weather permitting) or otherwise use the outside area?	Y N	Y N	Y N	Y N
Inside				
11. Is the lobby clean and well furnished?	Y N	Y N	Y N	Y N
12. Do residents use the lobby?	Y N	Y N	Y N	Y N
13. Are the corridors well lighted and wide enough for two wheelchairs to pass easily?	Y N	Y N	Y N	Y N
14. Does there seem to be enough room in general for the residents?	Y N	Y N	Y N	Y N
15. Are emergency exits well marked?	Y N	Y N	Y N	Y N
16. Is there an emergency lighting system?	Y N	Y N	Y N	Y N
17. Is there an actively functioning safety committee?	Y N	Y N	Y N	Y N
18. Is fire-fighting equipment (such as fire extinguishers) prominent?	Y N	Y N	Y N	Y N
19. Are there sufficient smoke detectors?	Y N	Y N	Y N	Y N

THE BUILDING AND GROUNDS	NURSING HOMES			
	A:	B:	C:	D:

Rooms

	A:	B:	C:	D:
1. Are the rooms neat and clean?	Y N	Y N	Y N	Y N
2. Is there sufficient light?	Y N	Y N	Y N	Y N
3. Are there curtains on the windows?	Y N	Y N	Y N	Y N
4. Do all the rooms open on a hallway?	Y N	Y N	Y N	Y N
5. Do residents hang their own pictures?	Y N	Y N	Y N	Y N
6. Is there sufficient closet space?	Y N	Y N	Y N	Y N
7. Does each resident have a sink and mirror?	Y N	Y N	Y N	Y N
8. Is there counter space for personal objects?	Y N	Y N	Y N	Y N
9. Is the room nicely furnished?	Y N	Y N	Y N	Y N
*10. Is the room air conditioned?	Y N	Y N	Y N	Y N
*11. Do the rooms have individual thermostats?	Y N	Y N	Y N	Y N
*12. Is there an adjoining bathroom?	Y N	Y N	Y N	Y N
*13. Are the bathrooms shared by no more than four residents?	Y N	Y N	Y N	Y N
*14. Do residents have a choice between single and jointly shared rooms?	Y N	Y N	Y N	Y N
15. In general, do residents have enough personal space?	Y N	Y N	Y N	Y N
*16. Are procedures for changing roommates liberal and clearly spelled out?	Y N	Y N	Y N	Y N
*17. If the rooms have television sets, are they equipped with earphones?	Y N	Y N	Y N	Y N
18. Do the beds have bedspreads?	Y N	Y N	Y N	Y N
19. Are there grab bars on the toilet and bathtub?	Y N	Y N	Y N	Y N
20. Do the tubs have nonslip surfaces?	Y N	Y N	Y N	Y N
21. Do bathrooms and toilet areas have sufficient privacy?	Y N	Y N	Y N	Y N
22. Do the rooms have private telephones?	Y N	Y N	Y N	Y N

Personnel

	A:	B:	C:	D:
* 1. Does the home's administrator have a current license?	Y N	Y N	Y N	Y N
2. Was the administrator or his or her representative courteous to you?	Y N	Y N	Y N	Y N
3. Did he or she see you promptly?	Y N	Y N	Y N	Y N
4. Were the home's administrative policies well explained?	Y N	Y N	Y N	Y N
5. Was the administrator open to your questions?	Y N	Y N	Y N	Y N
* 6. Does the home employ:				
a. a physical therapist?	Y N	Y N	Y N	Y N
b. an occupational therapist?	Y N	Y N	Y N	Y N
c. a speech pathologist?	Y N	Y N	Y N	Y N

THE BUILDING AND GROUNDS	NURSING HOMES			
	A:	B:	C:	D:
d. a dietitian?	Y N	Y N	Y N	Y N
e. a nurse practitioner?	Y N	Y N	Y N	Y N
* 7. Is the nursing supervisor an R.N.?	Y N	Y N	Y N	Y N
* 8. Are all the head nurses R.N.'s?	Y N	Y N	Y N	Y N
9. Do there seem to be enough nurses, nurse's aides, and orderlies on duty?	Y N	Y N	Y N	Y N
10. Was the staff generally friendly toward you?	Y N	Y N	Y N	Y N
11. Were they neatly dressed?	Y N	Y N	Y N	Y N
12. Did the residents seem at ease with the staff?	Y N	Y N	Y N	Y N
13. Did the staff speak to the residents in respectful, noncondescending terms?	Y N	Y N	Y N	Y N
14. Did the staff seem to like the residents?	Y N	Y N	Y N	Y N
15. Did the staff generally have pleasant expressions on their faces?	Y N	Y N	Y N	Y N

Medical/Nursing Care

	A:	B:	C:	D:
* 1. Is a physician on the premises for a fixed period of time each day?	Y N	Y N	Y N	Y N
* 2. Is a physician on call in case of emergency?	Y N	Y N	Y N	Y N
* 3. Is a registered nurse on duty during the day, seven days a week?	Y N	Y N	Y N	Y N
* 4. Is at least one R.N. or one L.P.N. on duty day and night?	Y N	Y N	Y N	Y N
* 5. Are dental services provided in the home itself?	Y N	Y N	Y N	Y N
* 6. Are there facilities outside of the residents' rooms for physical examinations?	Y N	Y N	Y N	Y N
* 7. May the resident select his or her own physician?	Y N	Y N	Y N	Y N
* 8. May the resident select his or her own hospital?	Y N	Y N	Y N	Y N
* 9. Does the home have a contract with an ambulance service?	Y N	Y N	Y N	Y N
*10. Does the home have access to a pharmacist who maintains records on each resident and reviews them when new medications are ordered?	Y N	Y N	Y N	Y N
*11. Is the family allowed to make alternative arrangements for purchasing prescription drugs?	Y N	Y N	Y N	Y N
*12. Are arrangements made for patients who wish to use alternative professional services such as podiatrists or chiropractors?	Y N	Y N	Y N	Y N
*13. Does the home make arrangements for private duty nurses when the family thinks one is required?	Y N	Y N	Y N	Y N
*14. Does the home have policies that severely restrict the use of physical restraints?	Y N	Y N	Y N	Y N
*15. Are the majority of the residents free of physical restraints?	Y N	Y N	Y N	Y N

THE BUILDING AND GROUNDS	NURSING HOMES			
	A:	B:	C:	D:
16. Are the rooms and halls free of any smell of human excrement?	Y N	Y N	Y N	Y N
17. Do they smell of heavy perfume?	Y N	Y N	Y N	Y N
18. Does each resident have a call button within easy reach?	Y N	Y N	Y N	Y N
19. Can it be turned off only at the patient's bed?	Y N	Y N	Y N	Y N
20. Are there call buttons in the bathrooms and bathing areas?	Y N	Y N	Y N	Y N
21. Does each resident have a water container and clean glass in his/or her room?	Y N	Y N	Y N	Y N
22. Are the more inactive residents' fingernails trimmed, and are the men cleanly shaved?	Y N	Y N	Y N	Y N
*23. Does the home keep its own medical records?	Y N	Y N	Y N	Y N
*24. Does the resident (or resident's family) have access to them?	Y N	Y N	Y N	Y N

Recreational/Social Arrangements

	A:	B:	C:	D:
* 1. Does the home employ a full-time social director?	Y N	Y N	Y N	Y N
* 2. Are residents permitted to entertain visitors in their rooms?	Y N	Y N	Y N	Y N
* 3. Are visiting hours liberal?	Y N	Y N	Y N	Y N
* 4. Are residents given reasonable leeway in establishing when they go to bed?	Y N	Y N	Y N	Y N
* 5. Are members of the opposite sex permitted to visit one another in their rooms with the doors closed?	Y N	Y N	Y N	Y N
* 6. Is alcohol permitted in the home?	Y N	Y N	Y N	Y N
* 7. Are there no limitations on outgoing or incoming telephone calls?	Y N	Y N	Y N	Y N
* 8. Do the published rules and regulations seem reasonable to you?	Y N	Y N	Y N	Y N
* 9. Are children permitted to visit?	Y N	Y N	Y N	Y N
10. Is there a quiet, private place where residents can entertain visitors?	Y N	Y N	Y N	Y N
11. Does there seem to be a wide range of recreational activities?	Y N	Y N	Y N	Y N
*12. Are residents included in this planning in some formal way?	Y N	Y N	Y N	Y N
*13. If there an actively functioning patient council?	Y N	Y N	Y N	Y N
14. Is there sufficient room for the residents to engage in recreational/social events?	Y N	Y N	Y N	Y N
15. Are calendars of such events posted in convenient places?	Y N	Y N	Y N	Y N
16. Did you observe a substantial number of patients engaging in recreational/social events?	Y N	Y N	Y N	Y N

THE BUILDING AND GROUNDS	NURSING HOMES			
	A:	B:	C:	D:
17. Is there a newsletter for families of residents?	Y N	Y N	Y N	Y N
*18. Are religious services held on the premises?	Y N	Y N	Y N	Y N
*19. Are arrangements made to allow patients to attend outside religious services if they wish?	Y N	Y N	Y N	Y N
20. Is there a library with recent magazine issues and a good selection of books?	Y N	Y N	Y N	Y N
21. Does the home sponsor frequent outings for those residents who are able to go?	Y N	Y N	Y N	Y N
22. Is there a canteen?	Y N	Y N	Y N	Y N
23. Do patients appear to socialize with one another?	Y N	Y N	Y N	Y N
*24. Does the home have any special programs with area schools to bring young people in to interact with the resident?	Y N	Y N	Y N	Y N
*25. Does the home subscribe to (and provide you with a copy of) a liberal Patient Bill of Rights?	Y N	Y N	Y N	Y N
*26. Is there a formal health education program for residents?	Y N	Y N	Y N	Y N
*27. Does the home provide frequent continuing education courses for its staff?	Y N	Y N	Y N	Y N

Food

	A:	B:	C:	D:
1. Are fresh fruits and vegetables served in season?	Y N	Y N	Y N	Y N
2. Does the home prepare meals from scratch rather than use frozen or prepackaged meals?	Y N	Y N	Y N	Y N
3. Do the residents have a choice in the selection of meals?	Y N	Y N	Y N	Y N
* 4. Are provisions for special diets made?	Y N	Y N	Y N	Y N
* 5. Is help available for residents requiring feeding assistance?	Y N	Y N	Y N	Y N
* 6. Is this help available both in the resident's room and in the dining area?	Y N	Y N	Y N	Y N
* 7. Are residents served in their rooms if they prefer?	Y N	Y N	Y N	Y N
* 8. Is there a reasonable amount of flexibility as to when residents can eat?	Y N	Y N	Y N	Y N
* 9. Are dining hours for the convenience of the residents rather than the staff?	Y N	Y N	Y N	Y N
10. Are residents given sufficient time to eat their meals?	Y N	Y N	Y N	Y N
11. Does the food appear appetizing to you?	Y N	Y N	Y N	Y N
*12. Can the kitchen accommodate special, nonmedically prescribed diets (e.g., for religious reasons)?	Y N	Y N	Y N	Y N
13. Is the kitchen basically clean by your standards?	Y N	Y N	Y N	Y N
14. Does the kitchen staff appear neat and clean?	Y N	Y N	Y N	Y N
15. Is the menu cycle adequately varied?	Y N	Y N	Y N	Y N

THE BUILDING AND GROUNDS	NURSING HOMES			
	A:	B:	C:	D:
16. Does the meal being served match the one on the menu?	Y N	Y N	Y N	Y N
17. Are the food carts closed for sanitation purposes?	Y N	Y N	Y N	Y N
18. Does the kitchen have a dishwashing machine?	Y N	Y N	Y N	Y N
*19. Are snacks available between meals and at bedtime?	Y N	Y N	Y N	Y N
*20. Do residents have access to a refrigerator to store their snacks?	Y N	Y N	Y N	Y N
21. Is the dining area clean and attractive?	Y N	Y N	Y N	Y N
22. Are the tables convenient for wheelchair use?	Y N	Y N	Y N	Y N

After the Visit

After you have completed the checklist, it may appear as though you have found out everything there is to know about the homes you have just visited. There is more to choosing a nursing home, however, than just answering questions. Your overall impression of each home is equally as important as its different services. One of the chief purposes of answering all these questions is to get this overall impression. (It is possible to have answered "yes" to all the questions in a particular category and still have a negative overall impression.) Therefore, we suggest that you do the following as soon after your visit as possible:

- Find a quiet place where you can work.
- Review the questions and answers under each of the six categories in the checklist.
- Attempt to rate each of the six categories on a scale of 1 to 5:
  1 Completely unsatisfactory
  2 Poor
  3 Adequate (barely)
  4 Good (improvement possible)
  5 Excellent
- Using these individual ratings, try to come up with an overall rating for each nursing home. Try to answer the following question:

Overall, how do you rate this facility as a potential nursing home for the person?
1 Completely unsatisfactory
2 Poor
3 Adequate
4 Good
5 Excellent

There is no magical way to come up with this important rating. In the final analysis, you (possibly with input from the potential resident if he or she is able to provide it) must decide how to weigh the different categories. A single "1", for example, on some categories might be enough to remove a home from serious consideration for most people. For others, the quality of the medical/nursing care provided, or even the recreational/social services provided, may completely overshadow all others.

- Finally, place all the ratings (individual and overall) in the Overall Ratings Chart on page 216. (You may prefer to write in the words instead of the number — for example, "poor" instead of "2".)

Overall Rating: This chart should now enable you to choose the best home from among the ones you visit. If it doesn't, go back to the original Nursing Home Checklist in this chapter and compare the homes question by question. If this still doesn't resolve the issue, try this next strategy.

A Final Strategy

If you still find it difficult to decide among the homes you visited, examine the reason for the problem. Is it because none is really suitable, and you have to choose among the least of several evils? If so, consider visiting some more homes, possibly making a more systematic effort to get recommendations from acquaintances and health professionals.

In the first strategy, you rated each home "Unsatisfactory" to "Excellent," or you may have used a one (1) to five (5) scale. If this did not produce one home that seemed to stand out from all the others, perhaps you should consider converting your responses into percentages. A score of 90 percent in a particular category, or 90 percent overall, may tell you more about a particular home than a rating of "Adequate."

If you decide to convert your responses into percentages, use the chart entitled Overall Ratings by Percentage of Responses on page 216 along with the following steps:

- Go back to the Nursing Home Checklist and for each category (taking each home separately) count the number of "yes" answers you have recorded (e.g., under Nursing Home A, in the category "Rooms" you have 12 "yes" answers). Place this number above the fraction bar in the appropriate cell in the Overall Ratings by Percentage of Responses Chart.

■ Now count the total number of questions you answered (both "yes" and "no") in a particular category (e.g., under Nursing Home A, in the category "Rooms," you answered 15 questions). Put this number below the fraction bar in the appropriate cell. Your numbers should look like this:

$$\frac{12}{15}$$

OVERALL RATINGS CHART

	NURSING HOMES			
	A:	B:	C:	D:
Name				
Address				
Telephone				
CHECKLIST CATEGORIES Building and grounds				
Rooms				
Personnel				
Medical/nursing care				
Recreational/social arrangements				
Food				
Overall Rating				

OVERALL RATINGS BY PERCENTAGE OF RESPONSES CHART

CHECKLIST CATEGORIES	NURSING HOMES			
	A:	B:	C:	D:
Building and grounds	___ ___%	___ ___%	___ ___%	___ ___%
Rooms	___ ___%	___ ___%	___ ___%	___ ___%
Personnel	___ ___%	___ ___%	___ ___%	___ ___%
Medical/nursing care	___ ___%	___ ___%	___ ___%	___ ___%
Recreational/social arrangements	___ ___%	___ ___%	___ ___%	___ ___%
Food	___ ___%	___ ___%	___ ___%	___ ___%
Overall Rating	___ ___%	___ ___%	___ ___%	___ ___%
	6	6	6	6

- At this point you have a fraction. You should now divide the bottom number into the top number. In our example, when you divide 15 into 12, you get a decimal of 0.8, which is then converted into a percentage by moving the decimal point two places to the right (0.8 = 80., or 80 percent). Or you could multiply the decimal by 100 (0.8 × 100 = 80 percent).

- You have now calculated the percentage response to your answers in one particular category. Now do this for the remaining categories.

- After determining the percentages in the remaining categories (remember, there are six), you can determine the overall percentage rating of a particular home. To do this, simply add the percentages determined in all six categories and divide by six (e.g., percentages 75 + 80 + 70 + 90 + 85 + 80 = 480 ÷ 6 = 80 percent).

Dealing with Problems that Arise in Nursing Home Care

It is difficult for nursing home residents to be effective advocates for themselves. If they are on Medicaid, they may have surrendered all their assets to obtain funding for their nursing home stay and may, in effect, be trapped in the home. They do not complain simply because they do not want to make a bad situation worse. The same applies, to a lesser degree, to just about everyone else. Even if they are economically able to move, there may be long waiting lists at the homes they want to move to.

On the other hand, some people have completely unrealistic expectations of nursing homes. No patient in a nursing home should expect the attention that a private duty nurse in a hospital can give. No nursing home can afford to provide that much service routinely. Even if the service is excellent, it may not be possible to accommodate all residents' wishes for particular services (such as bathing) when they want it.

But there's a minimum below which no nursing home should fall:

- No resident should be allowed to remain in a soiled bed a moment longer than absolutely necessary.
- It is close to impossible to prevent all pressure sores, but they should be small in size and promptly treated by positioning the patient, special mattresses, and attention by a doctor when needed.
- Food should be hot or cold as appropriate and of better-than-just-acceptable quality.

- Dehydration and malnutrition should *not* develop and should be promptly and vigorously treated if found.
- Medications should be given, and given reasonably close to the prescribed schedule. Drug reactions should be noted in writing and reported to the doctor quickly.

The best way to make sure that a friend or relative is getting the kind of services he or she should is by visiting frequently and randomly. It is good to arrange visits so that promised events can be checked on. If a particular program is scheduled, such as a movie, exercise, a walk, a presentation by a visiting speaker, visit when it is scheduled and make sure that it happens from time to time. Some cancellations are unavoidable due to weather and such, but the general program the home promises should be carried out.

Appendix L contains the Bill of Rights for Nursing Home Patients suggested by the **Health Care Financing Administration,** which runs Medicare and Medicaid. Real, serious violations of these rights should be reported to the state authorities listed in appendix K. You should also contact the state nursing home ombudsman's office; a list is provided in appendix O.

Generally, it is best to deal with problems by pointing them out, politely but firmly, to the appropriate person — the nurse, the administrator, the billing office. The approach of being firm but not antagonistic works best. Keep repeating, in a polite manner, the problem you see and the solution you want.

Example: *You discover that your mother has not had her heart medication for three days. You contact the nurse and tell her this. Ask why the problem occurred. Listen carefully. (If the answer is "She had a drug reaction, so we called Dr. Fanyatz, who said to stop the drug," the right thing, not the wrong thing, has probably been done.) Depending on the response, you may need to suggest that the doctor be called, or that the medicine be obtained from a local pharmacy while the nursing home's pharmacy is awaiting its order, and so on.*

An important point to remember is this: *Don't let the nursing home put the monkey on your back.* You do not have to solve, or even sympathize with, their difficulties. In some situations, the proper answer to "What would you suggest?" is "I don't have to suggest anything. *You* have to find a way to deliver the services you promised, even if the pharmacy order is late."

Finally, it is not useful to threaten to move the patient. Besides the antagonism this may create, it may carry no weight in some areas. Many nursing homes have waiting lists and are well aware of the difficulties that often occur with nursing home placement. If a move is clearly indicated, make the arrangements and carry them out.

Home Health Services

You may be able to stay out of a nursing home with the assistance of **home health care.** Home health care consists of the following services:

- Part-time or intermittent nursing care, provided by or under the supervision of a registered professional nurse (R.N.)
- Physical, occupational, or speech therapy
- Medical social services provided under the direction of a doctor
- Part-time or intermittent services of a home health aide
- Medical supplies (excluding drugs and biologicals) and **durable medical equipment**)
- If the **Home Health Agency (HHA)** is affiliated with or under the control of a hospital, services of interns or residents of the hospital.

Not covered under home health care are transportation, housekeeping services, and those services that are normally not covered if provided in a hospital.

To qualify for home health services, you must be one of the following:

- Confined to your home or to an institution that is not a skilled nursing facility or rehabilitation facility
- Under the care of a doctor who is a medical doctor, an osteopath, or a podiatrist
- In need of intermittent skilled nursing care, physical therapy, or speech therapy
- In need of occupational therapy *after* a period during which skilled nursing care, physical therapy, or speech therapy was needed. (In other words, needing *only* occupational therapy does not qualify you for home care, but needing occupational therapy *plus* another service, or after another service, does.)

You are entitled to an unlimited number of home visits, as long as you need the service. The HHA providing the services must be one that is Medicare-participating.

You can have home health care visits for up to thirty-eight consecutive days. After this, a gap of at least one day must follow before home health care visits can be prescribed again.

It is important to understand that home care under Medicare is composed of some (not all) *medical* services that will allow you to remain at home, rather than in a nursing home, *and these only*. It is not a "total care package" such as the social **health maintenance organization** experiments tried to provide.

Paying for Services Medicare Doesn't Cover

What can you do if you need services beyond what Medicare can offer? Many HHAs offer these. They may include services such as delivery of hot meals, homemaker assistance, and companions. Your supplemental insurance may cover some of these services, for a limited time. You will also find that the HHA is almost always willing to bill Medicare for the Medicare-covered services and bill you for the remainder. You may find that the charge for noncovered services, such as homemaker assistance, is affordable.

Many HHAs will help you assess your home to see if modifications will make it more suitable for home care. If what is needed falls under the category of **durable medical equipment** and a doctor prescribes it, Medicare usually will pay for all of the cost if it is provided under Part A and 80 percent of the cost under Part B. Regardless of the part of Medicare under which it is paid, Medicare pays 100 percent of the costs for used equipment. Many vendors of durable medical equipment know what Medicare covers and what it doesn't, and can tell you. You can also check with your Social Security district office.

Some Cautionary Notes About Home Care

First, when ordering medical equipment and having your home checked for suitability for home care, make sure there is a way for you to terminate the rental or return the item if it turns out that it is not Medicare-covered and you decide you cannot afford it. You may be stuck with large expenses otherwise.

Second — and we regret having to mention this — you should make sure your money and valuables are in a safe place that you control before the home health worker visits. You should treat a visit from the home health worker like any other instance in which a stranger enters your home. There have been many instances of theft. Even very reputable agencies cannot always control the behavior of the people they hire. You should ask the HHA about its policies in case of theft. Are they insured for theft by employees? What do they require in the way of proof? Is it enough to prove that no one other than the HHA worker was in your home?

Because of prejudices against older people, you may be told that a stolen item was not stolen and you simply forgot where you put it. (Of course, you should make sure that the item *was* stolen before you report it.) If something is stolen, report it to the police, to the HHA, and to your insurance agent, if you have homeowner's or renter's insurance.

Third, as with all services, *complain (politely) if you are unsatisfied.* HHAs cannot make up for all the burdens of being old and ill, but they should, at a minimum, provide the medical services that were prescribed and any services that you are paying for, and provide them well. The authorities regulating HHAs in the various states are listed in appendix M. Complain to them if your discussion with the HHA does not produce good results.

Hospice Care

Hospice care is care provided to those who are **terminally ill,** either in their homes or in a hospice facility. It is designed to help those who are dying do so with the greatest possible dignity and comfort, while avoiding treatment that will only prolong suffering. Hospice care is available on an unlimited basis, provided that a physician or the hospice director certifies that the person is still terminally ill.

Medicare covers hospice care. Your Medicare supplemental insurance may cover any charges that Medicare does not pay. Check with your Medicare supplemental insurer about coverage. We also suggest that you look at chapter 5, which contains information on care for the dying and representation.

Respite Care

The new Medicare catastrophic coverage law provides for up to eighty hours per year of care in the home for chronically ill individuals who have met either the drug deductible or the out-of-pocket cap for the year. This is really a benefit for the caregiver as much as for the person who is chronically ill. One must be dependent on a voluntary caregiver for assistance with at least two of the "activities of daily living," such as bathing, eating, dressing, or using the toilet.

In this chapter, we'll review: What to do when the system doesn't work ▪ How to appeal decisions involving your doctor ▪ How to protect your assets ▪ What to look for when purchasing insurance ▪ How to clarify problems when Medicare rejects a claim ▪ When to request a refund from a doctor for a service that wasn't medically necessary ▪ When and how to use the appeal process ▪ How to protect your rights

8. If It Can Go Wrong, It Will

The purpose of this chapter is to provide troubleshooting advice for dealing with the various things that can go wrong with the Medicare program. Medicare is so complicated that there are literally hundreds of reasons why a particular bill might not be paid.

The number of people and agencies who have a hand somewhere in the process is enormous. They include Congress, the Health Care Financing Administration, the various federal district courts, the Medicare carriers and intermediaries, your various doctors, the hospital utilization review committee, the peer review organizations, your employer's or former employer's health care insurer, the employer's review agent, home health agencies, nursing homes, and suppliers of medical equipment. Every one of them can do something, somewhere along the way, that can result in a medical expense you thought would be covered not being covered. It's a safe bet that in the vast majority of cases, you won't be told about it until you're informed that the bill isn't paid. And not having bills paid is just part of what can go wrong.

This chapter covers the most common problems under the following headings:

- Eligibility and Enrollment
- Hospitals
- Nursing Homes and Home Care
- Insurance

- Getting Bills Paid/Filing Claims
- Appeals
- Coordination with employers' health insurance and retirement plans

Most of the chapter is in question-and-answer format, but we depart from this when the information can best be presented in some other way. Most of the questions are ones that **People's Medical Society (PMS)** members have asked us over the years.

Three Important Points, Again

We'd like to emphasize three points that we raised earlier in this book but that are important enough to bear repeating:

- You are not responsible for any medical bill you could not reasonably have been expected to know was not covered. But *you* have to make the case that you did not know that the service or expense was not covered.

- Increasingly, rejections of claims and termination or denial of services under Medicare are being based on *medical necessity*. If payment is denied, you usually have nothing to worry about — see the section on claims below. For denials of admission to hospitals, in-patient surgery, and notices of noncoverage of further hospital or nursing home stays, you should work closely with your doctor — after all, it's *your doctor's* medical judgment that is being questioned.

- It is vitally important to *keep records* of your dealings with Medicare. We believe that the Claims Log, in appendix B, is the best way of doing this for routine bills. But for requests for reconsideration of denials, appeals, and the like, it is important to *keep copies* of correspondence. When the correspondence has to be sent by a certain date, we recommend that you send it *certified mail, return receipt requested,* so that you will have proof of mailing and proof of receipt. This is inexpensive, and the window clerks at any post office can show you how to do it.

You should also remember to *ask questions* of your local Social Security office if you have them. If the people there don't know the answer, they can refer you to someone who does. Keep asking until you get an answer, and until you're satisfied it's the right answer. Your local Social Security office *is* your Medicare office for many issues. You can always call them and receive help or be directed to the right place.

Eligibility and Enrollment

1. I've applied for Medicare and have been told that I'm ineligible. What should I do?

Find out exactly why you are ineligible. (If you filed an application, you should receive a letter telling you the reason.) If you do not meet one of the *categorical* requirements of the program — for example, you are not yet 65, or are under 65 and not disabled, or are not a U.S. citizen or an alien admitted for permanent residence — you should try to alter your status. (There's no way to be 65 faster, but you can consult a lawyer who specializes in disability cases, apply for citizenship or alien resident status, and — if you were found ineligible because you had not worked enough — check your earnings record.

If you feel that a clear error has been made and that it is not being corrected, you can appeal the finding of ineligibility.

You should also check to see if you are entitled on the basis of someone else's earnings. See chapter 2, which offers several examples. You may be eligible as the wife, widow, divorced wife, husband, widower, divorced husband, child, or parent of someone else.

2. I don't know when I should apply for Medicare.

To be safe, you should apply for both Part A (hospital insurance) and Part B (doctor insurance) three months before you turn 65. This will allow you time to gather the proofs of earnings, date of birth, and so on that you need, and for cleaning up of any errors in your earnings record. It will also avoid increases in your Part B premium due to late enrollment. Medicare and Social Security have been changing their procedures on automatic enrollment, and they may change them again. *If you want Medicare, apply for it.* Call your Social Security office for forms and procedures.

It is *very important* to remember that if you do not have forty quarters of coverage (are not "fully insured"), you may be covered on the basis of the work you have done in six of the last thirteen calendar quarters. This is a moving target, and eligibility on this basis ("currently insured status") can be lost if you quit work, you do not apply immediately, and sufficient time elapses so that you have not, in fact, worked in six of the last thirteen quarters.

3. I suspect my earnings record at Social Security is wrong, but I don't know how to check it.

Send a letter like the one illustrated in chapter 2 to the Social Security Administration, P.O. Box 57, Baltimore, MD 21203, and request a copy, or call your local Social Security office and request Form 7004PC, fill it out, and mail it in.

4. I applied on the basis of disability, and have been turned down. I want to appeal. What can I do?

Realistically, you have to hire a lawyer. Disability law is complicated, is affected variously by different precedents in different judicial districts, and changes constantly due to court decisions. Beware of lawyers who promise to get you disability benefits. No one can promise that; it depends on the facts of your case. Also, be aware that the federal regulations governing disability limit the fees the attorney may charge you for representation before the **Social Security Administration (SSA).** The fee is limited to the smallest of the following:

- Twenty-five percent of past-due benefits
- The fee you and the attorney agreed on
- The fee set by the Social Security Administration

If the case goes to a federal court, the court may award a fee higher than any of the above, but the amount the SSA will pay out of past-due benefits awarded is limited to the smallest of the three amounts. You are responsible for any fees above that amount that are awarded by the court. The SSA does not pay any fees if you lose, because in that case there are no past-due benefits to pay from. In other words, you always have to pay the attorney, but the fee is paid from past-due benefits if you win.

Before paying for an attorney, contact senior citizens' centers, area agencies on aging, and welfare rights projects that are listed in the phone book. No-cost or reduced-cost legal services may be available from them.

5. I now know that I am definitely not eligible for Medicare. What can I do?

Persons who are age 65 and do not otherwise qualify for Medicare can purchase Medicare coverage just like private insurance. This is expensive, running $189.90 per month for the combined hospital (Part A), doctor bill (part B) and catastrophic coverages, in 1989. If you purchase Medicare, you will still have to purchase supplemental insurance to have a package that really protects you against the financial effects of illness. You may find that it is cheaper to purchase individual coverage from a **health maintenance organization (HMO),** which offers very comprehensive benefits for one, fixed price, if an HMO is available where you live. See chapter 4.

You are permitted to purchase Part B of Medicare (insurance for doctor bills) if you are a resident of the United States, are 65 or over, and are either a citizen or an alien lawfully admitted for permanent residence who has resided in the United States for the last five years. (It is under this rule that *everyone* enrolls in Part B.) If you are not eligible for Part A of Medicare, enrolling for Part B entitles you to purchase it. So you have to buy Part B to get Part A.

6. How do I apply?

The first step is to telephone your local Social Security Office. These offices are commonly listed under the federal government section in the blue pages of your local telephone directory, and under "U. S. Government" in the white pages. If you can't find a listing, call the information operator and ask for any Social Security office. Calling one will enable you to find out which one you should go to.

Call that office. Tell them that you want to apply for Medicare (and Social Security if you are not already receiving it.) The SSA is making a determined effort to carry out as much business as possible over the phone. This is generally more efficient, and it saves you a visit to the Social Security office. At the same time, if you have trouble dealing with matters like this over the phone (if, for example, you have trouble hearing and don't have an amplified phone), you can insist on a face-to-face visit. (For more on this, see chapter 2.)

Whichever way you apply, the Social Security office representative will fill out most of the forms for you. This is done to ensure that the type of answers SSA needs to make a decision get answered on the forms involved. After the representative has filled out the forms, you should read them — and insist on the correction of any errors — before signing them. If you need special assistance — if, for example, you are blind, deaf, or illiterate — special help will be made available to you. You may have to go to another Social Security office to find the right person to help you. The representative at the first Social Security office you go to will give you instructions. If you think you will need special help, you should mention this when you first call.

The representative will ask you to bring certain documents when you come to the Social Security office, usually the following:

- Proof of age
- Records of earnings, such as W-2 forms (or tax returns for the self-employed) for the past two years
- Your Social Security card

If you are applying because you think you are disabled, you will be asked to bring some documents relating to your medical problems. The Social Security office representative will tell you what they are.

Keep your originals. Keep your originals. Keep your originals. More on the application process can be found in chapter 2.

7. I've lost my Social Security card and don't think I can remember the number. What can I do?

You need not worry if you have lost your Social Security card. If you can remember the number, you can apply for a duplicate. If you can't remember the number, it is likely to be on a number of other documents around your house, such as payroll stubs, credit card bills, and insurance policies. If all else fails, the Social Security office has access to a computer system that will retrieve your name or any that sound like it from the Social Security computer system. This considerably narrows the search for your number.

Hospitals

1. I want to visit my sister in Canada this summer and have some surgery done while we are together so she can take care of me. Will Medicare pay for a hospital stay outside the United States?

No. People think that Medicare pays for care anywhere in the world. It doesn't. Only care in hospitals in the fifty states and the District of Columbia, Puerto Rico, and the last two U.S. territories — Guam and the Virgin Islands — is paid for. Care you receive in Europe, Canada, Mexico, and the rest of the world is *not* covered. The only exceptions are situations in which you are close to the Mexican or Canadian borders and need emergency care, and the nearest hospital is a Mexican or Canadian one, or if the Mexican or Canadian hospital is much closer to your home than any American hospital and is accredited by the Joint Commission on Accreditation of Health Care Facilities or a comparable body in the foreign country. In these situations, Medicare will pay for services in a Mexican or Canadian hospital.

Please note that doctor's services outside the United States are covered only if they are given during an inpatient hospitalization that is paid for under the circumstances described above. *No other doctors services outside the United States are paid for by Medicare.*

2. I am worried that I will have to leave the hospital when my DRG runs out, even if I'm not well.

Don't be. It's illegal for the hospital even to suggest it. During the early days of the **diagnosis-related groups (DRG) system,** there were a number of instances of abuse. Patients were told that they had to leave the hospital "because your DRG has run out" or something similar. Discharging any patient who still needs hospital care because of financial considerations is a total violation of the hospital's contract with Medicare. The hospital has agreed to provide services to you as long as they are medically necessary.

Because of abuses observed, the **People's Medical Society (PMS)** and the **American Association for Retired Persons (AARP)** joined forces to ask Medicare to require hospitals to "mirandize" Medicare patients: just as persons being arrested are told of their constitutional rights. Medicare now requires *all* hospitals to provide Medicare beneficiaries with an *Important Message from Medicare* upon admission for *any* patient care. It appears on pages 229–231.

To sum up: the only reasons you can be discharged from a hospital under Medicare are *medical* ones. Even if Medicare is no longer paying, you should not be discharged for lack of ability to pay. The hospital's social service staff should explore your eligibility for **Medicaid** and see what alternative sources of care are available. State law in many states is rapidly evolving to the position that no patient who needs hospital care for *medical* reasons should ever be discharged or transferred for lack of ability to pay.

3. The hospital tells me that I have to leave because "my DRG has run out."

Telling you this is (a) untrue, and (b) a violation of the hospital's contract with Medicare. You are entitled to hospital services as long as they are medically necessary. The hospital can always apply for additional payment.

We suggest that you, or someone helping you, first write down the name and presumptive title of anyone who told you this. Then call the administrator's office. Tell them that you are aware that the hospital will be paid the full DRG for your admission. Tell them that you are aware that they can apply for **outlier** payments. Ask them if they have done so. Then tell them the only reason that you can be discharged is because you no longer need hospital care. Tell them that hospitals don't discharge people, doctors do. Ask which doctor made the deter-

AN IMPORTANT MESSAGE FROM MEDICARE

YOUR RIGHTS WHILE YOU ARE A MEDICARE HOSPITAL PATIENT

• You have the right to receive all the hospital care that is necessary for the proper diagnosis and treatment of your illness or injury. According to Federal law, **your discharge date must be determined solely by your medical needs,** not by "DRGs" or Medicare payments.

• You have the right to be fully informed about decisions affecting your Medicare coverage and payment for your hospital stay and for any post-hospital services.

• You have the right to request a review by a Peer Review Organization of any written Notice of Noncoverage that you receive from the hospital stating that Medicare will no longer pay for your hospital care. Peer Review Organizations (PROs) are groups of doctors who are paid by the Federal Government to review medical necessity, appropriateness and quality of hospital treatment furnished to Medicare patients. The phone number and address of the PRO for your area are:

_____

_____

TALK TO YOUR DOCTOR ABOUT YOUR STAY IN THE HOSPITAL

You and your doctor know more about your condition and your health needs than anyone else. Decisions about your medical treatment should be made between you and your doctor. **If you have any questions about your medical treatment, your need for continued hospital care, your discharge, or your need for possible post-hospital care, don't hesitate to ask your doctor.** The hospital's patient representative or social worker will also help you with your questions and concerns about hospital services.

IF YOU THINK YOU ARE BEING ASKED TO LEAVE THE HOSPITAL TOO SOON

• Ask a hospital representative for a written notice of explanation immediately, if you have not already received one. This notice is called a "Notice of Noncoverage." You must have this Notice of Noncoverage if you wish to exercise your right to request a review by the PRO.

• The Notice of Noncoverage will state either that your doctor or the PRO agrees with the hospital's decision that Medicare will no longer pay for your hospital care.

+ If the hospital and your doctor agree, the PRO does not review your case before a Notice of Noncoverage is issued. But the PRO will respond to your request for a review of your Notice of Noncoverage and seek your opinion. You cannot be made to pay for your hospital care until the PRO makes its decision, if you request the review by noon of the first work day after you receive the Notice of Noncoverage.

+ If the hospital and your doctor disagree, the hospital may request the PRO to review your case. If it does make such a request, the hospital is required to send you a notice to that effect. In this situation the PRO must agree with the hospital or the hospital cannot issue a Notice of Noncoverage. You may request that the PRO reconsider your case after you receive a Notice of Noncoverage but since the PRO has already reviewed your case once, you may have to pay for **at least one day of hospital care** before the PRO completes this reconsideration.

IF YOU **DO NOT** REQUEST A REVIEW, **THE HOSPITAL MAY BILL YOU** FOR ALL THE COSTS OF YOUR STAY BEGINNING WITH THE THIRD DAY AFTER YOU RECEIVE THE NOTICE OF NONCOVERAGE. THE HOSPITAL, HOWEVER, CANNOT CHARGE YOU FOR CARE UNLESS IT PROVIDES YOU WITH A NOTICE OF NONCOVERAGE.

HOW TO REQUEST A REVIEW OF THE NOTICE OF NONCOVERAGE

- If the Notice of Noncoverage states that your **physician agrees** with the hospital's decision:
  + You must make your request for review to the PRO by **noon of the first work day** after you receive the Notice of Noncoverage by contacting the PRO by phone or in writing.
  + The PRO must ask for your views about your case before making its decision. The PRO will inform you by phone and in writing of its decision on the review.
  + If the PRO agrees with the Notice of Noncoverage, you may be billed for all costs of your stay beginning at noon of the day **after** you receive the PRO's decision.
  + Thus, you will **not** be responsible for the cost of hospital care before you receive the PRO's decision.

- If the Notice of Noncoverage states that the PRO agrees with the hospital's decision:
  + You should make your request for reconsideration to the PRO **immediately** upon receipt of the Notice of Noncoverage by contacting the PRO by phone or in writing.
  + The PRO can take up to three working days from receipt of your request to complete the review. The PRO will inform you in writing of its decision on the review.
  + Since the PRO has already reviewed your case once, prior to the issuance of the Notice of Noncoverage, the hospital is permitted to begin billing you for the cost of your stay beginning with the third calendar day after you receive your Notice of Noncoverage even **if the PRO has not completed its review.**
  + Thus, if the PRO continues to agree with the Notice of Noncoverage, **you may have to pay for at least one day of hospital care.**

NOTE: The process described above is called "immediate review." If you miss the deadline for this immediate review while you are in the hospital, you may still request a review of Medicare's decision to no longer pay for your care at any point during your hospital stay or after you have left the hospital. The Notice of Noncoverage will tell you how to request this review.

POST-HOSPITAL CARE

When your doctor determines that you no longer need all the specialized services provided in a hospital, but you still require medical care, he or she may discharge you to a skilled nursing facility or home care. The discharge planner at the hospital will help arrange for the services you may need after your discharge. Medicare and supplemental insurance policies have limited coverage for skilled nursing facility care and home health care. Therefore, you should find out which services will or will not be covered and how payment will be made. Consult with your doctor, hospital discharge planner, patient representative and your family in making preparations for care after you leave the hospital. **Don't hesitate to ask questions.**

ACKNOWLEDGEMENT OF RECEIPT — My signature only acknowledges my receipt of this Message from (name of hospital) on (date) and does not waive any of my rights to request a review or make me liable for any payment.

_____

Signature of beneficiary or
person acting on behalf of beneficiary.

mination that you no longer needed hospital care. Write down all the answers you get from every person you talk to. Then call the Office of the Inspector General at Health and Human Services, 1–800–368–5779. Say that you want to report a case of abuse of the Medicare program. They'll take it from there.

4. I want to have an operation in the hospital, and Medicare has denied me, saying that I have to have it done in an outpatient facility. What can I do?

You can appeal, even though there is generally no problem with outpatient surgery and you may be at less risk than you would be in the hospital. Your proposed admission was turned down because the **peer review organization (PRO),** or the hospital's **utilization review committee (URC)** acting for the PRO, did not find it medically necessary. You can request a reconsideration of this decision, just as you can any other PRO decision. The procedure is given below. Please note that this is a generic procedure for the filing of requests for reconsideration and appeals. These are two different stages of the same process; we'll refer to them all as "appeals" except where that might be confusing.

How to Appeal (Request a Reconsideration) of a Peer Review Organization Decision

You can appeal the PRO decision by filing a request for reconsideration with the PRO itself, at the address for the PRO shown on the notice you received; at any Social Security office, or at a Railroad Retirement Board office, if you are a railroad retirement beneficiary.

Your doctor and the hospital also have the right to file an appeal. They do *not* have the right to an "expedited reconsideration" that you have.

Time to File the Request for Reconsideration

You must file your request for reconsideration within sixty days of the date you receive the Notice of Noncoverage. Unless you can prove otherwise, the notice is deemed to have been received by you five days after the date on it. (Example: The notice is dated January 5. You are deemed to have received it on January 10, unless you can prove you received it later. Your sixty-day period for appeal started on January 10. The last day you can file an appeal is March 10, the sixtieth day after the deemed receipt of the notice.)

"Good Cause" for Late Filing

Generally, you will be allowed to file late if there is what the PRO considers to be "good cause" for it. The regulations are very broad, and it is hard to see what exactly might count. The regulations give examples such as serious illness, a death in the family, failure to receive information you had requested before the sixty-day limit, a misunderstanding of what the PRO notice told you, and so on.

Obtaining Information

Both you and your doctor have a right to see the information on which the PRO based its decision. You should ask for this when you file your request for reconsideration. You may add to the information anything you or your doctor want to add.

Expedited Reconsideration and Time Limits

You can request that the PRO make an expedited reconsideration of the denial. How fast "expedited" has to be depends on the circumstances:

- Within three working days if you are still a patient in the hospital (this doesn't really apply here, of course, since you're trying to get it);
- Within three days if the initial determination was a denial of hospital admission and you are still in the hospital;
- Within ten working days if you are in a skilled nursing facility;
- Within thirty working days in all other situations, and in every situation where someone other than you files the appeal. Having expedited redetermination available is a very important reason for *you* to file the appeal and have the doctor or hospital submit information as part of an appeal.

What to Include

You should file your claim using HCFA Form 2649, which is shown on page 234. You can request an appeal with just a letter, but using the form will ensure that you include everything that is needed. You should ask your doctor to provide medical documentation. It is important for both you and your doctor to focus on the issue at hand, and not editorialize. The general issue you will be dealing with in PRO denials of admission is the *medical necessity* for you to be hospitalized at all, or to have a procedure done in the hospital or done at all. Keep the focus on these issues. They will boil down to appropriate medical judgment. Your doctor will probably want to submit information regarding your condition, plus evidence from the medical literature indicating that what the PRO wants done is unwise.

Notices and Appeals

When the PRO provides you with its reconsidered decision, it must do so *in writing* and inform you of the following:

- The decision
- The reasons for it

DEPARTMENT OF HEALTH, EDUCATION, AND WELFARE
HEALTH CARE FINANCING ADMINISTRATION

Form Approved.
OMB No. 066-R-0067

REQUEST FOR RECONSIDERATION OF PART A HEALTH INSURANCE BENEFITS

INSTRUCTIONS: *Please type or print firmly.* Leave the block empty if you cannot answer it. Take or mail the WHOLE form to your Social Security office which will be glad to help you. Please read the statement on the reverse side of page 2.

1. BENEFICIARY'S NAME	2. HEALTH INSURANCE CLAIM NUMBER

3. REPRESENTATIVE'S NAME, IF APPLICABLE

(☐ RELATIVE   ☐ ATTORNEY   ☐ OTHER PERSON)   ☐ PROVIDER FILING

4. PLEASE ATTACH A COPY OF THE NOTICE(S) YOU RECEIVED ABOUT YOUR CLAIM TO THIS FORM.

5. THIS CLAIM IS FOR

☐ INPATIENT HOSPITAL   ☐ SKILLED NURSING FACILITY (SNF)   ☐ HEALTH MAINTENANCE ORGANIZATION (HMO)
☐ EMERGENCY HOSPITAL   ☐ HOME HEALTH AGENCY (HHA)

6. NAME AND ADDRESS OF PROVIDER (Hospital, SNF, HHA, HMO)	CITY AND STATE	PROVIDER NUMBER

7. NAME OF INTERMEDIARY	CITY AND STATE	INTERMEDIARY NUMBER

8. DATE OF ADMISSION OR START OF SERVICES	9. DATE(S) OF THE NOTICE(S) YOU RECEIVED

10. I DO NOT AGREE WITH THE DETERMINATION ON MY CLAIM. PLEASE RECONSIDER MY CLAIM BECAUSE

11. YOU MUST OBTAIN ANY EVIDENCE *(For example, a letter from a doctor)* YOU WISH TO SUBMIT.

☐ I HAVE ATTACHED THE FOLLOWING EVIDENCE:

☐ I WILL SEND THIS EVIDENCE WITHIN 10 DAYS:

☐ I HAVE NO ADDITIONAL EVIDENCE OR OTHER INFORMATION TO SUBMIT WITH MY CLAIM.

12. IS THIS REQUEST FILED WITHIN 60 DAYS OF THE DATE OF YOUR NOTICE?

☐ YES   ☐ NO

IF YOU CHECKED "NO" ATTACH AN EXPLANATION OF THE REASON FOR THE DELAY TO THIS FORM.

13. ONLY ONE SIGNATURE IS NEEDED. THIS FORM IS SIGNED BY:

☐ BENEFICIARY   ☐ REPRESENTATIVE   ☐ PROVIDER REP.

SIGN HERE ▶

14. STREET ADDRESS

CITY, STATE, ZIP CODE

TELEPHONE	DATE

15. If this request is signed by mark (X), TWO WITNESSES who know the person requesting reconsideration must sign in the space provided on the reverse side of this page of the form.

DO NOT FILL IN BELOW THIS LINE — FOR SOCIAL SECURITY USE — THANK YOU

16. ROUTING

☐ INTERMEDIARY

☐ HCFA, RO-MEDICARE

☐ BSS, ODR

18. SSA OR INTERMEDIARY DATE STAMP

17. ADDITIONAL INFORMATION

FORM **HCFA-2649** (8-79 FORMERLY SSA-2649)
DESTROY PRIOR EDITIONS

INTERMEDIARY

Page 1 of 4

- A statement of the effect the decision has on what Medicare will pay for or has paid for
- A statement of your appeal rights, with complete instructions for filing the appeal

When you receive a notice of a reconsidered decision that is not in your favor, consider whether you want to request a hearing. A hearing is more formal than a reconsideration, and entitles you to appear before an **administrative law judge (ALJ)**. If you do request a hearing, it is wise to have a lawyer involved. Hearings can involve subpoenaing witnesses and other legal steps. It is less formal than a court case, but far more formal than a request for reconsideration.

Only you, not your doctor or the hospital, have this right. The rules for filing an appeal are exactly the same as for filing for reconsideration with the PRO — sixty days, counted from five days after the date of the notice, and all that. You should file your appeal on HCFA HA-501-US, unless the information you received with the PRO's Notice of Reconsideration tells you to do something else.

The first thing the ALJ will attempt to determine is whether or not the controversy involves at least $200 (with the price of health care these days, it almost surely will). If the ALJ determines that the amount is less than $200, he will notify you and any other concerned parties that he has determined this and that they have fifteen days to show why he is wrong. If no evidence is submitted within fifteen days, the request for a hearing is dismissed. (You will not have to worry about this if you don't receive such a notice.)

You will be notified by the ALJ of the date of the hearing at least ten days before it is filed.

If the ALJ's decision is unfavorable, you can appeal to the Social Security Appeals Council. Your attorney can tell you how to do this. The Appeals Council does not take all the appeals addressed to it. If $2,000 or more is involved, you can appeal an Appeals Council determination (or the ALJ's decision if the Appeals Council refused a hearing) to the federal courts. This must be done within sixty days of the date of the Appeals Council determination, or its decision not to hear your case.

5. My doctor wants to do my operation in the hospital, but the PRO says no. What can I do?

See the answer to the preceding question.

Nursing Homes and Home Care

1. I need to go to a nursing home, but I'm not sure Medicare will pay for it. How can I tell?

Medicare does not cover what people usually think of as "nursing home care." There are three levels of nursing home care:

- **Skilled nursing facilities** (SNFs) offer care delivered by registered and licensed practical nurses on the orders of an attending physician. They offer services such as oxygen therapy, intravenous and tube feedings, care of catheters and wound drains, and physical, occupational, and speech therapy.

- **Intermediate care facilities** (ICFs) provide less intensive care than do SNFs. Patients are generally more mobile, and rehabilitation therapies are stressed.

- **Sheltered**, or **custodial, care,** is nonmedical. Residents do not require constant attention from nurses and aides, but need assistance with one or more daily activities or no longer want to be bothered with keeping up a house. The social needs of residents are met in a safe, secure environment free of as many anxieties as possible.

Medicare covers nursing home care at the SNF level only. This coverage is intended for basically one situation: if you need more care to recuperate, but care that is less intense than that provided in a hospital. For the first 8 days of SNF care, a copayment ($22.00 per day in 1989) is required. Medicare covers the next 142 days in full. From the 151st day forward, Medicare pays nothing. You are once again eligible for another 150 days of SNF care in the next calendar year.

2. There should be no question that I need a nursing home and that Medicare will pay for it. After all, I can't do for myself a lot of the things that I used to. That's a health problem, and Medicare covers those — correct?

Not really. Nursing home care is covered only for a short time, and only if it will improve physical or mental functioning to a degree that makes the nursing home stay *medically* "reasonable and necessary." **Medical necessity** is *the* key issue in payment for SNF services. The SNF regulations go to great lengths to define what is and is not SNF.

The key is that care that is complex enough to require the services of a nurse or skilled rehabilitation personnel is covered; care that you could do yourself is not. But complications may require SNF-level care, even for situations that would normally not be covered. Basically, SNF care is rehabilitation; if your condition cannot be expected to improve as a result of SNF care *and* you do not need observation by skilled personnel, your care will not be covered. Obviously, what your doctor writes in the chart makes a big difference in what gets covered. If you are worried about coverage of SNF services, discuss this with her.

3. Is there anything I can do to stay out of a nursing home?

Yes. There are many alternatives that may enable you to stay out, depending on your level of functioning and the exact services you may need. Use the Health Status checklist in Chapter 7 to assess your needs.

For those who are not bedridden, adult day care, home health care, homemaker services, sharing a home with other elderly people, Meals on Wheels, shopping services, and adult foster care may be alternatives that will avoid a nursing home stay. For the availability of these services, you can check with your local agency on aging, the medical social services office of the hospital (if the person is in the hospital awaiting discharge), and departments of social services. Many are listed in the telephone book under the names we've used, for example, "shopping services."

4. What about home health care? What does Medicare cover?

Home health care consists of the following services:

- Part-time or intermittent nursing care provided by or under the supervision of a registered professional nurse (R.N.)
- Physical, occupational, or speech therapy
- Medical social services provided under the direction of a doctor
- Part-time or intermittent services of a home health aide
- Medical supplies (excluding drugs and biologicals) and **durable medical equipment**
- If the **Home Health Agency** (**HHA**) is affiliated with or under the control of a hospital, services of interns or residents of the hospital

Not covered under home health care are transportation, housekeeping services, and those services that are normally not covered if provided in a hospital.

To qualify for home health services, you must be one of the following:

- Confined to your home or to an institution that is not a SNF or rehabilitation facility

- Under the care of a doctor who is a medical doctor, an osteopath, or a podiatrist
- In need of intermittent skilled nursing care, physical therapy, or speech therapy
- In need of occupational therapy *after* a period during which skilled nursing care, physical therapy, or speech therapy were needed. (In other words, needing *only* occupational therapy does not qualify you for home care, but needing occupational therapy *plus* another service, or after another service, does.)

You are entitled to an unlimited number of home visits, as long as you need the service, but for no more than thirty-eight consecutive days. After that, a gap of at least one day must occur before you can receive home health services again. The HHA providing the services must be one that is Medicare-participating.

It is important to understand that home care under Medicare is composed of some (not all) *medical* services that will allow you to remain at home, rather than in a nursing home, *and these only*. It is not a "total care package."

5. Are there some things I should watch out for in regard to home care?

First, ordering medical equipment and when having your home checked for suitability for home care, make sure there is a way for you to terminate the rental or return the item if it turns out that it is not Medicare-covered and you decide you cannot afford it. You may be stuck with large expenses otherwise.

Second — and we regret having to mention this — you should make sure your money and valuables are in a safe place that you control before the home health worker visits. You should treat a visit from the home health worker like any other instance in which a stranger enters your home. There have been many instances of theft. Even very reputable agencies cannot always control the behavior of the people they hire. You should ask the HHA about its policies in case of theft. Are they insured for theft by employees? What do they require in the way of proof? Is it enough to prove that no one other than the HHA worker was in your home?

Because of prejudices against older people, you may be told that a stolen item was not stolen and you simply forgot where you put it. (Of course, you should make sure that the item *was* stolen before you report it.) If something is stolen, report it to the police, to the HHA, and to your insurance agent, if you have homeowner's or renter's insurance.

Third, as with all services, *complain (politely) if you are unsatisfied*. HHAs cannot make up for all the burdens of being old and ill, but they should, at a minimum, provide the medical services that were prescribed and any services that you are paying for, and provide them well. The authorities regulating HHAs in the various states are listed in appendix M. Complain to them if your discussion with the HHA does not produce good results.

6. I've considered every alternative to care in a nursing home that you listed in chapter 7, and I still find I need nursing home care. Medicare won't pay for it. What can I do?

The Medicaid program covers nursing home care. Medicaid is intended for the *very* poor who have nowhere else to turn, but not all of the very poor are covered. It is a state-run program that receives federal funds. States make most of the rules, and the trend in recent years has been to make Medicaid requirements more stringent. The old law virtually guaranteed that the spouse who stayed at home would have to impoverish him- or herself to pay for the care of the spouse in the nursing home.

The new Medicare catastrophic coverage provisions greatly reduce the burden but can still lead to a substantial loss of assets. Beginning January 1, 1989,

- In any month in which a married person is in a nursing home, no income of the at-home spouse is to be considered available to the spouse in the nursing home.

- Income is considered the property of the person to whom it is paid. Income paid to both spouses is attributed 50 percent to each.

- The home, household goods, and personal effects of both spouses are not counted in considering Medicaid eligibility.

- All assets other than these will be counted and divided in two. If the at-home spouse has less than $12,000, the spouse in the nursing home may transfer assets to him or her to make up to $12,000 available to the at-home spouse. (States may, at their option, raise this figure to any amount less than $60,000. The $12,000 amount will be indexed to inflation.)

- The assets that remain in the name of the spouse in the nursing home are considered available to pay for his or her nursing home care. All assets in excess of $60,000 are attributed to the spouse in the nursing home and are considered available to pay for nursing home care.

- States must allow nursing home residents to retain certain sums for medical expenses not covered by Medicare or Medicaid before contributing to the expense of their nursing home care. The states may place "reasonable limits" on the amounts spent.

Beginning September 30, 1989,

- The states must allow the at-home spouse sufficient income from the other spouse to bring total household income of the at-home spouse to at least 122 percent of the federal poverty level for a two-person household. In 1989, this will be $789 per month. On July 1, 1991, it will be raised to 133 percent of the poverty level, and to 150 percent on July 1, 1992. States will not be required to allow more than $1,500 per month, except by court order or change in regulations.

These requirements dramatically reduce the economic stress on the spouse who remains at home, but they still may require him or her to part with large amounts of income and assets. Your spouse and parents do not *actually* have to give anything toward the cost of your care, but your *eligibility* is determined as though they are. The exact requirements, as well as the amount of assets and income you may retain and still be eligible, vary from state to state. Check the list of state Medicaid offices in appendix N to find out where to call to determine the exact eligibility requirements for your state.

You are automatically eligible for Medicaid if you are eligible for, or receiving, *Supplemental Security Income (SSI)* payments for aged, blind, and disabled, but you must apply at a state welfare office. If you meet the requirements for SSI, there is little chance that you would have to give up additional income or assets to qualify for Medicaid.

If your income, less certain deductions and medical bills, is within certain (low) limits, you may be eligible for Medicaid as medically needy. You must "spend down" to pay medical bills to the point at which you are eligible; after that, Medicaid pays for all of them as long as you are eligible.

7. But I don't have the money to pay my medical bills *now*. You're telling me that I have to pay them all off in order to get Medicaid to pay for future ones?

No. This is a common misunderstanding. The requirement for the medically needy spend-down is that you have *incurred* enough medical bills so that your income, less allowances and the medical bills, is less than the income limit for eligibility. Medicaid pays all of the bills, both current and future, if you meet this test, have assets under the asset limit, and meet other requirements, such as age and residency, your particular state may impose.

8. I don't want to give up my home. Can't I transfer it and my other assets over the limit to my children, and continue to keep it?

You no longer have to give up your home to become eligible for Medicaid. The new Medicare catastrophic coverage law contains protection against impoverishment, under the following terms:
Beginning January 1, 1989,

- In any month in which a married person is in a nursing home, no income of the at-home spouse is to be considered available to the spouse in the nursing home.

- Income is considered the property of the person to whom it is paid. Income paid to both spouse is attributed 50 percent to each.

- The home, household goods, and personal effects of both spouses are not counted in considering Medicaid eligibility.

- All assets other than these will be counted and divided in two. If the at-home spouse has less than $12,000, the spouse in the nursing home may transfer assets to him or her to make up to $12,000 available to the at-home spouse. (States may, at their option, raise this figure to any amount less than $60,000. The $12,000 amount will be indexed to inflation.)

- The assets that remain in the name of the spouse in the nursing home are considered available to pay for his or her nursing home care. All assets in excess of $60,000 are attributed to the spouse in the nursing home and are considered available to pay for nursing home care.

- States must allow nursing home residents to retain certain sums for medical expenses not covered by Medicare or Medicaid before contributing to the expense of their nursing home care. The states may place "reasonable limits" on the amounts spent.

Beginning September 30, 1989,

- The states must allow the at-home spouse sufficient income from the other spouse to bring total household income of the at-home spouse to at least 122 percent of the federal poverty level for a two-person household. In 1989, this will be $789 per month. On July 1, 1991, it will be raised to 133 percent of the poverty level, and to 150 percent on July 1, 1992. States will not be required to allow more than $1,500 per month, except by court order or change in regulations.

You can transfer your assets to someone *other* than your spouse (for example, to a child) in order to become eligible for Medicaid, but you must have done so *more than two years* before you become eligible for Medicaid. If you want to transfer your assets in order to become eligible for nursing home coverage under Medicaid, *you should do so only with the services of a lawyer who understands the Medicaid program.* This is both to protect you and to ensure that you actually will be found eligible for Medicaid based on the action you took. There is no point in transferring assets only to find that you are still not eligible.

9. How do I apply for Medicaid?

Medicaid applications are taken at welfare offices, but many states also take them at senior citizens' centers, agencies on aging, and other locations. Call the Medicaid office for your state (listed in appendix N) to find out where you can apply in your area. When you call the office in your area, find out what you need to bring with you for the application process.

Generally, you should bring proof of age, financial status, and any disability you may have. The proof of financial status should include the last six months' bank statements for checking and savings accounts, rent or mortgage payment receipts, loan papers for your car or the title to it, any documents relating to stock or bond ownership, and check stubs for any regular payments you receive. You should also have the amount of your Social Security check, if you are currently receiving Social Security payments. You should always have your Social Security number. Bring your medical bills, or copies of them, for the last year.

10. How can I select a good nursing home?

You can begin the process of selecting a nursing home by eliminating those you know you don't want to use. Don't consider nursing homes that are as follows:

- Too far away to allow visiting by relatives and friends
- Too expensive
- Not properly certified or licensed
- Not offering the medical or other services needed
- Unsuitable for some other reason, such as being owned by a religious denomination with which you do not want to associate

You can find out whether or not a home is properly certified or licensed by contacting the state agencies regulating nursing homes that are listed in appendix K at the back of this book.

Chapter 7 contains a checklist, on pages 209–214, and several more suggestions for selecting a nursing home.

11. Now that I'm in the nursing home, I'm shocked by the conditions. What can I do about it?

It is difficult for nursing home residents to be effective advocates for themselves. If they are on Medicaid, they may have surrendered all their assets to obtain funding for their nursing home stay and may, in effect, be trapped in the home. They do not complain simply because they do not want to make a bad situation worse. The same applies, to a lesser degree, to just about everyone else. Even if they are economically able to move, there may be long waiting lists at the homes they want to move to.

On the other hand, some people have completely unrealistic expectations of nursing homes. No patient in a nursing home should expect the attention that a private duty nurse in a hospital can give. No nursing home can afford to provide that much service routinely. Even if the service is excellent, it may not be possible to accommodate all residents' wishes for particular services (such as bathing) exactly when they want it.

But there's a minimum below which no nursing home should fall:

- No resident should be allowed to remain in a soiled bed a moment longer than absolutely necessary.
- It is close to impossible to prevent all pressure sores for totally bedridden people, but they should be small in size and promptly treated by positioning the patient, special mattresses, and immediate attention by a doctor when needed.
- Food should be hot or cold as appropriate and of better-than-just-acceptable quality.
- Dehydration and malnutrition should *not* develop and should be promptly and vigorously treated if found.
- Medications should be given, and given reasonably close to the pre-

scribed schedule. Drug reactions should be noted in writing and reported to the doctor quickly.

The best way to make sure that a friend or relative is getting the kind of services he or she should is by visiting frequently and randomly. It is good to arrange visits so that promised events can be checked on. If a particular program is scheduled, such as a movie, exercise, a walk, a presentation by a visiting speaker, visit when it is scheduled and make sure that it happens from time to time. Some cancellations are unavoidable due to weather and such, but the general program the home promises should be carried out.

Appendix L contains the Bill of Rights for Nursing Home Patients suggested by the **Health Care Financing Administration,** which runs Medicare and Medicaid. Real, serious violations of these rights should be reported to the state authorities listed in appendix K. You should also contact the state nursing home ombudsman's office; a list is provided in appendix O.

Generally, it is best to deal with problems by pointing them out, politely but firmly, to the appropriate person — the nurse, the administrator, the billing office. The approach of being firm but not antagonistic works best. Keep repeating, in a polite manner, the problem you see and the solution you want.

An important point to remember is this: *Don't let the nursing home put the monkey on your back.* You do not have to solve, or even sympathize with, their difficulties. In some situations, the proper answer to "What would you suggest?" is "I don't have to suggest anything. *You* have to find a way to deliver the services you promised and are being paid for."

Finally, it is not useful to threaten to move a resident. Besides the antagonism this may create, it may carry no weight at all in some areas. Many nursing homes have waiting lists and are well aware of the difficulties that often occur with nursing home placement. If a move is clearly indicated, make the arrangements and carry them out.

Insurance

1. I want to buy insurance to supplement my Medicare. What should I look for?

We suggest that, at a minimum, you should purchase a policy that covers *all* the deductibles and copayments for hospital and doctor bills. This means that you will have to pay only what Medicare does not reimburse, which limits your expense to relatively minor items (with the exception of nursing home care). You should also check for coverage of amounts charged by physicians in excess of the Medicare approved charge. Policies that cover this expense typically do not pay unlimited amounts to doctors, but they will further limit your out-of-pocket expenses. The policy should also cover the copayment for the first eight days of skilled nursing facility care.

Some other features to look for are the following:

- Guaranteed renewability
- No restrictions on payment for pre-existing conditions
- No limitations to single diseases, such as cancer
- Payment for services in full, rather than payment of fixed money amounts
- No waiting periods for coverage

Chapter 4 provides more information about supplemental insurance and gives you a means of comparing policies.

Getting Bills Paid/Filing Claims

1. How do I file a Medicare claim?

Appendix D (How to File a Medicare Claim) explains how to file a claim. Utilize the Medicare Claims Log to help you keep track of the claims you file.

2. I followed your instructions to the letter and used all the right forms, filled out in all the right places. I'm sitting here at the kitchen table with a pile of rejected claims in front of me. What went wrong?

Well . . . what should be a simple, efficient process offering maximum speed of payment for providers and minimum worry for beneficiaries isn't. A large part of the reason is the number of hands spoiling the broth: the Part A intermediaries, the Part B carriers, the peer review organizations, Medicare itself, the billing agencies for doctors, and so on (and on, and on). Here are some suggestions for the situation you face, which is all too common. First, check the reason given on the **Explanation of Medicare Benefits (EOMB)** for rejection. It may well be some variation of some phrase that amounts to "claim already paid," "duplicate claim," or some such. A lot of claims are rejected for this reason. What happens is this:

- You promptly bill the Medicare carrier as soon as you get the bill from your doctor. (Your doctor must be one who does not take assignment, or is not taking it on this claim. Otherwise, there would be no bill to send in; you would just pay the 20 percent copayment or send a claim to your Medicare supplemental insurer.) Time passes, you do not get a check, he sends another bill and his collection agency calls, so you send in another claim, in the meantime the check is sent to you, and the carrier's computer rejects your claim because it's already been paid.

- You got the check for the claim from Medicare, but deposited it and did not mail the payment to the doctor; both you and he record it as unpaid, so you sent the claim in again, and the computer rejected it as already paid.

- He's a doctor who *does* take assignment (and therefore bills Medicare directly for 80 percent of the approved charge); his billing agency sent in a duplicate claim. Same situation, although here you don't even know that someone else's sending in a duplicate claim caused the rejection.

- Medicare has already paid its 80 percent of the approved fee on an assigned claim. You send Medicare a claim for the 20 percent copayment (which you must pay) instead of sending it to your Medicare supplemental insurer. Many carriers' computers often can't distinguish this situation from other duplicate claims, so you're told it's being rejected as duplicate, rather than being told that you're filing a claim for something that you or your insurer must pay.

- Medicare has already paid its 80 percent of the approved fee on an assigned claim. The doctor does not take assignment, or is not taking it on this claim, and is billing you for the difference between his *total* fee and 80 percent of the approved charge, under the same date and service code as were on the original bill. You are sending Medicare a claim for the difference between the total charge and 80 percent of the approved charge, plus the copayment of 20 percent of the approved charge, which you must pay. Many carriers' computers often can't distinguish this situation from other duplicate claims, so you're told it's being rejected as duplicate. Such claims should be sent instead to your Medicare supplemental insurer, which may cover costs over the Medicare approved charge.

Second, check for these other common reasons for claims rejection:

- Medicare had paid for the maximum number of services you can have. For example, Part A of Medicare pays for home health visits for thirty-eight consecutive days, but after that a gap of at least one day must elapse before more visits can be paid for.

- You sent Medicare a claim for a service that *is* covered under your Medicare supplemental policy but *not* under Medicare. Your Medicare supplemental insurer may maintain a help line (perhaps a toll-free number) that can help you determine where to file for what services. Also check your policy: it may provide a chart, or a simple English explanation, of what should be filed with it and what with Medicare.

- The claim, or part of it, was not paid because the money was needed to meet the Part A or Part B deductible.

- For psychiatric services, you have already received the maximum dollar value ($1,100 per year in 1989) for outpatient care or the lifetime maximum number (190) of inpatient days.

3. But my claim was rejected because the peer review organization (or the carrier, or the intermediary) found that it was not medically necessary. What should I do now?

You don't need to do anything unless the doctor (or some other Medicare provider) demands payment. Rejection of claims because the services the doctor rendered were not "reasonable and necessary" — which translates into *medically necessary* in the eyes of the PRO — is becoming more common. As we've noted repeatedly: *You are not required to pay for any service which you could not reasonably have been expected to know was not covered by Medicare. The only circumstance in which you are required to pay is one in which you were informed that no Medicare payment would be made for the specific service and you agreed to have the service performed in spite of this.* That a service (a course of treatment, a single treatment, a hospital stay) was not medically necessary is a judgment that the PRO is in most cases making after the fact. Hence, you're not required to pay: you cannot reasonably have been expected to know that the PRO, three months down the line, would find that the service you received wasn't needed. Does the PRO function of judging medical necessity mean that what Medicare routinely pays for on one side of some state or county line will be routinely rejected on the other? The answer is *yes*. This is, however, the nature of medical peer review. Groups of doctors in one part of the country don't necessarily always agree with groups of doctors in another.

How do you make use of this protection? Remember that in the vast majority of cases, you owe the doctor nothing. (You will probably get at least one bill, if the doctor's billing service is at all efficient, before you get the Explanation of Medicare Benefits [EOMB] with the rejection notice.) If you get a bill, send the doctor a *copy* of the EOMB (keep your original) together with the appropriate letter from pages 248–254.

Exactly how you make sure you don't have to pay, or get a refund if you have paid, is a bit complicated. The following letters cover all the situations you will encounter. The essence is this:

- For a participating or nonparticipating doctor whom you have not paid, you should pay nothing; just send the letter if the doctor bills you.

- For a participating or nonparticipating doctor whom you *have* paid, you are owed a refund within thirty days unless the doctor appeals, in which he must pay the refund within fifteen days after he receives the notice of the decision. If the decision is to pay him, you will receive a revised Explanation of Medicare Benefits.

For a Doctor Who Is a Medicare Participant or Who Accepted Assignment on the Rejected Claim, to Whom You *Have Not Paid* the 20 percent Copayment

Your name
Your street address
Your city, state, and ZIP code

The date [*Important!*]

Your doctor's name
His street address
His city, state, and ZIP code

Dear Doctor [*insert your doctor's name*]:

I recently received your bill for $ [*insert amount*] for [*insert name of service, such as "fulguration of warts," from bill or Explanation of Medicare Benefits*] rendered on [*insert date*].

As you can see from the enclosed copy of my Explanation of Medicare Benefits, Medicare has rejected this claim because the services were found not to be medically necessary. A notice to this effect should have been sent to you by Medicare.

I am sure that you always try to give me the best care you can, and that doctors may differ from time to time. It is important that you know that I am not required to pay the 20 percent Medicare copayment under these circumstances. Depending on the circumstances, you may or may not be paid by Medicare for the other 80 percent of the Medicare approved charge.

Please correct your records to show that I do not owe you anything for this service.

Thank you for your attention to this request.

Sincerely yours,
Your signature

For a Doctor Who is a Medicare Participant or Who Accepted Assignment on the Rejected Claim, to Whom You *Have Paid* the 20 percent Copayment

Your name
Your street address
Your city, state and ZIP code

The date [*Important!*]

Your doctor's name
His street address
His city, state, and ZIP code

Dear Doctor [*insert your doctor's name*]:

I recently received your bill for $[*insert amount*] for [*insert name of service, such as "fulguration of warts," from bill or Explanation of Medicare Benefits*] rendered on [*insert date*].

As you can see from the enclosed copy of my Explanation of Medicare Benefits, Medicare has rejected this claim because the services were found not to be medically necessary. A notice to this effect should have been sent to you by Medicare.

I am sure that you always try to give me the best care you can, and that doctors may differ from time to time. It is important that you know that I am not required to pay the 20 percent Medicare copayment under these circumstances. Depending on the circumstances, you may or may not be paid by Medicare for the other 80 percent of the Medicare-approved charge.

I would appreciate your refunding me the amount of $[*insert amount*], which I paid [*insert "by check number" and number if you paid by check, "by money order" and number if you paid by money order*] on [*insert date*].

Thank you for your attention to this request.

Sincerely yours,
Your signature

For a Doctor Who Is Not a Medicare Participant or Who Did Not Accept Assignment on the Rejected Claim, to Whom You *Have Not Paid* the 20 percent Copayment and Any Additional Amount

Your name
Your street address
Your city, state and ZIP code

The date [*Important!*]

Your doctor's name
His street address
His city, state, and ZIP code

Dear Doctor [*insert your doctor's name*]:

I recently received your bill for $[*insert amount*] for [*insert name of service, such as "fulguration of warts," from bill or Explanation of Medicare Benefits*] rendered on [*insert date*].

As you can see from the enclosed copy of my Explanation of Medicare Benefits, Medicare has rejected this claim because the services were found not to be medically necessary. A notice to this effect should have been sent to you by Medicare.

I am sure that you always try to give me the best care you can, and that doctors may differ from time to time. It is important that you know that I am not required to pay any of your bill under these circumstances. Depending on the circumstances, you may or may not be paid by Medicare for the other 80 percent of the Medicare approved charge.

Thank you for your attention to this request.

Sincerely yours,
Your signature

For a Doctor Who Is Not a Medicare Participant or Who Did Not Accept Assignment on The Rejected Claim, to Whom You *Have Paid* the 20 percent Copayment and Any Additional Amounts

Your name
Your street address
Your city, state and ZIP code

The date [*Important!*]

Your doctor's name
His street address
His city, state, and ZIP code

Dear Doctor [*insert your doctor's name*]:

I recently received your bill for $[*insert amount*] for [*insert name of service, such as "fulguration of warts," from bill or Explanation of Medicare Benefits*] rendered on [*insert date*].

As you can see from the enclosed copy of my Explanation of Medicare Benefits, Medicare has rejected this claim because the services were found not to be medically necessary. A notice to this effect should have been sent to you by Medicare.

I am sure that you always try to give me the best care you can, and that doctors may differ from time to time. It is important that you know that I am not required to pay the 20 percent Medicare copayment under these circumstances. Depending on the circumstances, you may or may not be paid by Medicare for the other 80 percent of the Medicare approved charge.

I would appreciate your refunding me the amount of $ [*insert amount*], which I paid [*insert "by check number" and number if you paid by check, "by money order" and number if you paid by money order*] on [*insert date*].

Thank you for your attention to this request.

Sincerely yours,
Your signature

4. My claim wasn't rejected totally, but I got a notice that it was reduced because of a judgment of medical necessity. What does that mean?

Essentially, the situation is exactly the same as for a rejected claim, but the PRO found that some other procedure, logically part of what the doctor did, *was* medically justified. For example, a charge for a lengthy office visit was changed to a charge for a brief office visit, and the doctor was paid 80 percent of the approved charge for that. You can use letters similar to the ones cited. Samples with the appropriate changes follow.

For a Doctor Who Is a Medicare Participant or Who Accepted Assignment on the Rejected Claim, to Whom You *Have Not Paid* the 20 percent Copayment

Your name
Your street address
Your city, state and ZIP code

The date [*Important!*]

Your doctor's name
His street address
His city, state, and ZIP code

Dear Doctor [*insert your doctor's name*]:

I recently received your bill for $[*insert amount*] for [*insert name of service, such as "fulguration of warts," from bill or*

Explanation of Medicare Benefits] rendered on [*insert date*].

As you can see from the enclosed copy of my Explanation of Medicare benefits, Medicare has reduced the charge for this claim because the services were found not to be medically necessary. A notice to this effect should have been sent to you by Medicare.

I am sure that you always try to give me the best care you can, and that doctors may differ from time to time. It is important that you know that I am not required to pay more than 20 percent Medicare copayment for the reduced claim under these circumstances.

Please correct your records to show that I do not owe you any more than this amount for this service.

Thank you for your attention to this request.

Sincerely yours,
Your signature

For a Doctor Who Is a Medicare Participant or Who Accepted Assignment on the Rejected Claim, to Whom You *Have Paid* the 20 percent Copayment

Your name
Your street address
Your city, state and ZIP code

The date [*Important!*]

Your doctor's name
His street address
His city, state, and ZIP code

Dear Doctor [*insert your doctor's name*]:

I recently received your bill for $[*insert amount*] for [*insert name of service, such as "fulguration of warts," from bill or Explanation of Medicare Benefits*] rendered on [*insert date*].

As you can see from the enclosed copy of my Explanation of Medicare Benefits, Medicare has reduced the charge for this claim because some of the services were found not to be medically necessary. A notice to this effect should have been sent to you by Medicare.

I am sure that you always try to give me the best care you can, and that doctors may differ from time to time. It is important that you know that I am not required to pay the 20 percent Medicare copayment for the reduced claim under these circumstances. Depending on the circumstances, you may or may not be paid by Medicare for the other 80 percent of the Medicare-approved charge.

I would appreciate your refunding me the amount of $[*insert amount*], which I paid [*insert "by check number" and number if you paid by check, "by money order" and number if you paid by money order*] on [*insert date*].

Thank you for your attention to this request.

Sincerely yours,
Your signature

For a Doctor Who Is Not a Medicare Participant or Who Did Not Accept Assignment on the Rejected Claim, to Whom You *Have Not Paid* 20 percent Copayment and Any Additional Amount

Your name
Your street address
Your city, state and ZIP code

The date [*Important!*]

Your doctor's name
His street address
His city, state, and ZIP code

Dear Doctor [*insert your doctor's name*]:

I recently received your bill for $[*insert amount*] for [*insert name of service, such as "fulguration of warts," from bill or Explanation of Medicare Benefits*] rendered on [*insert date*].

As you can see from the enclosed copy of my Explanation of Medicare Benefits, Medicare has reduced this claim because some of the services were found not to be medically necessary. A notice to this effect should have been sent to you by Medicare.

I am sure that you always try to give me the best care you can, and that doctors may differ from time to time. It is important that you know that I am not required to pay more than your Maximum Allowable Actual Charge, less 80 percent of the Medicare approved charges, under these circumstances.

Please correct your records to show that I do not owe you any more than this amount for this service.

Thank you for your attention to this request.

Sincerely yours,
Your signature

For a Doctor Who Is Not a Medicare Participant or Who Did Not Accept Assignment on the Rejected Claim, to Whom You *Have Paid* the 20 percent Copayment and Any Additional Amounts

Your name
Your street address
Your city, state and ZIP code

The date [*Important!*]

Your doctor's name
His street address
His city, state, and ZIP code

Dear Doctor [*insert your doctor's name*]:

I recently received your bill for $[*insert amount*] for [*insert name of service, such as "fulguration of warts," from bill or Explanation of Medicare Benefits*] rendered on [*insert date*].

As you can see from the enclosed copy of my Explanation of Medicare Benefits, Medicare has rejected this claim because the services were found not to be medically necessary. A notice to this effect should have been sent to you by Medicare.

I am sure that you always try to give me the best care you can, and that doctors may differ from time to time. It is important that you know that I am not required to pay more than your Maximum Allowable Actual Charge, less 80 percent of the Medicare approved charges, under these circumstances.

I would appreciate your refunding me the amount of $[*insert amount*], which I paid [*insert "by check number" and number if you paid by check, "by money order" and number if you paid by money order*] on [*insert date*].

Thank you for your attention to this request.

Sincerely yours,
Your signature

5. My doctor says she doesn't have to correct the bill, or pay the refund, because she has a sign in her waiting room that says that Medicare may not cover some services. Is she right?

No. Medicare has specifically ruled that the display of such a sign does *not* excuse the doctor from correcting bills, reducing charges, or paying refunds.

6. I've sent the letters you suggested, but my doctor is dunning me and I don't want my credit rating ruined. What should I do?

Review the situation to make sure that you are facing a claim that you don't have to pay. If you are reasonably certain, ask for assistance from the Medicare carrier or intermediary. If you have asked for assistance and have received none, call the Department of Health and Human Services Office of the Inspector General at 1-800-368-5779.

Appeals

There are basically three circumstances in which you will want to appeal. The first is that in which you are about to be admitted to a hospital or nursing home, or to have an inpatient or outpatient operation, and the PRO finds it medically unnecessary. The second is the one in which you are a patient, and the PRO or a review body, such as the hospital's utilization review committee (URC), determines that your stay is no longer medically necessary and determines that Medicare will no longer pay. The third is one in which a claim you have submitted for a service already received is denied.

We covered the first two circumstances in chapter 6. That material is repeated below. The procedure is generic for both hospitals and nursing homes. Before you decide to appeal a decision not to pay a claim, check the discussion about claims above to make sure that you do, in fact, have to pay something. If the claim is covered under Medicare's **waiver of liability** rules, your doctor usually has the right to appeal nonpayment and you don't have to pay anything. Appeal procedures for Part A and Part B bills follow.

Procedure for Appeals of Peer Review Organization Decisions

The procedure that follows is *generic*. It applies to *all* actions by the PROs. Only the evidence submitted would differ.

Notices: Your denial is called a Notice of Noncoverage, and it will explain why something is being denied.

How to Appeal (Request a Reconsideration) of a Peer Review Organization Decision: You can appeal the PRO decision by filing a request for reconsideration with the PRO itself, at the address for the PRO shown on the notice you received; at any Social Security office, or at a Railroad Retirement Board office, if you are a railroad retirement beneficiary.

Your doctor and the hospital also have the right to file an appeal. They do *not* have the right to an "expedited reconsideration" that you have.

Time to File the Request for Reconsideration: You must file your request for reconsideration within sixty days of the date you receive the

Notice of Noncoverage. Unless you can prove otherwise, the notice is deemed to have been received by you five days after the date on it. (Example: The notice is dated January 5. You are deemed to have received it on January 10, unless you can prove you received it later. Your sixty-day period for appeal started on January 10. The last day you can file an appeal is March 10, the sixtieth day after the deemed receipt of the notice.)

"Good Cause" for Late Filing: Generally, you will be allowed to file late if there is what the PRO considers to be "good cause" for it. The regulations are very broad, and it is hard to see what exactly might count. The regulations give examples such as serious illness, a death in the family, failure to receive information you had requested before the sixty-day limit, a misunderstanding of what the PRO notice told you, and so on.

Obtaining Information: Both you and your doctor have a right to see the information on which the PRO based its decision. You should ask for this when you file your request for reconsideration. You may add to the information anything you or your doctor want to add.

Expedited Reconsideration and Time Limits: You can request that the PRO make an expedited reconsideration of the denial. How fast "expedited" has to be depends on the circumstances.

- Within three working days if you are still a patient in the hospital (this doesn't really apply here, of course, since you're trying to get in)
- Within three days if the initial determination was a denial of hospital admission and you are still in the hospital
- Within ten working days if you are in a skilled nursing facility
- Within thirty working days in all other situations, and in every situation where someone other than you files the appeal. Having expedited redetermination available is a very important reason for *you* to file the appeal and have the doctor or hospital submit information as part of an appeal.

What to Include: You should file your claim using HCFA Form 2649, which is shown on page 257.

You can request an appeal with just a letter, but using the form will ensure that you include everything that is needed. You should ask your

Form Approved.
OMB No. 088-R-0087

REQUEST FOR RECONSIDERATION OF PART A HEALTH INSURANCE BENEFITS

INSTRUCTIONS: *Please type or print firmly.* Leave the block empty if you cannot answer it. Take or mail the WHOLE form to your Social Security office which will be glad to help you. Please read the statement on the reverse side of page 2.

1. BENEFICIARY'S NAME	2. HEALTH INSURANCE CLAIM NUMBER

3. REPRESENTATIVE'S NAME, IF APPLICABLE

☐ RELATIVE ☐ ATTORNEY ☐ OTHER PERSON) ☐ PROVIDER FILING

4. PLEASE ATTACH A COPY OF THE NOTICE(S) YOU RECEIVED ABOUT YOUR CLAIM TO THIS FORM.

5. THIS CLAIM IS FOR

☐ INPATIENT HOSPITAL   ☐ SKILLED NURSING FACILITY (SNF)   ☐ HEALTH MAINTENANCE ORGANIZATION (HMO)
☐ EMERGENCY HOSPITAL   ☐ HOME HEALTH AGENCY (HHA)

6. NAME AND ADDRESS OF PROVIDER *(Hospital, SNF, HHA, HMO)*	CITY AND STATE	PROVIDER NUMBER

7. NAME OF INTERMEDIARY	CITY AND STATE	INTERMEDIARY NUMBER

8. DATE OF ADMISSION OR START OF SERVICES	9. DATE(S) OF THE NOTICE(S) YOU RECEIVED

10. I DO NOT AGREE WITH THE DETERMINATION ON MY CLAIM. PLEASE RECONSIDER MY CLAIM BECAUSE

11. YOU MUST OBTAIN ANY EVIDENCE *(For example, a letter from a doctor)* YOU WISH TO SUBMIT.

☐ I HAVE ATTACHED THE FOLLOWING EVIDENCE:

☐ I WILL SEND THIS EVIDENCE WITHIN 10 DAYS:

☐ I HAVE NO ADDITIONAL EVIDENCE OR OTHER INFORMATION TO SUBMIT WITH MY CLAIM.

12. IS THIS REQUEST FILED WITHIN 60 DAYS OF THE DATE OF YOUR NOTICE?

☐ YES   ☐ NO

IF YOU CHECKED "NO" ATTACH AN EXPLANATION OF THE REASON FOR THE DELAY TO THIS FORM.

13. ONLY ONE SIGNATURE IS NEEDED. THIS FORM IS SIGNED BY:

☐ BENEFICIARY   ☐ REPRESENTATIVE   ☐ PROVIDER REP.

SIGN HERE ▶

14. STREET ADDRESS

CITY, STATE, ZIP CODE

TELEPHONE	DATE

15. If this request is signed by mark (X), TWO WITNESSES who know the person requesting reconsideration must sign in the space provided on the reverse side of this page of the form.

DO NOT FILL IN BELOW THIS LINE — FOR SOCIAL SECURITY USE — THANK YOU

16. ROUTING

☐ INTERMEDIARY

☐ HCFA, RO-MEDICARE

☐ BSS, ODR

18. SSA OR INTERMEDIARY DATE STAMP

17. ADDITIONAL INFORMATION

FORM HCFA-2649 (8-79 FORMERLY SSA-2649)
DESTROY PRIOR EDITIONS

INTERMEDIARY

Page 1 of 4

doctor to provide medical documentation. It is important for both you and your doctor to focus on the issue at hand, and not editorialize. The general issue you will be dealing with in PRO denials of admission is the *medical necessity* for you to be hospitalized at all, or to have a procedure done in the hospital or done at all. Keep the focus on these issues. They will boil down to appropriate medical judgment. Your doctor will probably want to submit information regarding your condition, plus evidence from the medical literature indicating that what the PRO wants done is unwise.

Notices and Appeals: When the PRO provides you with its reconsidered decision, it must do so *in writing* and inform you of the following:

- The decision
- The reasons for it
- A statement of the effect the decision has on what Medicare will pay for or has paid for
- A statement of your appeal rights, with complete instructions for filing the appeal
- When you receive a notice of a reconsidered decision that is not in your favor, you should consider whether you want to request a hearing. A hearing is more formal than a reconsideration, and it entitles you to appear before an **administrative law judge** (**ALJ**). If you do request a hearing, it is wise to have a lawyer involved. Hearings can involve subpoenaing witnesses and other legal steps. It is less formal than a court case, but far more formal than a request for reconsideration. Medicare is emphasizing doing all business possible, including hearings, over the phone. Although a hearing can be conducted over the phone, you should carefully consider appearing in person. It is sometimes easier to make your case in person, depending on the circumstances.
- Only you, not your doctor or the hospital, have this right. The rules for filing an appeal are exactly the same as for filing for reconsideration with the PRO — sixty days, counted from five days after the date of the notice, and all that. You should file your appeal on HCFA HA-501-US, unless the information you received with the PRO's Notice of Reconsideration tells you to do something else.
- The first thing the ALJ will attempt to determine is whether or not the controversy involves at least $200 (with the price of health care these days, it almost surely will). If the ALJ determines that the

amount is less than $200, he will notify you and any other concerned parties that he has determined this and that they have fifteen days to show why he is wrong. If no evidence is submitted within fifteen days, the request for a hearing is dismissed. (You will not have to worry about this if you don't receive such a notice.)

- You will be notified by the ALJ of the date of the hearing at least ten days before it is filed.
- If the ALJ's decision is unfavorable, you can appeal to the Social Security Appeals Council. Your attorney can tell you how to do this. The Appeals Council does not take all the appeals addressed to it. If $2,000 or more is at issue, you can appeal an Appeals Council decision, or the ALJ's decision if the Appeals Council refused a hearing, to the federal courts. This must be done within sixty days of the date of the Appeals Council decision on your case, or its decision not to hear it.

Requesting Reconsiderations (Appealing Decisions) on Payment of Claims

The procedures in this section apply to denial of payment for all services, other than doctors' services, after you have left the hospital. They also apply to notices regarding hospital care that you receive from the Medicare intermediary while you are in the hospital.

Notices: Your Notice of Noncoverage will come either in the form of an **Explanation of Medicare Benefits (EOMB)** or in the form of a letter. In any case, it must be in writing. It will explain the reason that something is being denied. A typical EOMB is shown on page 260.

How to Appeal (Request a Reconsideration) of a Payment Denial or Intermediary Determination that Care is Not Medically Necessary: You can appeal the PRO decision by filing a request for reconsideration with the intermediary itself, at the address shown on the EOMB, at any Social Security office, or a Railroad Retirement Board office, if you are a railroad retirement beneficiary, or at any office of the Health Care Financing Administration.

Your doctor and the hospital have the right to file an appeal only if you do not plan to do so and you certify this in writing on a form they will provide. They do *not* have the right to an "expedited reconsideration" that you have.

Time to File the Request for Reconsideration: You must file your request for reconsideration within sixty days of the date you receive the notice of denial. Unless you can prove otherwise, the notice is deemed

YOUR EXPLANATION OF MEDICARE BENEFITS
Read this notice carefully and keep it for your records.
This is not a bill.

This is your Part B Carrier. If you suspect a mistake, contact this office.

HEALTH CARE FINANCING ADMINISTRATION

Iphigenia Smith
4321 Edgar Allen Poe Drive
San Diego, CA 99110

Dec. 31, 1987
Need help? Contact:
TRANSAMERICA OCCIDENTAL
   LIFE INSURANCE
1149 South Broadway
Box 54905 Terminal Annex
Los Angeles, CA 90054
Phone: 213 Area: 748-2311
   Other Areas: 1-800-252-9020

This tells you if Assignment was taken and the dollar amount billed.

Assignment was taken on your claim for $45.00 from MIDWAY MEDICAL CLNC.
(See item 4 on back.)

This indicates the service and date provided.

		Billed	Approved
1 Office Service	Dec 05, 1987	$45.00	$40.00

Approved amount limited by item 5c on back.

This indicates amount Billed and Approved.

Total approved amount	$40.00
Medicare payment (80% of the approved amount minus 2.324%)	$31.26

This indicates the Approved amount and Medicare's 80 percent.

MIDWAY MEDICAL CLNC agreed to charge no more for the above approved services than the amount approved by Medicare. We are paying a total of $31.26 to MIDWAY MEDICAL CLNC.

This is what Medicare pays.

You are responsible to the physician / supplier for the difference of $8.00 between the approved amount and the Medicare payment. If you have other insurance, it may help with the part Medicare did not pay.

This explains what You pay.

A new law has reduced your Medicare payment by 2.324% for services from November 21, 1987 to March 31, 1988. You are not responsible for the 2.324% reduction on this assigned claim.

This explains any change in billing and what — if any — affect on you.

(You have met the deductible for 1987)

This indicates whether or not you have met the $75 deductible.

260

IMPORTANT: If you do not agree with the amounts approved you may ask for a review. To do this you must *write* to us before *Jun 31, 1988.* (See item 1 on the back.) — This gives you the time frame to file any appeal.

DO YOU HAVE A QUESTION ABOUT THIS NOTICE? If you believe Medicare paid for a service you did not receive, or there is an error, contact us immediately. Always give us the:

Medicare Claim No. 987 65 4321A   Claim Control No. 7350 316 290

Use these numbers when making any inquiry on your claim.

to have been received by you five days after the date on it. (Example: The notice is dated January 5. You are deemed to have received it on January 10. The last day you can file an appeal is March 10, the sixtieth day after the deemed receipt of the notice.)

Request for Extension of Time to File: If you need more than sixty days to file your appeal, you can request more time at any Social Security office, Medicare office, or the Railroad Retirement Board. You cannot file an extension request with an intermediary. You will be notified in writing of the time granted you.

"Good Cause" for Granting a Time Extension: Generally, you will be allowed to file late if there is what PRO considers to be "good cause" for it. The regulations are very broad and it is hard to see what exactly might count. The regulations give examples such as serious illness, a death in the family, failure to receive information you had requested before the sixty-day limit, a misunderstanding of what the PRO notice told you, and so on.

Obtaining Information: Both you and your doctor have a right to see the information on which the PRO based its decision. You should ask for this when you file your request for reconsideration. You may add to the information anything you or your doctor want to add.

Expedited Reconsideration: There is a procedure for expedited appeals under Part A (hospital insurance), but it may be used only if both the person appealing and the secretary of Health and Human Services (HHS) agree that the only issue is a constitutional one. This is a rare situation.

What to Include: You should file your claim using HCFA Form 2649. You can request an appeal with just a letter, but using the form will ensure that you include everything that is needed. You should ask your doctor to provide medical documentation. It is important for both you and your doctor to focus on the issue at hand, and not editorialize. The general issues you will be dealing with are as follows:

- The medical necessity of the service
- Whether or not Medicare covers it
- Whether or not you are entitled to it
- Whether or not the amount paid is what ought to have been paid

Medical necessity issues will boil down to appropriate medical judgment. Your doctor will probably want to submit information regarding your condition, plus evidence from the medical literature that indicates that the decision is unwise.

Time Limits: The regulations provide no time limit for a decision on a Part A request for reconsideration.

Notices and Appeals: When you are provided with the reconsidered decision, it will include, in writing, the following:

- The decision
- The reasons for it
- A statement of the effect the decision has on what Medicare will pay for, or has paid for
- A statement of your appeal rights, with complete instructions for filing the appeal

When you receive a notice of a reconsidered decision that is not in your favor, consider whether you want to request a hearing. A hearing is more formal than a reconsideration, and entitles you to appear before an ALJ. If you do request a hearing, it is wise to have a lawyer involved. Hearings can involve subpoenaing witnesses and other legal steps. It is less formal than a court case, but far more formal than a request for reconsideration.

Only you, not your doctor or the hospital, have this right. The rules for filing an appeal are exactly the same as for filing for reconsideration — sixty days, counted from five days after the date of the notice, and all that. You should file your appeal on HCFA HA-501-US, unless the information you received with the Notice of Reconsideration tells you to do something else.

You may request a hearing only if the amount in controversy is $100 or more.

You should also note that your request for a hearing will be deemed received *five days* after the date on it, unless you can show that it was received earlier. If you are within five days of the sixty-day limit, send it *certified mail, return receipt requested,* so you will have proof of the date it was actually received.

The first thing the ALJ will attempt to determine is whether or not the controversy involves at least $200 (with the price of health care these days, it almost surely will). If the ALJ determines that the amount is less than $200, he will notify you and any other concerned parties that he has determined this and that they have fifteen days to show why he is wrong. If no evidence is submitted within fifteen days, the request for a hearing is dismissed. (You will not have to worry about this if you don't receive such a notice.)

You will be notified by the ALJ of the date of the hearing at least ten days before it is filed.

If the ALJ's decision is unfavorable, you can appeal to the Social Security Appeals Council. Your attorney can tell you how to do this. The Appeals Council does not take all the appeals addressed to it. If $1,000 or more is at issue, you can appeal an Appeals Council decision, or the ALJ's decision if the Appeals Council refused a hearing, to the federal courts. This must be done within sixty days of the date of the Appeals Council decision on your case, or its decision not to hear it.

If you receive a favorable determination, Medicare will pay its usual amounts for the services rendered. If you do not receive a favorable determination, you pay.

Appeals of Health Maintenance Organization Decision

As a member of an health maintenance organization, you have all the appeal rights that Medicare beneficiaries have. In addition, Medicare requires that the HMO have a written appeals procedure for all members for matters within the HMO. Which one you should use depends on the circumstances. We suggest using the HMO appeals process for matters that can be resolved within the HMO (for example, you want a treatment and your doctor does not think it is medically indicated) and the Medicare process for matters you cannot resolve using the HMO procedure. Just keep in mind the time limits for Medicare appeals. Do not fail to file a Medicare appeal of a Notice of Noncoverage, for example, just because you are trying to work matters out with the HMO.

Coordination with Employers' Health Insurance and Retirement Plans

Plans are so varied, and changes so rapid, that it is hard to give specific advice. Keep in mind that employer-provided health insurance for persons over 65 who continue to work is now the *secondary* payer, with Medicare picking up the difference between what the plan doesn't pay and what Medicare does — *not* the difference between what the plan pays and what you are charged. Look carefully at the list of Medicare covered items in chapter 3, and if you think Medicare covers something that the employer plan does not cover (the most common example is likely to be skilled nursing facility services), make sure you file a claim with Medicare.

Also remember that many employer health plans are, in fact, health insurance purchased from a carrier for a group of employees and are regulated by the insurance commission or equivalent body in your state. Contact the insurance commission if you suspect you are not receiving fair treatment or the benefits to which you are entitled.

Appendix A: Medicare Intermediaries and Carriers

Note: The toll-free or 800 numbers listed below can be used only in the states or service areas indicated. Also listed are the local commercial numbers for some carriers.

Alabama
Medicare/Blue Cross–Blue Shield of
  Alabama
P.O. Box C-140
Birmingham, AL 35283
1-800-292-8855
205-988-2244

Alaska
Medicare/Aetna Life & Casualty
200 S.W. Market Street
P.O. Box 1998
Portland, OR 97207-1998
1-800-547-6333

Arizona
Medicare/Aetna Life & Casualty
P.O. Box 37200
Phoenix, AZ 85069
1-800-352-0411
602-861-1968

Arkansas
Medicare/Arkansas Blue Cross and
  Blue Shield
P.O. Box 1418
Little Rock, AR 72203
1-800-482-5525
501-378-2320

California
*Counties of Los Angeles, Orange, San
  Diego, Ventura, Imperial, San Luis
  Obispo, Santa Barbara:*
Medicare/Transamerica Occidental
  Life Insurance Co.
Box 54905 Terminal Annex
Los Angeles, CA 90054
1-800-252-9020
213-748-2311

Rest of state:
Medicare Claims Dept.
Blue Shield of California

Chico, CA 95976
(In area codes 209, 408, 415, 707,
  916)
1-800-952-8627
(In area codes 213, 619, 714, 805,
  818)
1-800-848-7713
714-824-0900

Colorado
Medicare/Blue Shield of Colorado
700 Broadway
Denver, CO 80273
1-800-332-6681
303-831-2661

Connecticut
Medicare/The Travelers Ins. Co.
P.O. Box 5005
Wallingford, CT 06493-5005
1-800-982-6819
(In Hartford) 203-728-6783

Delaware
Medicare/Pennsylvania Blue Shield
P.O. Box 65
Camp Hill, PA 17011
1-800-851-3535

District of Columbia
Medicare/Pennsylvania Blue Shield
P.O. Box 100
Camp Hill, PA 17011
1-800-233-1124

Florida
Medicare/Blue Shield of Fla. Inc.
P.O. Box 2525
Jacksonville, FL 32231
1-800-333-7586
904-355-3680

Georgia
Medicare/Aetna Life & Casualty
Medicare Administration

12052 Middleground Road
Suite A
Savannah, GA 31419-1699
912-927-0934

Hawaii
Medicare/Aetna Life & Casualty
P.O. Box 3947
Honolulu, HI 96812
1-800-272-5242
808-524-1240

Idaho
Medicare/Equicor–Equitable HCA
   Corp.
P.O. Box 8048
Boise, ID 83707
1-800-632-6574
208-342-7763

Illinois
Medicare Claims
Blue Cross and Blue Shield of Illinois
P.O. Box 4422
Marion, IL 62959
1-800-642-6930
312-938-8000

Indiana
Medicare Part B
Associated Ins. Companies, Inc.
P.O. Box 7073
Indianapolis, IN 46207
1-800-622-4792
317-842-4151

Iowa
Medicare/Blue Shield of Iowa
636 Grand
Des Moines, IA 50309
1-800-532-1285
515-245-4785

Kansas
Counties of Johnson, Wyandotte:
Medicare/Blue Shield of Kansas City
P.O. Box 169
Kansas City, MO 64141
1-800-892-5900
816-561-0900

Rest of state:
Medicare/Blue Shield of Kansas
P.O. Box 239

Topeka, KS 66601
1-800-432-3531
913-232-3773

Kentucky
Medicare Part B
Blue Cross and Blue Shield of KY
100 East Vine Street
Lexington, KY 40507
1-800-432-9255
606-233-1441

Louisiana
Blue Cross and Blue Shield of LA
7700 GSRI Avenue
Baton Rouge, LA 70820-7498
1-800-462-9666
(In New Orleans) 504-529-1494
(In Baton Rouge) 504-379-8400

Maine
Medicare/Blue Shield of
   Massachusetts/Tri-State
P.O. Box 1010
Biddeford, ME 04005
1-800-492-0919

Maryland
*Counties of Montgomery, Prince
   Georges:*
Medicare/Pennsylvania Blue Shield
P.O. Box 100
Camp Hill, PA 17011
1-800-233-1124

Rest of state:
Maryland Blue Shield, Inc.
700 E. Joppa Road
Towson, MD 21204
1-800-492-4795
301-561-4160

Massachusetts
Medicare/Blue Shield of
   Massachusetts, Inc.
55 Accord Park Drive
Rockland, MA 02371
1-800-882-1228

Michigan
Medicare Part B
Michigan Blue Cross and Blue Shield
P.O. Box 2201
Detroit, MI 48231-2201

(In area code 313) 1-800-482-4045
(In area code 517) 1-800-322-0607
(In area code 616) 1-800-442-8020
(In area code 906) 1-800-562-7802
(In Detroit) 313-225-8200

Minnesota
Counties of Anoka, Dakota, Filmore,
   Goodhue, Hennepin, Houston,
   Olmstead, Ramsey, Wabasha,
   Washington, Winona:
Medicare/The Travelers Ins. Co.
8120 Penn Avenue
South Bloomington, MN 55431
1-800-352-2762
612-884-7171

Rest of state:
Medicare/Blue Shield of Minnesota
P.O. Box 64357
St. Paul, MN 55164
1-800-392-0343
612-456-5070

Mississippi
Medicare/The Travelers Ins. Co.
P.O. Box 22545
Jackson, MS 39205
1-800-682-5417
601-982-9411

Missouri
Counties of Andrew, Atchison, Bates,
   Benton, Buchanan, Caldwell,
   Carroll, Cass, Clay, Clinton,
   Daviess, DeKalb, Gentry, Grundy,
   Harrison, Henry, Holt, Jackson,
   Johnson, Lafayette, Livingston,
   Mercer, Nodaway, Pettis, Platte,
   Ray, St. Clair, Saline, Vernon,
   Worth:
Medicare/Blue Shield of Kansas City
P.O. Box 169
Kansas City, MO 64141
1-800-892-5900
816-561-0900

Rest of state:
Medicare/General American Life
   Insurance Co.
P.O. Box 505
St. Louis, MO 63166

1-800-392-3070
314-843-8880

Montana
Medicare/Blue Shield of Montana, Inc.
P.O. Box 4310
Helena, MT 59601
1-800-332-6146
406-444-8350

Nebraska
Medicare/Blue Shield of Iowa
P.O. Box 10479
Des Moines, IA 50306
1-800-633-1113
420-397-9182

Nevada
Medicare/Aetna Life & Casualty
P.O. Box 37230
Phoenix, AZ 85069
1-800-528-0311

New Hampshire
Medicare/Blue Shield of
   Massachusetts/Tri-State
P.O. Box 1010
Biddeford, ME 04005
1-800-447-1142

New Jersey
Medicare/Pennsylvania Blue Shield
Box 65
Camp Hill, PA 17011
1-800-382-1274

New Mexico
Medicare/Aetna Life & Casualty
P.O. Box 25500
Oklahoma City, OK 73125-0500
1-800-423-2925
(In Albuquerque) 505-843-7771

New York
Counties of Bronx, Columbia,
   Delaware, Dutchess, Greene, Kings,
   Nassau, New York, Orange,
   Putnam, Richmond, Rockland,
   Suffolk, Sullivan, Ulster,
   Westchester:
Medicare/Empire Blue Cross and Blue
   Shield
P.O. Box 4840, Grand Central Station
New York, NY 10163

1-800-442-8430
201-490-4444

County of Queens:
Medicare/Group Health, Inc.
P.O. Box A966, Times Square Station
New York, NY 10036
212-760-6790

Rest of state:
Medicare/Blue Shield of Western
  New York
P.O. Box 5200
Binghamton, NY 13902-5200
607-772-9606
1-800-252-6550

North Carolina
Equicor Inc, Medicare Administration
1 Tried Center, Suite 240
7736 McClould Road
Greensboro, NC 27409
919-665-0341
919-665-0348
1-800-672-3071

North Dakota
Medicare/Blue Shield of North Dakota
4510 13th Avenue, S.W.
Fargo, ND 58121-0001
1-800-247-2267
701-282-0691

Ohio
Medicare/Nationwide Mutual Ins. Co.
P.O. Box 57
Columbus, OH 43216
1-800-282-0530
614-249-7157

Oklahoma
Medicare/Aetna Life & Casualty
701 N.W. 63d Street, Suite 300
Oklahoma City, OK 73116-7693
1-800-522-9079
405-848-7711

Oregon
Medicare/Aetna Life & Casualty
200 S.W. Market Street
P.O. Box 1997
Portland, OR 97207-1997
1-800-452-0125
503-222-6831

Pennsylvania
Medicare/Pennsylvania Blue Shield
Box 65
Camp Hill, PA 17011
1-800-382-1274

Rhode Island
Medicare/Blue Shield of Rhode Island
444 Westminster Mall
Providence, RI 02901
1-800-662-5170
401-861-2273

South Carolina
Medicare Part B
Blue Cross and Blue Shield of
  South Carolina
Fontaine Road Business Center
300 Arbor Lake Drive, Suite 1300
Columbia, SC 29223
1-800-922-2340
803-754-0639

South Dakota
Medicare Part B
Blue Shield of North Dakota
4510 13th Avenue, S.W.
Fargo, ND 58121-0001
1-800-437-4762

Tennessee
Medicare/The Equitable Life
  Assurance Society
P.O. Box 1465
Nashville, TN 37202
1-800-342-8900
615-244-5650

Texas
Medicare/Blue Cross and Blue Shield
  of Texas, Inc.
P.O. Box 660031
Dallas, TX 75266-0031
1-800-442-2620
214-647-2282

Utah
Medicare/Blue Shield of Utah
P.O. Box 30270
2455 Parley's Way
Salt Lake City, UT 84130-0270
1-800-662-3398
801-481-6196

Vermont
Medicare/Blue Shield of
   Massachusetts/Tri State
P.O. Box 1010
Biddeford, ME 04005
1-800-447-1142

Virginia
Counties of Arlington, Fairfax;
Cities of: Alexandria, Falls Church,
   Fairfax:
Medicare/Pennsylvania Blue Shield
P.O. Box 100
Camp Hill, PA 17011
1-800-233-1124

Rest of state:
Medicare/The Travelers Ins. Co.
P.O. Box 26463
Richmond, VA 23261
1-800-552-3423
804-254-4130

Washington
Medicare/Washington Physicians'
   Service
Mail to your local Medical Service
   Bureau
If you do not know which bureau
   handles your claim, mail to:

Medicare/Washington Physicians'
   Service
4th and Battery Bldg., 6th floor
2401 4th Avenue
Seattle, WA 98121

(In King County) 1-800-422-4087
                  206-464-3711
(In Spokane) 1-800-572-5256
                509-536-4550
(In Kitsap) 1-800-552-7114
              206-377-5576
(In Pierce) 206-597-6530

Others: Collect if out of call area.

Appendix B: Medicare Claims Log

			Medicare Claims Log, Parts A and B					
(1) DATE OF SERVICE	(2) NAME OF PROVIDER OR FACILITY	(3) MEDICARE CLAIM NUMBER	(4) CLAIM UNDER		(5) AMOUNT OF CLAIM		(6) DEDUCTIBLE MET	
			PART A	PART B	BILLED	APPROVED	PART A	PART B

(7) DATE CLAIM SUBMITTED TO CARRIER	(8) BALANCE OR COPAYMENT DUE	(9) AMOUNT CLAIMED	(10) AMOUNT RECEIVED	(11) OUT-OF-POCKET PAYMENT	(12) COMMENTS

Appendix C: State Insurance Offices

Alabama
Insurance Department
Retirement Systems Building
135 S. Union Street
Montgomery, AL 36130-3401
205-269-3550

Alaska
Division of Insurance
Department of Commerce &
    Economic Development
State Office Building
333 Willoughby Avenue
Mail to: P.O. Box D
Juneau, AK 99811
907-465-2515

Arizona
Insurance Department
801 E. Jefferson Street
Phoenix, AZ 85034
602-255-5400

Arkansas
Insurance Department
University Tower Building, Room 400
12th Street and University Avenue
Little Rock, AR 72204
501-371-1325

California
Department of Insurance
600 S. Commonwealth Avenue,
    14th floor
Los Angeles, CA 90005
213-736-2551

Colorado
Division of Insurance
Department of Regulatory Agencies
First Western Plaza Building,
    Room 500
303 W. Colfax Avenue
Denver, CO 80204
303-866-3201

Connecticut
Insurance Department
State Office Building, Room 425

165 Capitol Avenue
Hartford, CT 06106
203-566-2810

Delaware
Insurance Department
Rodney Building, Suite 100
841 Silver Lake Boulevard
Dover, DE 19903
302-736-4251
800-282-8611

District of Columbia
Insurance Administration
Department of Consumer and
    Regulatory Affairs
North Potomac Building, Room 516
614 H Street, N.W.
Washington, DC 20001
202-727-7419

Florida
Department of Insurance
The Capitol, Plaza Level II
Tallahassee, FL 32301
904-488-3440

Georgia
Office of Commissioner of Insurance
Floyd Memorial Building, West Tower
2 Martin Luther King, Jr. Drive
Atlanta, GA 30334
404-656-2056

Hawaii
Insurance Division
Department of Commerce and
    Consumer Affairs
1010 Richards Street
Mail to: P.O. Box 3614
Honolulu, HI 96811
808-548-6522

Idaho
Department of Insurance
State Capitol Building
700 W. State Street
Boise, ID 83720
208-334-2250

Illinois
Department of Insurance
Bicentennial Building
320 W. Washington Street
Springfield, IL 62767
217-782-4515

Indiana
Department of Insurance
311 W. Washington Street
Indianapolis, IN 46204
317-232-2386

Iowa
Division of Insurance
Department of Commerce
Lucas State Office Building
E. 12th and Grand Avenue
Des Moines, IA 50319
515-281-5705

Kansas
Insurance Department
420 W. 9th Street
Topeka, KS 66612
913-296-3071

Kentucky
Department of Insurance
Public Protection and Regulation
  Cabinet
Fitzgerald Building
229 W. Main Street
Mail to: P.O. Box 517
Frankfort, KY 40602
502-564-3630

Louisiana
Department of Insurance
Insurance Building
950 N. 5th Street
Mail to: P.O. Box 94214
Baton Rouge, LA 70804-9214
504-342-5322

Maine
Bureau of Insurance
Department of Professional and
  Financial Regulation
Hallowell Annex
Hallowell, ME 04347
207-289-3101
Mail to: State House, Station 34
Augusta, ME 04333

Maryland
Insurance Division
Department of Licensing and
  Regulation
Stanbalt Building
501 St. Paul Place
Baltimore, MD 21202
301-659-6300

Massachusetts
Division of Insurance
Department of Banking and Insurance
Leverett Saltonstall State Office
  Building
100 Cambridge Street
Boston, MA 02202
617-727-3333

Michigan
Insurance Bureau
Department of Licensing and
  Regulation
Ottawa Building North
611 W. Ottawa Street
Mail to: P.O. Box 30220
Lansing, MI 48909
517-373-9273

Minnesota
Department of Commerce
Metro Square Building, Room 500
7th and Robert Streets
St. Paul, MN 55101
612-296-4026 & 296-6848

Mississippi
Insurance Department
Walter Sillers State Office Building,
  Room 1804
550 High Street
Mail to: P.O. Box 79
Jackson, MS 39205
601-359-3569

Missouri
Company Regulations
Division of Insurance
Department of Economic
  Development
Harry S Truman State Office Building,
  Room 630
301 W. High Street
Mail to: P.O. Box 690

Jefferson City, MO 65102
314-751-4126

Montana
State Auditor Office
Mail to: P.O. Box 4009
Helena, MT 59604
406-444-2040

Nebraska
Department of Insurance
State Office Building
301 Centennial Mall, South
Mail to: P.O. Box 94699
Lincoln, NE 68509
402-471-2201

Nevada
Insurance Division
Department of Commerce
Nye Building
201 S. Fall Street
Mail to: Capitol Complex
Carson City, NV 89710
702-885-4270

New Hampshire
Insurance Department
169 Manchester Street
Concord, NH 03301
603-271-2261

New Jersey
Division of Administration
Department of Insurance
Arnold Constable Building, Room 307
201 E. State Street
Trenton, NJ 08625
609-292-5360

New Mexico
Department of Insurance
PERA Building, Room 428
Old Santa Fe Trail
Pasco de Peralta
Mail to: P.O. Drawer 1269
Santa Fe, NM 87504-1269
505-827-4500

New York
Insurance Department
160 W. Broadway
New York, NY 10013
212-602-0429

North Carolina
Agent Services and Consumer Division
Department of Insurance
Dobbs Building
430 N. Salisbury Street
Mail to: P.O. Box 26387
Raleigh, NC 27611
919-733-4935

North Dakota
Insurance Department
State Capitol, 5th Floor
Bismarck, ND 58505
701-224-2440

Ohio
Department of Insurance
2100 Stella Court
Columbus, OH 43215
614-481-5728

Oklahoma
Insurance Department
State Insurance Building
1901 N. Walnut Boulevard
Mail to: P.O. Box 53408
Oklahoma City, OK 73152-3408
405-521-2828

Oregon
Insurance Division
Department of Commerce
Commerce Building
158 12th Street, N.E.
Salem, OR 97310
503-378-4474

Pennsylvania
Division of Consumer Affairs and
    Enforcement
Department of Insurance
1321 Strawberry Square
Harrisburg, PA 17120
717-787-1972

Rhode Island
Director and Insurance Commissioner
Department of Business Regulation
100 N. Main Street
Providence, RI 02903
401-277-2246

South Carolina
Department of Insurance
1612 Marion Street

Mail to: P.O. Box 100105
Columbia, SC 29202-3105
803-737-6268

South Dakota
Division of Insurance
Department of Commerce and
    Regulation
State Capitol
500 E. Capitol Avenue
Pierre, SD 57501
605-773-3563

Tennessee
Department of Commerce and
    Insurance
1808 West End Building, Suite 1400
Nashville, TN 37219
615-741-2241

Texas
State Board of Insurance
State Insurance Building
1110 San Jacinto Boulevard
Austin, TX 78701-1998
512-463-6464

Utah
Insurance Department
Heber M. Wells Building
160 E. 300 South
Mail to: P.O. Box 45803
Salt Lake City, UT 84145
801-530-6400

Vermont
Department of Banking and Insurance
State Office Building
120 State Street
Montpelier, VT 05602
802-828-3301

Virginia
Bureau of Insurance
State Corporation Commission
Jefferson Building
1220 Bank Street
Mail to: P.O. Box 1157

Richmond, VA 23209
804-786-3741

Washington
Office of the Insurance Commissioner
Insurance Building, Room 200
Mail to: Mail Stop AQ-21
Olympia, WA 98504
206-753-7301

West Virginia
Department of Insurance
2100 Washington Street, E.
Charleston, WV 25305
304-348-3394

Wisconsin
Office of the Commissioner of
    Insurance
Loraine Building
123 W. Washington Avenue
Mail to: P.O. Box 7873
Madison, WI 53707
608-266-3585

Wyoming
Insurance Department
Herschler Building, 3rd Floor
122 W. 25th Street
Cheyenne, WY 82002
307-777-7401

Puerto Rico
Office of the Insurance Commissioner
Cobian's Plaza
1607 Ponce de Leon Avenue, Stop 23
Mail to: P.O. Box 8330, Fernandez
    Juncos Station
Santurce, PR 00910
809-722-8686

Virgin Islands
Office of the Lieutenant Governor
Lieutenant Governor's Office Building
18 Kongen Gade
Charlotte Amalie
St. Thomas, VI 00802
809-774-2991

Appendix D: How To File A Medicare Claim

PATIENT'S REQUEST FOR MEDICAL PAYMENT

IMPORTANT—SEE OTHER SIDE FOR INSTRUCTIONS

PLEASE TYPE OR PRINT INFORMATION | MEDICAL INSURANCE BENEFITS SOCIAL SECURITY ACT

NOTICE: Anyone who misrepresents or falsifies essential information requested by this form may upon conviction be subject to fine and imprisonment under Federal Law. No Part B Medicare benefits may be paid unless this form is received as required by existing law and regulations (20 CFR 422.510).

1 Name of Beneficiary from Health Insurance Card
(Last)   (First)   (Middle)

SEND COMPLETED FORM TO:

The Part B Carrier for your state will be listed in this space.

2 Claim Number from Health Insurance Card

Patient's Sex
☐ Male
☐ Female

3 Patient's Mailing Address (City, State, Zip Code)
Check here if this is a new address ⟶ ☐

_____
(Street or P.O. Box — Include Apartment Number)

_____
(City)   (State)   (Zip)

3b Telephone Number (Include Area Code)

(___ ___ ___)

___ ___ ___ — ___ ___ ___ ___

4 Describe the Illness or Injury for which Patient Received Treatment

4b Was condition related to:
A. Patient's employment
☐ Yes   ☐ No

B. Accident
☐ Auto   ☐ Other

4c Was patient being treated with chronic dialysis or kidney transplant?
☐ Yes   ☐ No

5
a. Are you employed and covered under an employee health plan?
☐ Yes   ☐ No

b. Is your spouse employed and are you covered under your spouse's employee health plan?
☐ Yes   ☐ No

c. If you have any medical coverage other than Medicare, such as private insurance, employment related insurance, State Agency (Medicaid), or the VA, complete:
Name and Address of other insurance, State Agency (Medicaid), or VA office

Policy or Medical Assistance No.

Policyholders Name:

NOTE: If you DO NOT want payment information on this claim released, put an (X) here ⟶ ☐

6 I AUTHORIZE ANY HOLDER OF MEDICAL OR OTHER INFORMATION ABOUT ME TO RELEASE TO THE SOCIAL SECURITY ADMINISTRATION AND HEALTH CARE FINANCING ADMINISTRATION OR ITS INTERMEDIARIES OR CARRIERS ANY INFORMATION NEEDED FOR THIS OR A RELATED MEDICARE CLAIM. I PERMIT A COPY OF THIS AUTHORIZATION TO BE USED IN PLACE OF THE ORIGINAL, AND REQUEST PAYMENT OF MEDICAL INSURANCE BENEFITS TO ME.

Signature of Patient (If patient is unable to sign, see Block 6 on reverse)

6b Date signed

IMPORTANT
ATTACH ITEMIZED BILLS FROM YOUR DOCTOR(S) OR SUPPLIER(S) TO THE BACK OF THIS FORM

Form HCFA-1490S (SC) (2-87) | DEPARTMENT OF HEALTH AND HUMAN SERVICES—HEALTH CARE FINANCING ADMINISTRATION

HOW TO FILL OUT THIS MEDICARE FORM

Medicare will pay you directly when you complete this form and attach an itemized bill from your doctor or supplier. Your bill does not have to be paid before you submit this claim for payment, but you MUST attach an itemized bill in order for Medicare to process this claim.

FOLLOW THESE INSTRUCTIONS CAREFULLY:

A. Completion of this form.

Block 1.   Print your name shown on your Medicare Card. (Last Name, First Name, Middle Name)

Block 2.   Print your Health Insurance Claim Number including the letter at the end **exactly** as it is shown on your Medicare card. Check the appropriate box for the patient's sex.

Block 3.   Furnish your mailing address and include your telephone number in Block 3b.

Block 4.   Describe the illness or injury for which you received treatment. Check the appropriate box in Blocks 4b and 4c.

Block 5a.   Complete this Block if you are age 65 or older and enrolled in a health insurance plan where you are currently working.

Block 5b.   Complete this Block if you are age 65 or older and enrolled in a health insurance plan where your spouse is currently working.

Block 5c.   Complete this Block if you have any medical coverage other than Medicare. Be sure to provide the Policy or Medical Assistance Number. You may check the box provided if you do not wish payment information from this claim released to your other insurer.

Block 6.   Be sure to sign your name. If you cannot write your name, make an (X) mark. Then have a witness sign his or her name and address in Block 6 too.

   If you are completing this form for another Medicare patient you should write (By) and sign your name and address in Block 6. You also should show your relationship to the patient and briefly explain why the patient cannot sign.

Block 6b.   Print the date you completed this form.

B. Each itemized bill MUST show all of the following information:

* Date of each service

* Place of each service   —Doctor's Office   —Independent Laboratory
                           —Outpatient Hospital   —Nursing Home
                           —Patient's Home   —Inpatient Hospital

* Description of each surgical or medical service or supply furnished.

* Charge for EACH service.

* Doctor's or supplier's name and address. Many times a bill will show the names of several doctors or suppliers. IT IS VERY IMPORTANT THE ONE WHO TREATED YOU BE IDENTIFIED. Simply circle his/her name on the bill.

* It is helpful if the diagnosis is shown on the physician's bill. If not, be sure you have completed Block 4 of this form.

* Mark out any services on the bill(s) you are attaching for which you have already filed a Medicare claim.

* If the patient is deceased please contact your Social Security office for instructions on how to file a claim.

* Attach an Explanation of Medicare Benefits notice from the other insurer if you are also requesting Medicare payment.

COLLECTION AND USE OF MEDICARE INFORMATION

We are authorized by the Health Care Financing Administration to ask you for information needed in the administration of the Medicare program. Authority to collect information is in section 205 (a), 1872 and 1875 of the Social Security Act, as amended.

The information we obtain to complete your Medicare claim is used to identify you and to determine your eligibility. It is also used to decide if the services and supplies you received are covered by Medicare and to insure that proper payment is made.

The information may also be given to other providers of services, carriers, intermediaries, medical review boards, and other organizations as necessary to administer the Medicare program. For example, it may be necessary to disclose information about the Medicare benefits you have used to a hospital or doctor.

With one exception, which is discussed below, there are no penalties under social security law for refusing to supply information. However, failure to furnish information regarding the medical services rendered or the amount charged would prevent payment of the claim. Failure to furnish any other information, such as name or claim number, would delay payment of the claim.

It is mandatory that you tell us if you are being treated for a work related injury so we can determine whether worker's compensation will pay for the treatment. Section 1877 (a) (3) of the Social Security Act provides criminal penalties for withholding this information.

✿ U.S. GOVERNMENT PRINTING OFFICE: 1987-706-734

Appendix E: Sample Explanation of Medicare Benefits

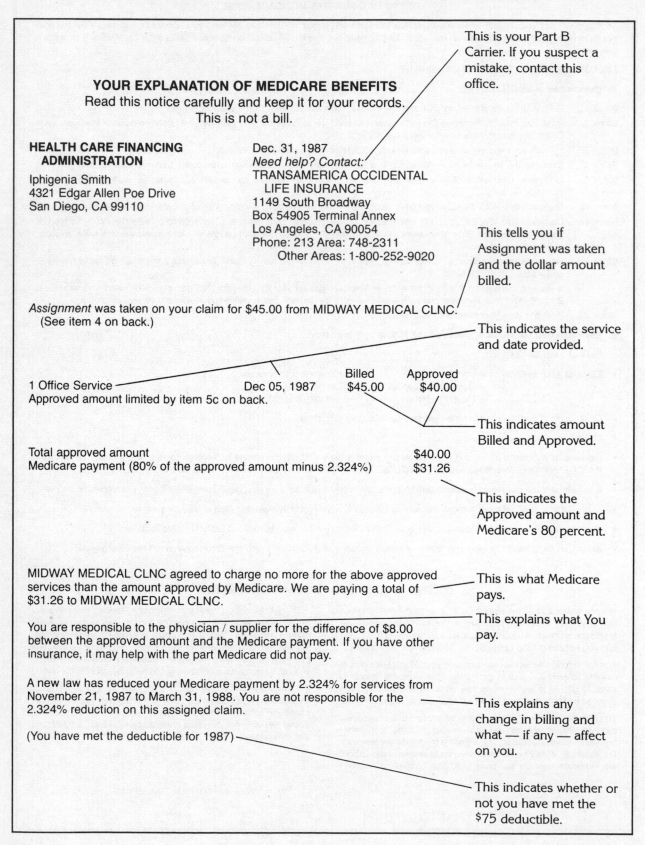

This is your Part B Carrier. If you suspect a mistake, contact this office.

YOUR EXPLANATION OF MEDICARE BENEFITS
Read this notice carefully and keep it for your records.
This is not a bill.

HEALTH CARE FINANCING ADMINISTRATION

Iphigenia Smith
4321 Edgar Allen Poe Drive
San Diego, CA 99110

Dec. 31, 1987
Need help? Contact:
TRANSAMERICA OCCIDENTAL LIFE INSURANCE
1149 South Broadway
Box 54905 Terminal Annex
Los Angeles, CA 90054
Phone: 213 Area: 748-2311
    Other Areas: 1-800-252-9020

This tells you if Assignment was taken and the dollar amount billed.

Assignment was taken on your claim for $45.00 from MIDWAY MEDICAL CLNC.
    (See item 4 on back.)

This indicates the service and date provided.

		Billed	Approved
1 Office Service	Dec 05, 1987	$45.00	$40.00

Approved amount limited by item 5c on back.

This indicates amount Billed and Approved.

Total approved amount	$40.00
Medicare payment (80% of the approved amount minus 2.324%)	$31.26

This indicates the Approved amount and Medicare's 80 percent.

MIDWAY MEDICAL CLNC agreed to charge no more for the above approved services than the amount approved by Medicare. We are paying a total of $31.26 to MIDWAY MEDICAL CLNC.

This is what Medicare pays.

You are responsible to the physician / supplier for the difference of $8.00 between the approved amount and the Medicare payment. If you have other insurance, it may help with the part Medicare did not pay.

This explains what You pay.

A new law has reduced your Medicare payment by 2.324% for services from November 21, 1987 to March 31, 1988. You are not responsible for the 2.324% reduction on this assigned claim.

This explains any change in billing and what — if any — affect on you.

(You have met the deductible for 1987)

This indicates whether or not you have met the $75 deductible.

IMPORTANT: If you do not agree with the amounts approved you may ask for a review. To do this you must *write* to us before *Jun 31, 1988.* (See item 1 on the back.)

— This gives you the time frame to file any appeal.

DO YOU HAVE A QUESTION ABOUT THIS NOTICE? If you believe Medicare paid for a service you did not receive, or there is an error, contact us immediately. Always give us the:

Medicare Claim No. 987 65 4321A   Claim Control No. 7350 316 290

Use these numbers when making any inquiry on your claim.

CODE
—of—
PRACTICE

As a PMS Code of Practice practitioner, I will assist you in finding information resources, support groups and health care providers to help you maintain and improve your health. When you seek my care for specific problems, I will abide by the following Code of Practice:

Office Procedures

1. I will post or provide a printed schedule of my fees for office visits, procedures, testing and surgery, and provide itemized bills.

2. I will provide certain hours each week when I will be available for non-emergency telephone consultation.

3. I will schedule appointments to allow the necessary time to see you with minimal waiting. I will promptly report test results to you and return phone calls.

4. I will allow and encourage you to bring a friend or relative into the examining room with you.

5. I will facilitate your getting your medical and hospital records, and will provide you with copies of your test results.

Choice in Diagnosis and Treatment

6. I will let you know your prognosis, including whether your condition is terminal or will cause disability or pain, and will explain why I believe further diagnostic activity or treatment is necessary.

7. I will discuss diagnostic, treatment and medication options for your particular problem with you (including the option of no treatment) and describe in understandable terms the risk of each alternative, the chances of success, the possibility of pain, the effect on your functioning, the number of visits each would entail, and the cost of each alternative.

8. I will describe my qualifications to perform the proposed diagnostic measures or treatments.

9. I will let you know of organizations, support groups, and medical and lay publications that can assist you in understanding, monitoring and treating your problem.

10. I will not proceed until you are satisfied that you understand the benefits and risks of each alternative and I have your agreement on a particular course of action.

≡People's Medical Society®
14 E. Minor Street • Emmaus, PA 18049

Appendix G: Books for a People's Medical Library

This list is a suggestion of what a basic People's Medical Library might contain.

Advanced First Aid and Emergency Care. The American Red Cross. New York: Doubleday and Company, 1986.

Advice for the Patient: Drug Information in Lay Language, 8th edition. Rockville, Md.: United States Pharmacopeial Convention, Inc., 1988.

American Medical Directory, 30th edition. Chicago, Ill.: American Medical Association, 1988.

Cancer: Principles and Practice of Oncology, 2d revised edition, edited by Vincent T. Devita, Jr., et al. Philadelphia: J. B. Lippincott, 1985.

Cancer Book. The American Cancer Society. New York: Doubleday & Company, 1986.

Caring for Your Parents, by H. MacLean. New York: Doubleday & Company, 1987.

Cecil Textbook of Medicine, 17th edition, edited by James Wyngaarden and Lloyd Smith. Philadelphia: W. B. Saunders, 1985.

Chemotherapy and You. National Cancer Institute. Bethesda, Md.: U.S. Department of Health and Human Services, 1987.

Choices: Realistic Alternatives in Cancer Treatment, revised and updated, by Marion Morra and Eve Potts. New York: Avon Books, 1987.

Coming Back: A Guide to Recovering from Heart Attack, by K. Cohn and D. Duke. Reading, Mass.: Addison-Wesley Publishing Co., 1987.

Conquering AIDS Now with Natural Treatment: A Non-Drug Approach, by B. Leonard and S. Gregory. New York: Warner Books, 1986.

Current Medical Diagnosis and Treatment, 26th edition, by Marcus Krupp and Milton L. Chatton. Los Altos, Calif.: Appleton-Lange, 1987.

Current Obstetric and Gynecologic Diagnosis and Treatment, 6th edition, by Ralph C. Benson and Matin Pernoll. Los Altos, Calif.: Appleton-Lange, 1987.

Current Surgical Diagnosis and Treatment, 7th edition, by L. W. Way. Los Altos, Calif.: Appleton-Lange, 1985.

Dermatology, 2d edition, by Samuel L. Moschella et al. Philadelphia: W. B. Saunders, 1985.

Directory of Medical Specialists, 23d edition. Chicago: Marquis Who's Who, 1987.

Do-It-Yourself Medical Testing, by Cathey and Edward Pinckney. New York: Facts on File, 1983.

Dorland's Illustrated Medical Dictionary, 26th edition, Philadelphia: W. B. Saunders, 1985.

Drug Information for the Consumer. Mount Vernon, N.Y.: Consumer Reports' Books, 1987.

General Ophthalmology, 11th edition, by Daniel Vaughn and Taylor Asbury. Los Altos, Calif.: Appleton-Lange, 1986.

Harrison's Principles of Internal Medicine, 11th edition, by Paul I. Jagger and Eugene Brauwald. New York: McGraw-Hill, 1987.

Health Care U.S.A.: Where to Find the Best Answers to Your Family Medical Health Problems, by J. Carper. New York: Prentice Hall Press, 1987.

Heart Attacks, Hypertension and Heart Drugs, by G. Kahn. Emmaus, Penn.: Rodale Press, 1986.

How to Avoid a Hysterectomy, by Lynn Payer. New York: Pantheon Books, 1987.

How to Evaluate and Select a Nursing Home, by R. Barker Bausell, Ph.D., Michael A. Rooney, M.P.A., and Charles B. Inlander. Reading, Mass.: Addison-Wesley, 1988.

How to Keep Your Child Fit from Birth to Six, by Bonnie Prudden. New York: Ballantine Books, 1986.

Living with Chronic Illness, by C. Register. New York: Free Press, 1987.

Mastering Pain, by R. Sternbach. New York: G. P. Putnam's Sons, 1987.

Mayo Clinic Diet Manual: A Handbook of Dietary Practices, 5th edition. Philadelphia: W. B. Saunders, 1981.

Medical Self-Care and Assessment, by Brent Q. Hafen, Molly J. Brog, and Kathryn J. Fransden. Englewood, Colo.: Morton, 1983.

Medical Self-Care Book of Women's Health, by Sadja Greenwood and Michael Castleman. Garden City, N.Y.: Doubleday, 1987.

Medicine on Trial, by Charles B. Inlander, Lowell Levin, Ed.D., and Ed Weiner. New York: Prentice-Hall, 1988.

Merck Manual of Diagnosis and Treatment, 15th edition, edited by Robert Berkow, M.D., et al. Rahway, N.J.: Merck, Sharp and Dohme, 1987.

Multiple Sclerosis: New Hope and Practical Advice for People with Multiple Sclerosis and Their Families, by L. Rosner and S. Ross. New York: Prentice Hall Press, 1987.

People's Book of Medical Tests, by Tom Ferguson, M.D., and David Sobel, M.D. New York: Summit Books, 1985.

Rodale's Encyclopedia of Natural Home Remedies, by Mark Bricklin. Emmaus, Penn.: Rodale Press, 1982.

Standard First Aid and Personal Safety. The American Red Cross. New York: Doubleday & Company, 1986.

Staying Healthy Without Medicine, by Daniel P. Marshall, J. Gregory Rabold, and Edgar S. Wilson. Chicago: Nelson Hall, 1983.

Take Care of Yourself: A Consumer's Guide to Medical Care, 3d edition, by Donald M. Vickery, M.D., and James F. Fries, M.D. Reading, Mass.: Addison-Wesley, 1986.

Take this Book to the Hospital with You, by Charles B. Inlander and Ed Weiner. Emmaus, Penn.: Rodale Press, 1985.

The American Medical Association Family Medical Guide, revised edition, edited by Jeffery R. Kuntz et al. New York: Random House 1987.

The American Medical Association Home Medical Adviser, edited by Charles Clayman, M.D., et al. New York: Random House, 1988.

The Columbia University College of Physicians and Surgeons Complete Home Medical Guide, edited by Donald F. Tapley, M.D., et al. New York: Crown Publishers, Inc., 1985.

The Essential Guide to Prescription Drugs, 6th edition, by James W. Long. New York: Harper & Row, 1988.

The Family Handbook of Medical Tests, by C. Eron and C. Horn. New York: Perigee Books, 1985.

The Food and Drug Interaction Books, by B. Morgan. New York: Simon & Schuster, 1986.

The Layman's Guide to Acupuncture, by Y. Manaka and I. Urguahart. New York: Weatherhill Press, 1986.

The New People's Pharmacy Book: A Guide to Prescription Drugs, by Joe Graedon. New York: Bantam Books, 1985.

The Older People's Pharmacy, by Joe Graedon. New York: Bantam Books, 1988.

The Patient's Guide to Medical Tests, 3rd revised and expanded edition, by Cathey and Edward Pinckney. New York: Facts on File, 1987.

The People's Medical Manual, by Howard R. and Martha E. Lewis. Garden City, N.Y.: Doubleday & Company, 1986.

The Practical Encyclopedia of Natural Healing, revised edition by Mark Bricklin. Emmaus, Penn.: Rodale Press, 1987.

Third Opinion, by John M. Fink. Garden City, N.Y.: 1988.

When Someone You Know Has AIDS, A Practical Guide, by L. Matelli and F. Peltz. New York: Crown Publishers, 1987.

Womancare: A Gynecological Guide to Your Body, by Linda Madras and Jane Patterson. New York: Avon Books, 1984.

Appendix H: Durable Power of Attorney Forms and Living Wills

| STATE | DURABLE POWER OF ATTORNEY (DPA) STATUTE | | OTHER STATUTES |
	CITATION	APPLIES TO HEALTH-CARE DECISIONS, EXPRESSLY OR BY INTERPRETATION	CF = PROVISIONS ALLOWING PERSONAL NOMINATION OF COURT-APPOINTED FIDUCIARIES[1] LW = PROVISIONS IN LIVING WILL STATUTES SPECIFYING HEALTH-CARE PROXY[2]
AL	Ala. Code §26-1-2 (Repl. 1986)		CF Ala. Code §26-1-2(c)(2) (Repl. 1986)
AK	Alaska Stat. §§13.26.325, 13.26.330 (1985)		CF Alaska Stat. §13.26.145(d)(1) (1985)
AZ	Ariz. Rev. Stat. Ann. §§14-5501, 14-5502 (1975)	Treatment wishes might be shown in DPA or proxy appointment. *Rasmusssen v. Fleming,* No. CV-86-0450-PR, slip op. at 26-27 n. 21 (Ariz. July 23, 1987)	
AR	Ark. Stat. Ann. §§58-501 to 58-511 (Repl. 1971 & Supp. 1985), §§58-701 to 58-704 (Supp. 1985)		CF Ark. Stat. Ann. §58-703(b) (Supp. 1985) LW 1987 Ark. Acts 713 §§1(10), 2
CA	Cal. Civ. Code §§2400-07, 2430-44, 2450-57, 2460-73, 2500-08, 2510-13 (West Supp. 1987)	DPA specifies that proxy may consent to or refuse medical treatment. See §§2410(b), 2411(h), 2411(i), 2412.5, 2417(h), 2421(c), 2421(d), 2430-44, 2500-08 (West Supp. 1987)	CF Cal. Civ. Code 22402(b) (West Supp. 1987)
CO	Colo. Rev. Stat. §§15-14-501, 15-14-502 (Supp. 1986)	DPA "may relate to any . . . matter . . . including by way of illustration but not limitation . . . power to consent to . . . any medical . . . treatment." Colo. Rev. Stat. §15-14-501 (Suppl. 1986) DPA may authorize proxy to refuse treatment. *In re Rodas,* No. 86PR139, slip op. at 34-35, 38 (Colo. Dist. Ct. Mesa County Jan. 22, 1987)	CF Colo. Rev. Stat. §14-14-311(2)(b) (1973 & Supp. 1986) LW Attorney-in-fact under DPA statute should, under certain circumstances, be notified that "certificate of terminal condition" is signed. Colo. Rev. Stat. §15-18-107 (Supp. 1986)
CT	Conn. Gen. Stat. Ann. §§1-42 to 1-56 (West 1969); §45-69o (West Supp. 1987)	DPA "may be persuasive relative to surrogate decision-making, [but] it is not . . . dispositive. Such factors as the nature of the	CF Conn. Gen. Stat. §45-70 (West Supp. 1987)

| STATE | DURABLE POWER OF ATTORNEY (DPA) STATUTE | | OTHER STATUTES |
	CITATION	APPLIES TO HEALTH-CARE DECISIONS, EXPRESSLY OR BY INTERPRETATION	CF = PROVISIONS ALLOWING PERSONAL NOMINATION OF COURT-APPOINTED FIDUCIARIES[1] LW = PROVISIONS IN LIVING WILL STATUTES SPECIFYING HEALTH-CARE PROXY[2]
		relationship between the patient and the surrogate, the type of medical treatment (or nontreatment) at issue, prior expressions if any, by the patient, to name a few, would be taken into account before honoring a surrogate-medical request by an individual named in a durable power of attorney." 9/3/86 letter from Assistant Attorney General	
DE	Del. Code Ann. tit. 12, §§4901 to 4905 (Supp. 1986)		CF Del. Code Ann. tit. 12, §4903(a) (Supp. 1986) LW Del. Code Ann. tit. 16, §2502(b) (Repl. 1983)
DC	D.C. Code Ann. §§21-2081 to 21-2085 (Supp. 1987)		CF D.C. Code Ann. §§21-2043(b), 21-2083(b) (Supp. 1987)
FL	Fla. Stat. Ann. §709.08 (West Supp. 1987)		LW Fla. Stat. Ann. §765.05(2) (1986)
GA	Ga. Code. Ann. §§10-6-5, 10-6-36 (1982)		CF Ga. Code Ann. §29-5-2(c)(1) (1986)
HI	Hawaii Rev. Stat. §§560:5-501, 5-502 (Repl. 1987)	No health-care language in DPA but living will statute refers to DPA as document of intent	LW Hawaii Rev. Stat. §327D-26 (Supp. 1986)
ID	Idaho Code §§15-5-501 to 15-5-507 (Supp. 1987), §§39-4502 to 39-4506 (Supp. 1986)	No health-care language in DPA statute, but living will statute amended to allow DPA for health care[3]	CF Idaho Code §15-5-503(2) (Supp. 1987) LW Idaho Code §§39-4502 to 39-4506 (Supp. 1986)[3]
IL	1987 Ill. Pub. Act No. 85-704	DPA can be used to delegate power to consent, refuse consent, or withdraw consent to treatment. 1987 Ill. Pub. Act No. 85-701, Article IV	CF Ill. Ann. Stat. ch. 110 1/2, §11a-6 (Smith-Hurd Supp. 1987)
IN	Ind. Code Ann. §§30-2-11-1 to 30-2-11-7 (Burns Supp. 1986)		CF Ind. Code Ann. §30-2-11(3)(b) (Burns Supp. 1986) LW Ind. Code Ann. §16-8-11-14(g)(2) (Burns Supp. 1986)[4]
IA	Iowa Code Ann. §§633.705, 633.706 (West Supp. 1987)	No health-care language in DPA statute, but explicitly in living will statute[4]	IW Iowa Code Ann. §144.A.7(1)(a) (Supp. 1986)[4]

| STATE | DURABLE POWER OF ATTORNEY (DPA) STATUTE | | OTHER STATUTES |
	CITATION	APPLIES TO HEALTH-CARE DECISIONS, EXPRESSLY OR BY INTERPRETATION	CF = PROVISIONS ALLOWING PERSONAL NOMINATION OF COURT-APPOINTED FIDUCIARIES[1] LW = PROVISIONS IN LIVING WILL STATUTES SPECIFYING HEALTH-CARE PROXY[2]
KS	Kan. Stat. Ann. §§58-610 to 58-617 (1983)		CF Kan. Stat. Ann. §58-612(b) (1983)
KY	Ky. Rev. Stat. Ann. §386.093 (Michie 1984)		CF Ky. Rev. Stat. §387.600(2) (Michie 1984)
LA	La. Civ. Code Ann. art. 3027 (West Supp. 1987)		CF La. Code Civ. Proc. Ann. art. 4550 (West Supp. 1987) LW La. Rev. Stat. Ann. §40:1299.58.3(c)(1) (West Supp. 1987)
ME	Me. Rev. Stat. Ann. tit. 18-A, §§5-501, 5-502 (1981 & Supp. 1986)	DPA authority includes power to withhold consent to any medical treatment. Me. Rev. Stat. Ann. tit. 18-A, §5-501 (Supp. 1986)	CF Me. Rev. Stat. Ann. tit. 18-A, §5-311(b)(1) (1981)
MD	Md. Est. & Trust Code Ann. §§13-601 to 13-603 (1974)	Health-care reference contained in Md. Health General Code Ann. §20-107(d) (Supp. 1986)[5]	CF Md. Est. & Trust §13-707(a)(1) (West 1987)
MA	Mass. Gen. Laws Ann. ch. 201B §§1 to 7 (West Supp. 1987)		CF Mass. Gen. Laws Ann. ch. 201B, §3(b) (West Supp. 1987)
MI	Mich. Comp. Laws Ann. §700.495 (West 1980)		CF Mich. Comp. Laws Ann. §700.454(2) (West 1987)
MN	Minn. Stat. Ann. §§523.01 to 523.25 (West Supp. 1987)		CF Minn. Stat. Ann. §525.544(1) (West Supp. 1987) "interested person" can seek to enforce patient rights, including right to refuse treatment; patient can choose representative to participate in planning treatment. Minn. Stat. Ann. §144.651(1), (9), (11), (19), §144.335(a) (Supp. 1987)
MS	Miss. Code Ann. §87-3-13 (Supp. 1986)		
MO	Mo. Ann Stat. §§486.550 to 486.595 (Vernon Supp. 1987)		CF Mo. Stat. Ann. §475.050(1) (Vernon Supp. 1987)
MT	Mont. Code Ann. §§72-5-501, 72-5-502 (1985)		CF Mont. Code Ann. §§72-5-312(2)(a), 72-5-501(2) (1985)
NE	Neb. Rev. Stat. §§30-2664 to 30-2675 (1985)		CF Neb. Rev. Stat. §30-2667(2) (1985)

| STATE | DURABLE POWER OF ATTORNEY (DPA) STATUTE | | OTHER STATUTES |
	CITATION	APPLIES TO HEALTH-CARE DECISIONS, EXPRESSLY OR BY INTERPRETATION	CF = PROVISIONS ALLOWING PERSONAL NOMINATION OF COURT-APPOINTED FIDUCIARIES[1] LW = PROVISIONS IN LIVING WILL STATUTES SPECIFYING HEALTH-CARE PROXY[2]
NV	Nev. Rev. Stat. §§111.460, 111.470 (1986)	DPA can be used to delegate power to consent, refuse consent, or withdraw consent to any treatment. 1987 Nev. Stat. ch. 396	CF Nev. Rev. Stat. §159.061(1) (1986)
NH	N.H. Rev. Stat. Ann. §506:6 (Supp. 1986)		
NJ	N.J. Stat. Ann. §§46:2B-8, 2B-9 (West Supp. 1987)	General DPA statutes can be used to delegate all-health care decisions, including termination-of-treatment decisions. *In re Peter,* slip op. at 13-14, to be reported at 108 N.J. 365, 529 A.2d 419 (1987)	
NM	N.M. Stat. Ann. §§45-5-501, 45-5-502 (1978)		
NY	N.Y. Gen. Oblig. Law §§5-1501 to 5-1601 (McKinney 1978 & Supp. 1986)	Medical proxies may decline treatment for patients with unambiguous living wills. *Evans v. Bellevue Hosp.,* No. 16536/87, slip op. at 2, 8 (N.Y. Sup. Ct. N.Y. County July 27, 1987) DPA can be used to specifically delegate the responsibility to communicate a person's decision to decline treatment under defined circumstances but not to generally delegate medical decisions (absent legislation). Op. Att. Gen. 84-F16 (Dec. 1984) N.Y. Task Force on Life and the Law supports act authorizing medical agents to consent, withhold consent, and withdraw consent to treatment (1987)	CF N.Y. Mental Hyg. Law §78.05 (McKinney 1978) proxy appointments authorized for "do not resuscitate" decisions. N.Y. Pub. Health Law §2965(b), 1987 N.Y. Laws Ch. 818
NC	N.C. Gen. Stat. §§32A-1 to 32A-14 (1984 Supp. 1985)	DPA short forms can be used for "personal relations and affairs," including principal health care. N.C. Gen. Stat. §§32A-1(9), 32A-2(9) (1984)	CF N.C. Gen. Stat. §32A-10(b) (1984)
ND	N.D. Cent. Code §§30.1-30-01 to 30.1-30-05 (Supp. 1987)		CF N.D. Cent. Code §§30.1-30-03.2 (Supp. 1987)

| STATE | DURABLE POWER OF ATTORNEY (DPA) STATUTE | | OTHER STATUTES |
	CITATION	APPLIES TO HEALTH-CARE DECISIONS, EXPRESSLY OR BY INTERPRETATION	CF = PROVISIONS ALLOWING PERSONAL NOMINATION OF COURT-APPOINTED FIDUCIARIES[1] LW = PROVISIONS IN LIVING WILL STATUTES SPECIFYING HEALTH-CARE PROXY[2]
OH	Ohio Rev. Code Ann. §§1337.09, 1337.091 (Page Supp. 1986)		CF Ohio Rev. Code Ann. §§1337.09(B), 2111.02, 2111.121(A) (Page Supp. 1986)
OK	Okla. Stat. Ann. tit. 58, §§1051 to 1062 (West Supp. 1987)		CF Okla. Stat. Ann. tit. 58, §896 (West 1965)
OR	Or. Rev. Stat. §§126.407, 126.413 (Repl. 1985)		CF Or. Rev. Stat. §126.035(1) (Repl. 1985)
PA	Pa. Stat. Ann. tit. 20, §§5601 to 5607 (Purdon Supp. 1987)	DPA can be used to authorize consent to medical procedures. Pa. Stat. Ann. tit. 20, §§5602(a)(9), 5603(h) (Purdon Supp. 1987)	CF Pa. Stat. Ann. tit. 20, §5604(c)(2) (Purdon Supp. 1987)
RI	R.I. Gen. Laws §34-22-6.1 (1984), §§23-4.10-1 to 23-4.10-2 (Supp. 1986)	Statutory form authorizes authority to consent, to refuse to consent, or to withdraw consent to any care, treatment, service, or procedure to maintain, diagnose, or treat a physical or mental condition, subject to declarant's desires and limitations expressed in the document. R.I. Gen. Laws §23-4.10-2 (Supp. 1986)	
SC	S.C. Code Ann. §§62-5-501, 62-5-502 (1987)		CF S.C. Code Ann. §62-5-311(5), 62-5-410(2) (1987)
SD	S.D. Codified Laws Ann. §§59-7-2.1 to 59-7-2.4 (Repl. 1978)		CF S.D. Codified Laws Ann. §30-27-25 (Repl. 1984)
TN	Tenn. Code Ann. §§34-6-101 to 34-6-107 (Repl. 1984)		CF Tenn. Code Ann. §34-6-104(b) (Repl. 1984)
TX	Tex. Prob. Code Ann. §36A (Vernon 1980)	Power of attorney signed by the patient with "appropriate formalities" is one of the "most probative" forms of evidence of the patient's wishes. *Newman v. William Beaumont Army Medical Center,* No. EP-86-CA-276, slip op. at 7 (W.D. Tex. Oct. 30, 1986)	CF Tex. Prob. Code Ann. §118A (Vernon Supp. 1987) LW Tex. Rev. Civ. Stat. Ann. art. §4590h(3)(e) (Vernon Supp. 1987)
UT	Utah Code Ann. §§75-5-5-1, 75-5-502 (Repl. 1978)		LW Utah Code Ann. §75-2-1106 (Supp. 1986)[6]

| STATE | DURABLE POWER OF ATTORNEY (DPA) STATUTE | | OTHER STATUTES |
	CITATION	APPLIES TO HEALTH-CARE DECISIONS, EXPRESSLY OR BY INTERPRETATION	CF = PROVISIONS ALLOWING PERSONAL NOMINATION OF COURT-APPOINTED FIDUCIARIES[1] LW = PROVISIONS IN LIVING WILL STATUTES SPECIFYING HEALTH-CARE PROXY[2]
VT	Vt. Stat. Ann. tit. 14, §§3051, 3052 (Supp. 1986)		CF Vt. Stat. Ann. tit. 14, §3072(b) (Supp. 1986)
VA	Va. Code §§11-9.1 to 11-9.4 (Repl. 1984 & Supp. 1987)	"[W]ithout express language in a durable power of attorney document delegating the decision-making in a manner conforming with the express provisions of the Natural Death Act, a durable power of attorney would probably have no effect." 8/7/86 letter from Assistant Attorney General	LW Va. Code §§54-325:8:4, 54-325:8:6.2 (Supp. 1986)
WA	Wash. Rev. Code Ann. §§11.94.010 to 11.94.900 (Supp. 1987)		CF Wash. Rev. Code Ann. §11.94.010(1) (Supp. 1987) DPA which "encompasses the authority to make health-care decisions" can consent to health care. 1987 Wash. Laws Ch. 162 §(1)(b)
WV	W. Va. Code §§39-4-1 to 39-4-7 (Supp. 1987)		CF W. Va. Code §39-4-3(b) (Supp. 1987)
WI	Wis. Stat. Ann. §243.07 (West Supp. 1986)		CF Wis. Stat. Ann. §243.07(3)(b) (West Supp. 1986)
WY	Wyo. Stat. §§3-5-101 to 3-5-103 (Supp. 1985)		LW Wyo. Stat. §33-26-145(d) (Supp. 1986)

Notes for chart

1. "Fiduciaries" includes guardians, conservators, committees, or trustees. Some of the statutes allow people to make nominations before any court action is commenced, while others allow the people subject to the action to provide information about their fiduciary preferences once the proceedings begin. Specific family consent and fiduciary laws in each state should also be consulted to determine whether they affect the ability of these people to make medical treatment decisions.

2. "Living will" legislation is a generic term (also called "natural death," "rights of the terminally ill" and "right-to-die" legislation) applied to statutes providing for patients to execute advance directives for health-care decisions. The majority of living will laws allow people to individualize their instructions; this may permit proxy appointments.

3. Idaho legislators recently amended the state's natural death statute, apparently intending to authorize durable powers of attorney for health care. However, the declaration form in the amended law, which must be precisely followed, does not include a means of naming a specific proxy. Until the legislature corrects this error, the best way for Idaho residents to designate a health-care proxy may still be the Idaho durable power form.

4. Indiana statute does not directly address proxy appointment, but by providing for consultation between attending physician and patient's representative under specified circumstances, statute by inference provides for proxy appointment. Iowa Code §144.A.7(1)(a) explicitly provides that under certain circumstances an attorney-in-fact designated to make health-care decisions under the durable power statute should be consulted if there is no living will.

5. This "substituted consent" law for disabled individuals states that "in the absence of a durable power of attorney that relates to medical care and is executed under [the durable power statute, specified] individuals may give a substituted consent for furnishing medical . . . treatment to a disabled individual."

6. Statute contains Special Power of Attorney form, to be substantially followed, which must be executed before notary public.

Health-care power of attorney forms specifically authorized by statute or case law; advance declaration forms that specifically comply with the 39 living will statutes enacted to date; and Living Will Declaration form offered to residents of states lacking living will legislation are available on request from Society for the Right to Die, 250 West 57th Street, New York, NY 10107.

**Society for the
Right to Die**

250 West 57th Street/New York, NY 10107

Living Will Declaration

*INSTRUCTIONS
Consult this column for help and
guidance.*

To My Family, Doctors, and All Those Concerned with My Care

I, _____, being of sound mind,
make this statement as a directive to be followed if I become unable to
participate in decisions regarding my medical care.

*This declaration sets forth your
directions regarding medical
treatment.*

If I should be in an incurable or irreversible mental or physical condition
with no reasonable expectation of recovery, I direct my attending physician
to withhold or withdraw treatment that merely prolongs my dying. I further
direct that treatment be limited to measures to keep me comfortable and to
relieve pain.

*You have the right to refuse
treatment you do not want, and
you may request the care you
do want.*

These directions express my legal right to refuse treatment. Therefore I
expect my family, doctors, and everyone concerned with my care to regard
themselves as legally and morally bound to act in accord with my wishes,
and in so doing to be free of any legal liability for having followed my
directions.

*You may list specific treatment
you do not want. For example:*

   *Cardiac resuscitation
   Mechanical respiration
   Artificial feeding/fluids by tubes*

*Otherwise, your general
statement, top right, will stand
for your wishes.*

I especially do not want: _____
_____
_____
_____
_____
_____

*You may want to add
instructions for care you do
want—for example, pain
medication; or that you prefer
to die at home if possible.*

Other instructions/comments: _____
_____
_____
_____

*If you want, you can name
someone to see that your wishes
are carried out, but you do not
have to do this.*

Proxy Designation Clause: Should I become unable to communicate my instructions as stated above, I designate the following person to act in my behalf:

Name_____

Address_____

If the person I have named above is unable to act in my behalf, I authorize the
following person to do so:

Name_____

Address_____

*Sign and date here in the
presence of two adult witnesses,
who should also sign.*

Signed: _____ Date: _____

Witness: _____ Witness: _____

*Keep the signed original with your personal papers at home. Give signed copies
to doctors, family, and proxy. Review your Declaration from time to time; initial
and date it to show it still expresses your intent.*

- -

Tear off and mail to: Society for the Right to Die, 250 West 57th Street, New York, NY 10107.

The Annual Report of the Society for the Right to Die is available from NY State Dept. of State, Office of Charitable Contributions, 162 Washington Ave., Albany, NY 12230

Please send me   additional copies of the Living Will Declaration.
☐ I am enclosing my tax-deductible dues/contribution in support of the Society's program.
   (Please make check payable to Society for the Right to Die. Minimum annual membership dues: $15.)
     ☐ $15   ☐ $35   ☐ $100   ☐ Other $

Name

Street Address

City   State   Zip

☐ I am enclosing names and addresses of others to receive information from the Society.

Sample of document distributed in states with living will laws.

DECLARATION

Declaration made this _____ day of _____ (month, year).

I, _____, being of sound mind, willfully and voluntarily direct that my dying shall not be artificially prolonged under the circumstances set forth in this declaration.

If at any time I should have an incurable injury, disease, or illness certified to be a terminal condition by two (2) physicians who have personally examined me, one (1) of whom shall be my attending physician, and the physicians have determined that my death is imminent and will occur whether or not life-sustaining procedures are utilized and where the application of such procedures would serve only to artificially prolong the dying process, I direct that such procedures be withheld or withdrawn, and that I be permitted to die naturally with only the administration of medication, the administration of food and water, and the performance of any medical procedure that is necessary to provide comfort care or alleviate pain. In the absence of my ability to give directions regarding the use of such life-sustaining procedures, it is my intention that this declaration shall be honored by my family and physician(s) as the final expression of my right to control my medical care and treatment.

Other instructions :

I am legally competent to make this declaration, and I understand its full import.

Signed _____

Address _____

Under penalty of perjury, we state that this declaration was signed by

_____ in the presence of the undersigned who, at his/her request, in his/her presence, and in the presence of each other, have hereunto signed our names and witnessed this _____ day of _____, 19_____. Further each of us, individually, states that: The declarant is known to me, and I believe the declarant to be of sound mind. I did not sign the declarant's signature to this declaration. Based upon information and belief, I am not related to the declarant by blood or marriage, a creditor of the declarant, entitled to any portion of the estate of the declarant under any existing testamentary instrument of the declarant, entitled to any financial benefit by reason of the death of the declarant, financially or otherwise responsible for the declarant's medical care, or an employee of any such person or institution.

_____ Address _____
_____
_____ Address _____
_____

1086

Courtesy of Society for the Right to Die, 250 West 57 Street, New York, NY 10107.

- -

Tear off and mail to: Society for the Right to Die, 250 West 57 Street, New York, NY 10107.

The Annual Report of Society for the Right to Die is available from NY State Dept. of State, Office of Charitable Contributions, 162 Washington Ave., Albany, NY 12230.

Please send me _____ additional copies of the Maryland Declaration.

☐ I am enclosing my tax-deductible dues/contribution in support of the Society's program.
       (Please make check payable to Society for the Right to Die. Minimum annual membership dues: $15.)
              ☐ $15   ☐ $35   ☐ $100   ☐ Other $_____

Name _____

Street Address _____

City _____ State _____ Zip _____

☐ I am enclosing names and addresses of others to receive information from the Society.

294

Appendix I: Hospital Patient's Bill of Rights

The American Hospital Association presents *A Patient's Bill of Rights* with the expectation that observance of these rights will contribute to more effective patient care and greater satisfaction for the patient, his physician, and the hospital organization. Further, the Association presents these rights in the expectation that they will be supported by the hospital on behalf of its patients as an integral part of the healing process. It is recognized that a personal relationship between the physician and the patient is essential for the provision of proper medical care.

The traditional physician-patient relationship takes on a new dimension when care is rendered within an organizational structure. Legal precedent has established that the institution itself also has a responsibility to the patient. It is in recognition of these factors that these rights are affirmed.

1. The patient has the right to considerate and respectful care.

2. The patient has the right to obtain from his physician complete current information concerning his diagnosis, treatment, and prognosis in terms the patient can be reasonably expected to understand. When it is not medically advisable to give such information to the patient, the information should be made available to an appropriate person in his behalf. He has the right to know, by name, the physician responsible for coordinating his care.

3. The patient has the right to receive from his physician information necessary to give informed consent prior to the start of any procedure and/or treatment. Except in emergencies, such information for informed consent should include, but not necessarily be limited to, the specific procedure and/or treatment, the medically significant risks involved, and the probable duration of incapacitation. Where medically significant alternatives for care or treatment exist, or when the patient requests information concerning medical alternatives, the patient has the right to such information. The patient also has the right to know the name of the person responsible for the procedures and/or treatment.

4. The patient has the right to refuse treatment to the extent permitted by law and to be informed of the medical consequences of his action.

5. The patient has the right to every consideration of his privacy concerning his own medical care program. Case discussion, consultation, examination, and treatment are confidential and should be conducted discreetly. Those not directly involved in his care must have the permission of the patient to be present.

6. The patient has the right to expect that all communications and records pertaining to his care should be treated as confidential.

7. The patient has the right to expect that within its capacity a hospital must make reasonable response to the request of a patient for services. The hospital must provide evaluation, service, and/or referral as indicated by the urgency of the case. When medically permissible, a patient may be transferred to another facility only after he has received complete information and explanation concerning the needs for and alternatives to such a transfer. The institution to which the patient is to be transferred must first have accepted the patient for transfer.

8. The patient has the right to obtain information as to any relationship of his hospital to other health care and educational institutions insofar as his care is concerned. The patient has the right to obtain information as to the existence of any professional relationships among individuals, by name, who are treating him.

9. The patient has the right to be advised if the hospital proposes to engage in or perform human experimentation affecting his care or treatment. The patient has the right to refuse to participate in such research projects.

10. The patient has the right to expect reasonable continuity of care. He has the right to know in advance what appointment times and physicians are available and where. The patient has the right to expect that the hospital will provide a mechanism whereby he is informed by his physician or a delegate of the physician of the patient's continuing health care requirements following discharge.

11. The patient has the right to examine and receive an explanation of his bill, regardless of source of payment.

12. The patient has the right to know what hospital rules and regulations apply to his conduct as a patient.

No catalog of rights can guarantee for the patient the kind of treatment he has a right to expect. A hospital has many functions to perform, including the prevention and treatment of disease, the education of both health professionals and patients, and the conduct of clinical research. All these activities must be conducted with an overriding concern for the patient, and, above all, the recognition of his dignity as a human being. Success in achieving this recognition ensures success in the defense of the rights of the patient.

Appendix J: State Peer Review Organizations

Alabama
Alabama Quality Assurance
    Foundation
236 Goodwin Crest Drive, Suite 300
Twin Towers East Building
Birmingham, AL 35209
205-942-0785

Alaska
Professional Review Organization for
    Washington
(see Washington)

Arizona
Health Services Advisory Group
301 E. Bethany Home Road
Suite B-157
P.O. Box 16731
Phoenix, AZ 85014
602-264-6382

Arkansas
Arkansas Foundation for Medical
    Care
P.O. Box 1508
809 Garrison Avenue
Fort Smith, AR 72902
501-785-2471

California
California Medical Review, Inc.
1388 Sutter Street, Suite 1100
San Francisco, CA 94109
415-923-2000

Colorado
Colorado Foundation for Medical
    Care
Suite 400, Building 2
6825 East Tennessee Avenue
Denver, CO 80224
303-321-8642

Connecticut
Connecticut Peer Review
    Organization
384 Pratt Street
Meriden, CT 06450
203-237-2773

District of Columbia
Delmarva Foundation for Medical
    Care
341-B North Aurora Street
Easton, MD 21601
301-822-0697

Delaware
West Virginia Medical Institute
(see West Virginia)

Florida
Professional Foundation for Health
    Care
2907 Bay to Bay Boulevard, Suite 100
Tampa, FL 33629
813-831-6273

Georgia
Georgia Medical Care Foundation
4 Executive Park Drive, N.E.
Suite 1300
Atlanta, GA 30329
404-982-6500

Hawaii
Hawaii Medical Services Association
818 Keeaumoku Street
P.O. Box 860
Honolulu, HI 96808
808-944-2110

Idaho
Professional Review Organization for
    Washington
(see Washington)

Illinois
Crescent Counties Foundation for
    Medical Care
350 Shuman Boulevard, Suite 240
Naperville, IL 60540
312-876-0652

Indiana
Peerview, Inc.
501 Congressional Boulevard
Suite 200
Carmel, IN 46032
317-573-6888

Iowa
Iowa Foundation for Medical Care
Colony Park Building
3737 Woodland Avenue, Suite 500
West Des Moines, IA 50265
515-223-2900

Kansas
Kansas Foundation for Medical Care
2947 S.W. Wanamaker Drive
Topeka, KS 66614
913-273-2552

Kentucky
Peerview, Inc.
10300 Linn Station Road
Suite 100
Louisville, KY 40223
502-429-0995

Louisiana
Louisiana Health Care Review
9357 Interline Avenue, Suite 200
Baton Rouge, LA 70809
504-926-6353

Maine
Health Care Review, Inc. (Maine)
(see Rhode Island)

Maryland
Delmarva Foundation for Medical
Care
(see District of Columbia)

Massachusetts
Massachusetts Peer Review
Organization
300 Bearhill Road
Waltham, MA 02154
617-890-0011

Michigan
Michigan Peer Review Organization
40500 Ann Arbor Road, Suite 200
Plymouth, MI 48170
313-459-0900

Minnesota
Foundation for Health Care
Evaluation
One Appletree Square, Suite 700
Minneapolis, MN 55420
612-854-3306

Mississippi
Mississippi Foundation for Medical
Care
P.O. Box 4665
1900 North West Street
Jackson, MS 39216
601-948-8894

Missouri
Missouri Patient Care Review
Foundation
311 Ellis Boulevard, Suite A
Jefferson City, MO 65101
314-634-4441

Montana
Montana-Wyoming Foundation for
Medical Care
P.O. Box 5117
21 North Main
Helena, MT 59604
406-443-4020

Nebraska
Iowa Foundation for Medical Care
(see Iowa)

Nevada
Nevada Physicians Review
Organization
4600 Kietzke Lane
Building A, Suite 108
Reno, NV 89502
702-826-1996

New Hampshire
New Hampshire Foundation for
Medical Care
P.O. Box 578
110 Locust Street
Dover, NH 03820
603-749-1641

New Jersey
Peer Review Organization of New
Jersey
Central Division
Brier Hill Court, Building J
East Brunswick, NJ 08816
201-238-5570

New Mexico
New Mexico Medical Review
Association
707 Broadway N.E., Suite 200

P.O. Box 9900
Albuquerque, NM 87106
505-842-6236

New York
Empire State Medical, Scientific and
   Educational Foundation
420 Lakeview Road, Box 5434
Lake Success, NY 11042
516-437-8134

North Carolina
Medical Review of North Carolina
Suite 200, P.O. Box 37309
1011 Schaub Drive
Raleigh, NC 27627
919-851-2955

North Dakota
North Dakota Health Care Review
900 North Broadway, Suite 212
Minot, ND 58701
701-852-4231

Ohio
Peer Review Systems, Inc.
3700 Corporate Drive, Suite 250
Columbus, OH 43229
614-895-9900

Oklahoma
Oklahoma Foundation for Peer
   Review
5801 Broadway Extension
Suite 400, The Paragon Building
Oklahoma City, OK 73118
405-840-2891

Oregon
Oregon Medical Professional Review
   Organization
1220 Southwest Morrison, Suite 300
Portland, OR 97205
503-243-1151

Pennsylvania
Keystone Peer Review Organization
645 North 12th Street
P.O. Box 618
Lemoyne, PA 17043
717-975-9600

Puerto Rico
Puerto Rico Foundation for Medical
   Care
Suite 605, Mercantile Plaza

Hato Ray, PR 00918
809-753-6805

Rhode Island
Health Care Review, Inc.
The Weld Building
345 Blackstone Boulevard
Providence, RI 02906
401-331-6661

South Carolina
Metrolina Medical Foundation
3000 Charlottetown Center
Charlotte, NC 28204
704-373-1545

South Dakota
South Dakota Foundation for Medical
   Care
1323 South Minnesota Avenue
Sioux Falls, SD 57105
605-336-3505

Tennessee
Mid-South Foundation for Medical
   Care
6401 Poplar Avenue, Suite 400
Memphis, TN 38119
901-682-0381

Texas
Texas Medical Foundation
Barton Oaks Plaza Two, Suite 200
901 Mopac Expressway South
Austin, TX 78746
512-329-6610

Utah
Utah Professional Standard Review
   Organization
540 East 5th South Street, Suite 200
Salt Lake City, UT 84102
801-532-7545

Vermont
New Hampshire Foundation for
   Medical Care
(see New Hampshire)

Virgin Islands
Virgin Islands Medical Institute
P.O. Box 1556
Christiansted
St. Croix, U.S. Virgin Islands 00820
809-778-6470

Virginia
Medical Society of Virginia Review
   Organization
1904 Byrd Avenue, Room 120
P.O. Box 6569
Richmond, VA 23230
804-289-5320

Washington
Professional Review Organization for
   Washington
2150 North 107th Street, Suite 200
Seattle, WA 98133
206-364-9700

West Virginia
West Virginia Medical Institute
3412 Chesterfield Avenue, S.E.
Charleston, WV 25304
304-925-0461

Wisconsin
Wisconsin Peer Review Organization
2001 West Beltline Highway
Madison, WI 53713
608-274-1940

Wyoming
Montana-Wyoming Foundation for
   Medical Care
(see Montana)

Appendix K: State Nursing Home Licensure Offices

State Nursing Home Licensure offices inspect institutions to assure a basic standard of care for the resident. They issue certification for institutions that qualify for federal programs: Medicare and Medicaid. These regulations are standard throughout the country. In addition, they issue state licensure for all long-term care institutions. These regulations vary from state to state. Copies of all regulations should be available from these offices.

Alabama
Nursing Home Licensure Office
Division of Licensure and
  Certification
Alabama Dept. of Health
Room 654, State Office Building
Montgomery, AL 36103-1701
205-261-5113

Alaska
Nursing Home Licensure Office
Dept. of Health and Social Services
Health Facilities Certification and
  Licensing
4041 B Street, Suite 101
Anchorage, AK 99503
907-561-2171

Arizona
Dept. of Health Services
Office of Health Care Licensure
411 North 24th Street
Phoenix, AZ 85008
602-220-6407

Arkansas
Arkansas Dept. of Health
Certification and Licensure Section
Office of Long Term Care
P.O. Box 1437
Little Rock, AR 72203
501-371-8143

California
Nursing Home Licensure Office
Licensure and Certification Division
Facilities Licensing Section
714 P Street, Room 823
Sacramento, CA 95814
916-445-3281

Colorado
Nursing Home Licensure Office
Colorado Dept. of Health
Health Facilities Division
Evaluation and Licensure Section
4210 East 11th Avenue, Room 254
Denver, CO 80220
303-331-4930

Connecticut
Nursing Home Licensure Office
Connecticut State Dept. of Health
Division of Hospital and Medical
  Care
150 Washington Street
Hartford, CT 06106
205-566-5758

Delaware
Office of Health Facility Licensing and
  Certification
Nursing Home Division
Division of Public Health
3000 Newport Gap Pike
Wilmington, DE 19808
302-571-3499

District of Columbia
Office of Licensing and Certification
Nursing Home Division
Dept. of Human Services
614 H Street, N.W., Suite 1014
Washington, DC 20001
202-727-7190

Florida
Nursing Home Licensure Office
Licensure and Certification Branch
Division of Health
Dept. of Rehabilitation Services
2727 Mahan Drive

Tallahassee, FL 32308
904-487-3513

Georgia
Nursing Home Licensure Office
Standards and Licensure Unit
Office of Regulatory Services
878 Peachtree Street NE
Suite 803
Atlanta, GA 30309
404-894-5137

Hawaii
Nursing Home Licensure Office
Hospital and Medical Facility Branch
Hawaii State Dept. of Health
P.O. Box 3378
Honolulu, HI 96801
808-548-5935

Idaho
Nursing Home Licensure Office
Facilities Standards and Development
Idaho Dept. of Health and Welfare
420 West Washington Street
Boise, ID 83720
208-334-4167

Illinois
Nursing Home Licensure Office
Illinois Dept. of Public Health
Health Facilities and Quality of Care
525 West Jefferson, Fourth Floor
Springfield, IL 62721
217-782-5180

Indiana
Nursing Home Licensure Office
Division of Health Facilities
Indiana State Board of Health
1330 West Michigan Street
P.O. Box 1964
Indianapolis, IN 46206-1964
317-633-8442

Iowa
Nursing Home Licensure Office
State Dept. of Health
Division of Health Facilities
Lucas State Office Building
Des Moines, IA 50319
515-281-4115 or 800-523-3213

Kansas
Kansas Dept. of Health and
  Environment
Bureau of Adult and Child Homes
Landon State Office Building, Tenth
  Floor
Topeka, KS 66602-0001
913-296-1240

Kentucky
Nursing Home Licensure Office
Division for Licensing and Regulation
Office of the Inspector General
CHR Building, Fourth Floor East
275 East Main Street
Frankfort, KY 40621
502-564-2800

Louisiana
Nursing Home Licensure Office
Dept. of Health and Human
  Resources
Division of Licensure and
  Certification
P.O. Box 3767
Baton Rouge, LA 70821
504-342-5774

Maryland
Office of Licensing and Certification
  Program
Dept. of Health and Mental Hygiene
201 West Preston Street, Room 106
Baltimore, MD 21201
301-225-5430

Maine
Nursing Home Licensure Office
Division of Licensure and
  Certification
249 Western Avenue
State House Station 11
Augusta, ME 04333
207-289-2606

Massachusetts
Nursing Home Licensure Office
Long-Term Care Facilities Program
Dept. of Public Health
80 Boylston Street, Eleventh Floor
Boston, MA 02116
617-727-5864

Michigan
Nursing Home Licensure Office
Bureau of Health Care Administration
Dept. of Public Health
3500 North Logan Street
Lansing, MI 48909
517-335-8505

Minnesota
Nursing Home Licensure Office
Minnesota Dept. of Health
Survey and Compliance Section
717 Southeast Delaware Street
P.O. Box 9441
Minneapolis, MN 55440
612-623-5426

Mississippi
Nursing Home Licensure Office
Health Facilities Certification and
  Licensure
Mississippi State Board of Health
P.O. Box 1700
Jackson, MS 39215
601-960-7769

Missouri
Missouri Dept. of Social Services
Division of Aging
P.O. Box 1337
1440 Aaron Court
Jefferson City, MO 65101
314-751-2712

Montana
Montana Dept. of Health and
  Environmental Services
Bureau of Licensing and Certification
Cogswell Building
Helena, MT 59620
406-444-2037

Nebraska
Division of Licensure and Standards
Nursing Home Division
Dept. of Health
301 Centennial Mall South
P.O. Box 95007
Lincoln, NE 68509
402-471-2946

Nevada
Nursing Home Licensure Office
Bureau of Regulatory Health Services

505 East King Street
Carson City, NV 89710
702-885-4475

New Hampshire
Dept. of Health and Human Services
Division of Public Health
Bureau of Health Facilities
  Administration
Six Hazen Drive
Concord, NH 03301
603-271-4592

New Jersey
Nursing Home Licensure Office
New Jersey State Dept. of Health
Licensing, Certification and Standards
CN 367
Trenton, NJ 08625-0367
609-292-5764

New Mexico
Nursing Home Licensure Office
Health and Social Services Dept.
4125 Carlisle, Northeast
Santa Fe, NM 87107
505-841-6524

New York
Bureau of Long Term Care Services
Corning, Second Tower
Empire State Plaza
Albany, NY 12237
518-473-1564

North Carolina
Nursing Home Licensure Office
Licensure and Certification Section
Health Care Facilities Branch
701 Barbour Drive
Raleigh, NC 27603
919-733-2786

North Dakota
Division of Health Facilities
State Dept. of Health
Nursing Home Division
State Capitol
Bismarck, ND 58505
701-224-2352

Ohio
Nursing Home Licensure Office
Medical Services

Licensing and Certification Division
Ohio Dept. of Health
246 North High Street
Eighth Floor
Columbus, OH 43216
614-466-2070

Oklahoma
Nursing Home Licensure Office
Licensure and Certification Division
Oklahoma State Dept. of Health
P.O. Box 53551
Oklahoma City, OK 73152
405-271-5116

Oregon
Senior Services Division
Long Term Care Licensing
Licensing and Certification
313 Public Service Building
Salem, OR 97310
503-378-3751

Pennsylvania
Nursing Home Licensure Office
Commonwealth of Pennsylvania
Division of Long-Term Care
Health and Welfare Building
Room 526
Harrisburg, PA 17120
717-787-1816

Rhode Island
Nursing Home Licensure Office
Rhode Island Dept. of Health
Division of Facilities Regulation
75 Davis Street
Providence, RI 02908
401-277-2566

South Carolina
Nursing Home Licensure Office
Division of Health Facilities and
   Services
Dept. of Health Licensing
2600 Bull Street
Columbia, SC 29101
803-734-4680

South Dakota
Dept. of Health
Division of Licensure and
   Certification
523 East Capitol Street

Pierre, SD 57501
605-773-3364

Tennessee
Dept. of Health and Environment
Board for Licensing Health Care
   Facilities
283 Plus Park Boulevard
Nashville, TN 37219-5407
615-371-6316

Texas
Nursing Home Licensure Office
Texas Dept. of Health
Quality Standards Division
1100 West 49th Street, Room 202
Austin, TX 78756-3188
512-458-7490

Utah
Nursing Home Licensure Office
Utah Dept. of Health
Bureau of Health Facilities Licensing
P.O. Box 16660
Salt Lake City, UT 84116-0660
801-538-6152

Vermont
Nursing Home Licensure Office
Vermont Dept. of Health
Medical Regulation
60 Main Street, P.O. Box 70
Burlington, VT 05402
802-863-7250

Virginia
Nursing Home Licensure Office
Division of Licensure and
   Certification
1013 Madison Building
109 Governor Street
Richmond, VA 23219
804-786-2081

Washington
Nursing Home Licensure Office
DSHS-Health Services Division
Aging and Adult Services
   Administration
623 8th Avenue, Southeast
Mail Stop HB-11
Olympia, WA 98504-0095
206-753-5840

West Virginia
Nursing Home Licensure Office
Health Facilities and Certification
  Section
P and G Building
1800 East Washington Street
Charleston, WV 25305
304-348-0050

Wisconsin
Dept. of Health and Social Services
Division of Health
Bureau of Quality Compliance

One West Wilson Street
Room 150, P.O. Box 309
Madison, WI 53701
608-266-3024

Wyoming
Dept. of Health and Social Services
Division of Health and Medical
  Services
Medical Facilities
Hathaway Building, Fourth Floor
Cheyenne, WY 82002-0717
307-777-7121

Appendix L: Nursing Home Patient Bill of Rights

Under federal regulations, nursing homes must have written policies covering the rights of patients. These rights must be posted where residents and visitors can easily see them. A Patient Bill of Rights ensures that each person admitted to a facility will have his/her rights protected. Flagrant violations of these rights should be reported to the proper state authorities.

A Patient:

1. is fully informed as evidenced by the resident's written acknowledgment of these rights and of all rules and regulations governing the exercise of these rights.

2. is fully informed of services available in the facility and of related charges for services not covered under Medicare/Medicaid, or not covered by the facility's basic daily rate.

3. is fully informed of his or her medical condition unless the physician notes in the medical record that it is not in the patient's interest to be told, and is afforded the opportunity to participate in the planning of his or her medical treatment and to refuse to participate in experimental research.

4. is transferred or discharged only for medical reasons, or for his or her welfare or that of other residents, and is given reasonable advance notice to ensure orderly transfer or discharge.

5. is encouraged and assisted, through his or her period of stay to exercise his or her rights as a resident and as a free citizen. To this end he or she may voice grievances and recommend changes in policies and services to facility staff and/or outside representatives of his or her choice without fear of coercion, discrimination, or reprisal.

6. may manage his or her personal financial affairs, or is given at least a quarterly accounting of financial transactions made on his or her behalf if the facility accepts the responsibility to safeguard the funds.

7. is free from mental and physical abuse, and free from chemical and physicial restraints except as authorized in writing by a physician for a specified and limited period of time or when necessary to protect patients from injury to themselves or others.

8. is assured confidential treatment of his or her personal and medical records and may approve or refuse their release to any individual outside facility.

Source: Suggested by the Health Care Financing Administration, U.S. Department of Health and Human Services, Washington, D.C.

9. is treated with consideration, respect, and full recognition of his or her dignity and individuality, including privacy in treatment and in care of his or her personal needs.

10. is not required to perform services for the facility that are not included for therapeutic purposes in this plan of care.

11. may associate and communicate privately with persons of his or her choice, and send and receive his or her personal mail unopened.

12. may meet with, and participate in activities of social, religious, and community groups at his or her discretion.

13. may retain and use his or her personal clothing and possessions as space permits, unless to do so would infringe upon rights of other patients, or constitute a hazard of safety.

14. is assured privacy for visits by his or her spouse; if both are inpatients in the facility, they are permitted to share a room.

Appendix M: State Agencies Regulating Home Health Care

Alabama
Department of Public Health
State Office Building, Room 381
501 Dexter Avenue
Montgomery, AL 36130-1701

Alaska
Department of Health and Social
  Services
Alaska Office Building, Room 503
350 Main Street
Mail To: Pouch H-06
Juneau, AK 99811-0610
097-465-3030

Arizona
Department of Health Services
1740 W. Adams Street
Phoenix, AZ 85007
602-255-1024

Arkansas
Department of Health
State Health Building
4815 W. Markham Street
Little Rock, AR 72205-3867
501-661-2112

California
Department of Health Services
714 P Street, Room 1253
Sacramento, CA 95814
916-445-1248

Colorado
Department of Health
4210 E. 11th Avenue
Denver, CO 80220
303-331-4602

Connecticut
Department of Health Services
150 Washington Street
Hartford, CT 06106
203-566-2038

Delaware
Division of Public Health
Department of Health and Social
  Services

Robbins Building
802 Silver Lake Boulevard
Mail to: P.O. Box 637
Dover, DE 19901
302-736-4701

District of Columbia
Commission of Public Health
Department of Human Services
Universal North Building, Room 825
1875 Connecticut Avenue, NW
Washington, DC 20009
202-673-7700

Florida
Health Program Office
Department of Health and
  Rehabilitative Services
Building I, Room 115
1323 Winewood Boulevard
Tallahassee, FL 32301
904-488-4115

Georgia
Division of Public Health
Department of Human Resources
878 Peachtree Street, N.E., Suite 201
Altanta, GA 30309
404-894-7505

Hawaii
Department of Health
Kinau Hale
1250 Punchbowl Street
Mail to: P.O. Box 3378
Honolulu, HI 96801
808-548-6505

Idaho
Bureau of Preventive Medicine
Division of Health
Department of Health and Welfare
Towers Building, 4th Floor
450 W. State Street
Boise, ID 83720
208-334-5930

Illinois
Department of Public Health
535 W. Jefferson Street

Springfield, IL 62761
217-782-4977

Indiana
State Board of Health
1330 W. Michigan Street
Mail to: P.O. Box 1964
Indianapolis, IN 46206-1964
317-633-8400

Iowa
Department of Public Health
Lucas State Office Building
E. 12th and Walnut Streets
Des Moines, IA 50319
515-281-5605

Kansas
Division of Health
Department of Health and
  Environment
Building 740
Forbes Field
Topeka, KS 66620
913-862-9360

Kentucky
Department for Health Services
Cabinet for Human Resources
Health Services Building, 1st Floor
275 E. Main Street
Frankfort, KY 40621
502-564-3970

Louisiana
Office of Preventive and Public Health
  Services
Department of Health and Human
  Resources
325 Loyola Avenue
Mail to: P.O. Box 60630
New Orleans, LA 70160
504-568-5052

Maine
Bureau of Health
Department of Human Services
157 Capitol Street
Mail to: State House, Station 11
Augusta, ME 04333
207-289-3201

Maryland
Department of Health and Mental
  Hygiene

Herbert R. O'Conor State Office
  Building
201 W. Preston Street
Baltimore, MD 21201
301-225-6500

Massachusetts
Department of Public Health
150 Tremont Street
Boston, MA 02111
617-727-0201

Michigan
Department of Public Health
Baker-Olin West Building
3500 N. Logan Street
Mail to: P.O. Box 30035
Lansing, MI 48909
517-373-8024

Minnesota
Department of Health
717 Delaware Street, S.E.
Mail to: P.O. Box 9441
Minneapolis, MN 55440
612-623-5460

Mississippi
Department of Health
2423 N. State Street
Mail to: P.O. Box 1700
Jackson, MS 39215-1700
601-354-6646

Missouri
Department of Health
Mail to: P.O. Box 570
Jefferson City, MO 65102
314-751-6001

Montana
Department of Health and
  Environmental Sciences
Cogswell Building, Room C108
Helena, MT 59620
406-444-2544

Nebraska
Department of Health
State Office Building
301 Centennial Mall, South
Mail to: P.O. Box 95007
Lincoln, NE 68509
402-471-2133

Nevada
Health Division
Department of Human Resources
Kinkead Building
505 E. King Street
Mail to: Capitol Complex
Carson City, NV 89710
702-885-4740

New Hampshire
Division of Public Health Services
Department of Health and Human
 Services
Health and Human Services Building
6 Hazen Drive
Concord, NH 03301-6527
603-271-4501

New Jersey
Department of Health
Health and Agriculture Building
John Fitch Plaza
Mail to: CN 360
Trenton, NJ 08625
609-292-7837

New Mexico
Health Services Division
Health and Environment Department
Harold Runnels Building
1190 St. Francis Drive
Mail to: P.O. Box 968
Santa Fe, NM 87504-0968
505-827-0020

New York
Department of Health
Corning Tower, Room 1408
Empire State Plaza
Albany, NY 12237
518-474-2011

North Carolina
Division of Health Services
Department of Human Resources
Cooper Memorial Health Building
225 N. McDowell Street
Mail to: P.O. Box 2091
Raleigh, NC 26702
919-733-3446

North Dakota
Department of Health
State Capitol

Bismarck, ND 58505
701-224-2372

Ohio
Department of Health
246 N. High Street
Columbus, OH 43226-0588
614-466-3543

Oklahoma
Department of Health
1000 N.E. 10th Street
Mail to: P.O. Box 53551
Oklahoma City, OK 73152
405-271-4200

Oregon
Health Division
Department of Human Resources
State Office Building, Room 811
1400 S.W. 5th Avenue
Mail to: P.O. Box 231
Portland, OR 97207
503-229-5032

Pennsylvania
Department of Health
Health and Welfare Building, Room
 802
Commonwealth Avenue and Forster
 Street
Mail to: P.O. Box 90
Harrisburg, PA 17108
717-787-6436

Rhode Island
Department of Health
Cannon Building, Room 401
75 Davis Street
Providence, RI 02908
401-277-2231

South Carolina
Department of Health and
 Environmental Control
R. J. Aycock Building
2600 Bull Street
Columbia, SC 29201
803-734-4880

South Dakota
Department of Health
Joe Foss Building
523 E. Capitol Avenue

Pierre, SD 57501
605-773-3361

Tennessee
Department of Health and
 Environment
Cordell Hull Building, Room 344
436 6th Avenue, North
Nashville, TN 37219-5402
615-741-3111

Texas
Department of Health
1100 W. 49th Street
Austin, TX 78756-3199
512-458-7375

Utah
Department of Health
288 N. 1460 West
Salt Lake City, UT 84116-0700
801-538-6101

Vermont
Department of Health
Agency of Human Services
60 Main Street
Mail to: P.O. Box 70
Burlington, VT 05402
802-863-7280

Virginia
Department of Health
James Madison Building
109 Governor Street
Richmond, VA 23219
804-786-3561

Washington
Division of Health
Department of Social and Health
 Services
1112 S. Quince Street
Mail to: Mail Stop ET-21
Olympia, WA 98504
206-753-5871

West Virginia
Department of Health
State Office Building 3, Room 206
1800 Washington Street, E.
Charleston, WV 25305
304-348-2971

Wisconsin
Division of Health
Department of Health and Social
 Services
Wilson Street State Office Building,
 Room 218
One W. Wilson Street
Mail to: P.O. Box 309
Madison, WI 53701-0309
608-266-1511

Wyoming
Department of Health and Social
 Services
Hathaway Building
2300 Capitol Avenue
Cheyenne, WY 82002-0710
307-777-7656

Appendix N: State Medicaid Offices

Note: Some telephone numbers may have changed; please consult your local directory.

Welfare Departments

Alabama
Alabama Medicaid Agency
2500 Fairlane Drive
Montgomery, AL 36130
205-277-2710

Alaska
Alaska Department of Health and
Social Services
Division of Medical Assistance
P.O. Box H-07
Juneau, AK 99811
907-465-3355

Arizona
Arizona Health Care Cost
Containment System
801 East Jefferson Street
Phoenix, AZ 85034
602-234-3655

Arkansas
Department of Human Services
Information and Referral
P.O. Box 1437
Little Rock, AR 72203-1437
501-682-1001

California
Department of Health Services
Referral Office for Medi-Cal
714-744 "P" Street
P.O. Box 942732
Sacramento, CA 94234-7320
916-445-4171

Colorado
Colorado Department of Social
Services
Division of Medical Services
Division of Programs-Long Term Care
Section
717 Seventeenth Street

Denver, CO 80218
303-294-5700

Connecticut
Connecticut Department of Human
Resources
Bureau of Field Operations
1049 Asylum Avenue
Hartford, CT 06105
203-566-4580

Delaware
Delaware Department of Health and
Social Services
Division of Economic Services
Biggs Building
Delaware State Hospital
P.O. Box 906
New Castle, DE 19720
302-421-6139

District of Columbia
Long Term Care Administration
Department of Human Services
Commission of Public Health
Central Referral Bureau
Two DC Village Lane, Infirmary
Washington, DC 20032
202-767-8356

Florida
Florida Department of Health and
Rehabilitative Services
Medicaid Program Office
Provider and Consumer Relations
Office
Building 6, Room 260
1317 Winewood Boulevard
Tallahassee, FL 32399
904-488-8291

Georgia
Georgia Department of Medical
Assistance

West Tower
Two Martin Luther King Drive, S.E.
Atlanta, GA 30334
404-656-4479

Hawaii
Department of Human Services
Health Care Administration Division
820 Milileni Street, Room 817
Honolulu, HI 96813
808-548-3855

Idaho
Idaho Department of Health and
    Welfare
Bureau of Medical Assistance
450 West State Street, Sixth Floor
Boise, ID 83720
202-334-5794

Illinois
Illinois Department of Public Aid
Division of Medical Programs
628 East Adams Street, Third Floor
Springfield, IL 62762
217 782 2550

Indiana
Indiana Department of Public Welfare
Medical Assistance Unit
100 North Senate Avenue
Room 702
Indianapolis, IN 46204
317-232-4324

Iowa
Bureau of Medical Services
Department of Human Services
Hoover State Office Building
Des Moines, IA 50319-0114
515-281-8621

Kansas
Kansas Department of Social and
    Rehabilitation Services
Division of Income Maintenance
Docking State Office Building, Room
    624 South
Topeka, KS 66612
913-296-3349

Kentucky
Cabinet for Human Resources
Department for Medicaid Services

275 East Main Street
Frankfort, KY 40621
502-564-4321

Louisiana
Louisiana Department of Health and
    Human Resources
Office of Family Security
P.O. Box 94065
Baton Rouge, LA 70804-9065
504-342-3950

Maine
Maine Department of Human Services
State House Station 11
Augusta, ME 04333
207-289-2736

Maryland
Medical Assistance Division
Office of Income Maintenance
Department of Human Resources
311 West Saratoga Street
Baltimore, MD 21201
301-576-5461

Massachusetts
Massachusetts Department of Public
    Welfare
180 Tremont Street
Boston, Massachusetts 02111
617-574-0100

Michigan
Michigan Department of Social
    Services
Citizen's and Legislative Inquiry
517-373-0707
1 + 800-638-6414
For referral to local agency

Minnesota
Minnesota Department of Human
    Services
Health Care and Residential Programs
444 Lafayette Road
St. Paul, MN 55155
612-296-2766

Mississippi
Mississippi Department of Public
    Welfare
Division of Medicaid
4785 Interstate 55 North

Jackson, MS 39236
601-981-4507

Missouri
Missouri Department of Social
   Services
Division of Family Services
P.O. Box 88
Jefferson City, MO 65103
1+800-392-1261 or 314-751-4247

Montana
Montana Department of Social and
   Rehabilitation Services
Economic Assistance Division
111 Sanders Street
P.O. Box 4210
Helena, MT 59604
406-444-4540

Nebraska
Nebraska Department of Social
   Services
301 Centennial Mall South, Fifth
   Floor
Lincoln, NE 68509
402-471-3121

Nevada
Department of Human Resources
Nevada Welfare Division
Medicaid Section
2527 North Carson Street
Carson City, NV 89710
702-885-4698

New Hampshire
New Hampshire Division of Health
   and Human Services
Department of Human Services-Office
   of Economic Services
Six Hazen Drive
Concord, NH 03301
1+800-852-3345 or 603-271-4321

New Jersey
New Jersey Department of Human
   Services
Division of Medical Assistance and
   Health Services
Seven Quakerbridge Plaza
Trenton, NJ 08625
609-588-2600 or 588-2602

New Mexico
New Mexico Department of Human
   Services
Medical Assistance Division
PERA Building, Room 524
P.O. Box 2348
Santa Fe, NM 87504-2348
505-827-4315

New York
New York State Department of Social
   Services
Division of Medical Assistance
40 North Pearl Street
Albany, NY 12243
1+800-342-3715 or 518-474-9475

North Carolina
North Carolina Department of
   Human Resources
Division of Medical Assistance
1985 Umstead Drive
Raleigh, NC 27603
919-733-4600

North Dakota
North Dakota Department of Human
   Services
Medical Services
State Capitol
Bismarck, ND 58505
701-224-2321

Ohio
Department of Human Services
Benefits Administration
Thirty East Broad Street
Thirty-First Floor
Columbus, OH 43216
614-466-3196

Oklahoma
Department of Human Services
Medical Services Division
P.O. Box 25352
Oklahoma City, OK 73125
405-557-2540

Oregon
Oregon Department of Human
   Resources
Senior Services Division
313 Public Service Building

Salem, OR 97310
503-378-4728

Pennsylvania
Pennsylvania Department of Public
Welfare
Health and Welfare Building
Room 515
Harrisburg, PA 17120
717-787-1870

Rhode Island
Rhode Island Department of Human
Services
Division of Medical Services
600 New London Avenue
Cranston, RI 02902
401-464-2178

South Carolina
South Carolina Department of Social
Services
Division of Medicaid Eligibility
P.O. Box 1520
Columbia, SC 29202-1520
803-734-5760

South Dakota
South Dakota Department of Social
Services
Office of Medical Services
700 Governor's Drive
Pierre, SD 57501
605-773-3495

Tennessee
Department of Health and
Environment
Bureau of Medicaid
729 Church Street
Nashville, TN 37219
615-741-0213

Texas
Texas Department of Human Services
Office of Services to the Aged and
Disabled
P.O. Box 2960
Austin, TX 78769
512-450-3192

Utah
Utah Department of Health
Bureau of Medical Payments

Medicaid Information Unit
288 North 1460 West
Salt Lake City, UT 84116
538-6155 (Salt Lake area)
1 + 800-662-9651

Vermont
Vermont Agency of Human Services
103 South Main Street
Waterbury, VT 05676
802-241-2852 or 241-2220

Virginia
Department of Medical Services
Division of Medical Social Services
Eligibility and Appeals Section
600 East Broad Street, Suite 1300
Richmond, VA 23219
804-786-6145

Washington
Washington Department of Social and
Health Services
Community Services Offices
*See local telephone directory for local
listing of office. Numbers are in
blue pages of telephone directory.*

West Virginia
West Virginia Department of Human
Services
Client Services
1900 Washington Street, E.
Charleston, WV 25305
304-348-2400

Wisconsin
All inquiries should be to
County Department of Social Services
*Consult blue pages of telephone
directory for local numbers.*
Recipient Hotline 1 + 800-362-3002;
Madison area 266-4279

Wyoming
Wyoming Department of Health and
Social Services
Division of Public Assistance and
Social Services
Hathaway Building, Third Floor
Cheyenne, WY 82002
307-777-7561

Appendix O: Nursing Home Ombudsman Offices

Alabama
Commission on Aging
136 Cotoma Street
Montgomery, AL 36130
205-261-5743

Alaska
Older Alaskan's Commission
Department of Administration
2600 Denali Street, Suite 403
Anchorage, AK 99503
907-279-2232

Arizona
Aging and Adult Services
Department of Economic Security
P.O. Box 6123-950 A
Phoenix, AZ 85007
602-255-4446

Arkansas
Division of Aging and Adult Services
Department of Human Services
Donaghey Building
Seventh and Main Streets
Little Rock, AR 72201
501-371-2441

California
California Department of Aging
Office of the Long-Term Care
  Ombudsman
1600 K Street
Sacramento, CA 95814
1 + 800-231-4024

Colorado
Colorado State Ombudsman Program
1565 Clarkson Street
Denver, CO 80218
1 + 800-582-7410
303-830-7744

Connecticut
Department on Aging
175 Main Street
Hartford, CT 06115
203-566-7770

Delaware (Northern)
Division on Aging
Delaware State Hospital
1901 North DuPont Highway
New Castle, DE 19720
302-421-6791

Delaware (Southern)
Division of Aging
Milford State Services Center
11-13 Church Street
Milford, DE 19963
302-422-1386

District of Columbia
Office on Aging
1424 K Street, N.W.
Second Floor
Washington, DC 20005
202-724-5622

Florida
State Long-Term Care Ombudsman
  Council
1317 Winewood Boulevard
Building One, Room 308
Tallahassee, FL 32399-0700
904-488-6190

Georgia
Office of Aging
Department of Human Resources
878 Peachtree Street, N.E.
Room 642
Atlanta, GA 30309
404-894-5336

Hawaii
Executive Office on Aging
Office of the Governor
335 Merchant Street, Room 241
Honolulu, HI 96813
808-548-2593

Idaho
Idaho Office on Aging
Statehouse, Room 114
Boise, ID 83720
208-334-3833

Illinois
Department on Aging
421 East Capitol Avenue
Springfield, IL 62701
217-785-3140

Indiana
Department of Human Services
251 North Illinois
P.O. Box 7083
Indianapolis, IN 46207-7083
1 + 800-622-4484 (Indiana only)

Iowa
Department of Elder Affairs
914 Grand
236 Jewett Building
Des Moines, IA 50319
515-281-5187

Kansas
Department on Aging
610 West Tenth
Topeka, KS 66612
913-296-4986

Kentucky
Department of Social Services
Division of Aging Services
CHR Building, 6 West
275 East Main Street
Frankfort, KY 40621
502-564-6930

Louisiana
Governor's Office of Elderly Affairs
P.O. Box 80374
Baton Rouge, LA 70898-0374
504-925-1700

Maine
Long Term Care Ombudsman
  Program
Maine Committee on Aging
State House Station 127
Augusta, ME 04333
1 + 800-452-1912
207-289-3658

Maryland
Office on Aging
301 West Preston Street
Room 104
Baltimore, MD 21201
301-225-1100

Massachusetts
Executive Offices-Elder Affairs
38 Chauncy Street
Boston, MA 02111
617-727-7750

Michigan
Citizens for Better Care
1553 Woodward, Suite 525
David Whitney Building
Detroit, MI 48226
313-962-5968

Minnesota
Minnesota Board on Aging
121 East Seventh Street
Suite 204 Metro Square Building
St. Paul, MN 55101
612-296-2770

Mississippi
Mississippi Council on Aging
301 West Pearl Street
Jackson, MS 39203-3092
601-949-2029

Missouri
Missouri Division of Aging
Department of Social Services
2701 West Main Street
Jefferson City, MO 65102
314-751-3082

Montana
Seniors Office — Legal and
  Ombudsman Services
P.O. Box 232
Capitol Station
Helena, MT 59620
406-444-4676

Nebraska
Nebraska Department on Aging
P.O. Box 95044
Lincoln, NE 68509
402-471-2307

Nevada
Division for Aging Services
505 East King Street
Kinkead Building, Room 101
Carson City, NV 89710
702-885-4210

New Hampshire
New Hampshire Long Term Care
  Ombudsman Program
Department of Elderly and Adult
  Services
Third Floor East
Six Hazen Drive
Concord, NH 03301-6508
603-271-4375

New Jersey
Ombudsman for the Institutionalized
  Elderly
28 West State Street, Room 305
Trenton, NJ 08625
1+800-624-4262
609-292-8016

New Mexico
State Agency on Aging
224 East Palace Avenue
Fourth Floor
Santa Fe, NM 87501
505-827-7640
1+800-432-2080

New York
New York State Office for Aging
Agency Building Number Two, Second
  Floor
Empire State Plaza
Albany, NY 12227
518-474-7329

North Carolina
Division of Aging
1985 Umstead Drive
Raleigh, NC 27603
919-733-3983

North Dakota
Long Term Care Ombudsman
Aging Services Division
State Capitol
Bismarck, ND 58505
701-224-2577

Ohio
Ohio Department on Aging
State Ombudsman
50 West Broad Street, Ninth Floor
Columbus, OH 43266-0501
1+800-282-1206
614-466-1220

Oklahoma
Department of Human Services
Office of Client Advocacy
Long Term Care Ombudsman
P.O. Box 25352
Oklahoma City, OK 73125
405-521-3731; 521-3737

Oregon
Long Term Care Ombudsman's Office
2475 Lancaster Drive
Building B, Suite Nine
Salem, OR 97305
1+800-522-2602
503-378-6533

Pennsylvania
Department of Aging
Bureau of Advocacy
231 State Street
Harrisburg, PA 17101
717-783-7247

Rhode Island
Department of Elderly Affairs
79 Washington Street
Providence, RI 02903
401-277-2894

South Carolina
Governor's Office Ombudsman
  Division
1205 Pendletown Street
Edgar A. Brown Building
Columbia, SC 29201
803-734-0457

South Dakota
Office of Adult Services and Aging
State Ombudsman
700 Governor's Drive
Pierre, SD 57501
605-773-3656

Tennessee
Commission on Aging
706 Church Street
Nashville, TN 37219
615-741-2056

Texas
Texas Department on Aging
P.O. Box 12786
Austin, TX 78711
512-444-2727

Utah
State Division of Aging and Adult
    Services
Long Term Care Ombudsman
120 North 200 West, Fourth Floor
Salt Lake City, UT 84145-0500
801-538-3929

Vermont
Vermont Office on Aging
Long Term Care Ombudsman
    Program
103 South Main Street
Waterbury, VT 05676
1+800-642-5119

Virginia
Virginia Department for the Aging
James Madison Building
18th Floor
101 North Fourteenth Street
Richmond, VA 23219
1+800-552-3402

Washington
State Long Term Care Ombudsman
Legislative and Constituent Services
Mail Stop OB-44Y
Olympia, WA 98504
206-753-0401

West Virginia
Commission on Aging
State Capitol Complex
Charleston, WV 25305
304-348-3317

Wisconsin
Governor's Ombudsman Program for
    the Aging and Disabled
819 North Sixth
Milwaukee, WI 53203
414-227-4386

Wyoming
Wyoming Nursing Home
    Ombudsman
P.O. Box 94
Wheatlyn, WY 82201
307-322-5553

Glossary

Administrative law judge (ALJ)   An official charged with making decisions in matters of administrative, as opposed to civil or criminal, law.

Ambulatory surgery   A large, although limited, range of procedures using operative and anesthesia techniques that allow the patient to recuperate at home, rather than in the hospital, immediately following the operation.

American Association of Retired Persons   A service and lobbying group composed of people age 50 and over that has the Medicare program among its concerns.

American Medical Association (AMA)   The largest, although not the only, trade association of American doctors.

Anesthesiologist or **anesthetist**   A person who administers anesthetics for surgery and diagnostic procedures. An anesthesiologist is always a holder of the M.D. or D.O. degree; an anesthetist may be a nurse-anesthetist or an anesthesia technician.

Approved charge   The amount that Medicare has determined is appropriate for payment to a physician for a service, based on his and his colleagues' histories of charge. See *Usual, customary, and reasonable reimbursement system* below.

Assignment   A process in which a Medicare beneficiary agrees to have Medicare's share of the cost of a service paid directly to a doctor or other provider, and the provider agrees to accept the Medicare approved charge as payment in full. Medicare pays 80 percent of the cost, the beneficiary 20 percent, for most services.

Attending physician   A doctor with staff privileges at a hospital who treats patients there. Usually applied to physicians on the staff of a teaching hospital who have a role in teaching and supervising interns and residents.

Biologicals   Drugs produced by extraction from plant or animal tissue, rather than chemical synthesis. For example, gamma globulin from horse serum, human growth hormone.

Brain stem   A portion of the brain involved in controlling basic bodily functions.

Cancer   A malignant tumor of potentially unlimited growth that expands locally by invading surrounding normal tissues and systemically by metastasis.

Cardio-pulmonary resuscitation (CPR)   A set of treatments and procedures used to restart or stabilize heart and lung function when either one ceases.

Carriers   Private organizations, usually insurance companies, that have contracts with the Health Care Financing Administration to process claims under Part B (doctor insurance) of Medicare.

Case law   The body of court decisions that establish binding interpretations of the law passed by legislative bodies.

Catastrophic illness   Any unusually expensive or lengthy illness that greatly exceeds an individual's ability to pay.

Catheters   Tubes used to drain various hollow cavities of the body.

Chemotherapy   Generally, the treatment of any disease by drugs; usually used to mean drug therapy for cancer using powerful agents that are toxic to both cancerous and noncancerous cells, but more so to the former.

Chiropractor   A holder of the degree of doctor of chiropractic (D.C.). Chiropractors treat disorders of location and relationship of bones and joints. Some hold that this type of treatment has positive effects on organ systems other than the musculoskeletal system, others do not. See Doctor of Chiropractic.

Competitive medical plan (CMP) An arrangement for prepaid care that is not as restricted as a health maintenance organization in benefits offered, premium calculation, and the like.

Congressional Budget Office The agency of Congress that prepares analyses of various national budget alternatives and studies budget-related issues for Congress.

Coordination of benefits A process in which insurers cooperate to make sure that they do not, together, pay more than the maximum benefit available from any of them.

Copayments Portions of the cost of care an insured person is required to pay, while the insurance usually, but not always, pays for the major part of the cost.

Deductibles Amounts that must be paid by an insured person before an insurance plan pays for any portion of the cost.

Dentist A holder of the degree of Doctor of Dental Medicine (D.D.M.), or doctor of Dental Surgery (D.D.S.), concerned with care of the teeth, gums, and associated structures.

Department of Health and Human Services The federal department charged generally with the administration of national welfare programs. Formed from the old Department of Health, Education, and Welfare when the Department of Education was split off.

Diagnosis-Related Groups (DRG) system A method of paying hospitals based on the average cost of treating patients with statistically similar conditions.

Diagnostic workup The process of testing and checking various hypotheses about possible conditions a patient may have when this cannot be immediately established from symptoms, history, or routine tests.

Dialysis Use of a machine to remove waste products or toxins from the blood to assist or replace kidney function.

Doctor of Chiropractic A holder of the degree of Doctor of Chiropractic, a school of medicine that places almost exclusive reliance on manipulation for alignment of the skeleton, plus exercise and nutrition.

Doctor of Medicine (M.D.) A holder of the degree of Medical Doctor, the dominant school of medicine in the United States, which is committed to allopathic medicine, that is, treatment agents that produce effects different from the symptoms of the disease they are intended to treat, foreign to the body or by high concentrations of naturally occurring agents, and surgery; conventional American medicine.

Doctor of Osteopathy (D.O.) A holder of the degree of Doctor of Osteopathy, a school of medicine that places emphasis, but not exclusive emphasis, on proper alignment of the skeleton.

Durable medical equipment Medical equipment that is intended to be used over and over again, usually by the patient or a caregiver, rather than being used once or a few times and discarded. Examples include wheelchairs, hospital beds, and oxygen tanks.

Durable power of attorney A delegation of some authority to another, which lasts until revoked. See power of attorney.

Earnings record The record of amounts earned by each individual for whom Social Security taxes were paid. Maintained by the Social Security Administration.

Elective surgery or procedure A surgery or procedure that, given the patient's diagnosis and condition, can be performed at any convenient time. Contrast with urgent procedure, one that must be done very soon, and emergency procedure, one that must be done immediately.

Electrocardiogram (EKG)   A medical test to measure the electrical activity of the heart, for diagnosis and therapy.

Electrolytes   Ions of sodium, potassium, and calcium in the blood that are intimately involved in regulating muscle contraction and heartbeat.

Emergency   A situation requiring immediate care to prevent death, serious injury, or deformity; contrast with urgent.

End stage renal disease   Kidney disease that is severe enough to require lifetime dialysis or a kidney transplant. End stage renal disease patients are eligible for Medicare and may be eligible for Social Security payments if found to be disabled.

Executive departments   The various entities within the federal government that ultimately report to the President (as opposed to Congress or to the Supreme Court).

Explanation of Medicare Benefits (EOMB)   A form sent to a Medicare beneficiary after a claim is paid, indicating what Medicare has paid for and why.

Face sheet   The top document in a patient's hospital chart, which the doctor attests is correct as to conditions and procedures to obtain payment from Medicare under the DRG system.

Family practice/Family practitioner   Delivery of primary health care to all members of families by a physician trained in general practice plus elements of pediatrics and obstetrics and gynecology; one who delivers such care.

Federal judicial districts   Major divisions of the United States that are under the jurisdiction of a single federal appeals court. The federal district courts make laws that establish precedents that the Social Security Administration and Medicare must follow, but these precedents have binding force only within the judicial district unless Congress aligns laws with them or the Supreme Court makes them the law of the land by upholding them when an appeal from the federal district court decision is filed.

Fee-for-service system   A system of payment for medical services in which each service rendered is charged for individually after the fact; the classic American way of paying for medical care; opposite of prepayment.

Food and Drug Administration (FDA)   A part of the Department of Health and Human Services that is charged with administering the Pure Food and Drug Act and various other laws that relate to prescription and veterinary drug production and sales.

Freedom of choice options   Arrangements under which members of a health maintenance organization or other prepaid plan can use physicians who are outside the panel of participating doctors, if they wish to do so. Additional payment is usually involved.

General enrollment period   The time from January 1 to March 31 of each year when anyone eligible for Part B of Medicare can enroll in it.

General medical/surgical floors   The areas of a hospital in which patients who do not require special treatment are cared for.

Group model health maintenance organization   A health maintenance organization that is staffed by the doctors in a group practice, who may or may not have ownership interest or control.

Group practice   A situation in which a group of doctors shares facilities and support staff, and often makes an attempt to offer patients of the group a range of specialties.

General Practice/General Practitioner The delivery of a wide range of primary care services by an M.D. or D.O.; one who delivers them. See Family Practice.

Gynecological problems Conditions and diseases peculiar to women. There is much current controversy about the best ways to treat many of these conditions and about whether some of them are properly considered diseases at all.

Health Care Financing Administration (HCFA) The part of the Department of Health and Human Services that operates Medicare and, together with the states, Medicaid.

Health maintenance organizations (HMOs) Entities that combine the functions of insurer and provider of care, giving most necessary care for a prepaid fee and placing an emphasis on prevention and careful assessment of medical necessity.

Home health agency (HHA) An agency approved by Medicare for the delivery of home health services to Medicare beneficiaries.

Home health care Care rendered in a patient's residence by employees of a home health agency or other approved provider of home health care.

Hormones Naturally occurring chemicals that regulate functions of the body when carried through the bloodstream.

Hospital-based physicians Term for doctors who treat patients exclusively or almost exclusively in hospitals and so use the hospital as their office, the place of primary contact with patients. Often the hospital bills for their services and pays them a salary.

House staff Doctors in training in a hospital, plus hospital-based physicians, who are the primary physicians for patients who do not have personal physicians and assist in the care of those who do.

Hydration Various treatments used to make sure that the body contains adequate water; also, the body's state of water balance. Compare dehydration.

Hyperalimentation Total nutrition via a tube placed in a vein. Proteins, fats, electrolytes, and carbohydrates are all provided, in contrast to shorter-term administration of intravenous solutions that contain only electrolytes and sugars. Also called total parenteral nutrition (TPN).

Iatrogenesis Causation of illness by a doctor in the course of treating another real or putative illness.

Immigration and naturalization records Records maintained by, or issued by, the Departments of State and Interior that show that an alien has legally entered the United States or become a citizen.

Immunosuppressive drug A drug given to control the immune system to keep it from damaging a transplanted organ or causing additional damage to normal tissues in an autoimmune disease.

Individual enrollment period The time, running from three months before one's sixty-fifth birthday to three months after, during which one can enroll in Part B of Medicare without a premium increase for delayed enrollment.

Individual practice association (IPA) health maintenance organization A health maintenance organization that is staffed by physicians in private practice who continue to maintain their own offices and see both HMO and non-HMO patients.

Inpatient Someone admitted to a hospital for care; an adjective applying to care given in a hospital.

Inpatient hospital care Care that is rendered in a hospital to someone who has been formally admitted and temporarily lives in the hospital while receiving treatment.

Intensive care unit A part of a hospital in which people whose life support requires constant monitoring, or who require close and constant observation, are cared for.

Intermediaries Private organizations, usually insurance companies, that have contracts with the Health Care Financing Administration to process claims under Part A (hospital insurance) of Medicare.

Intermediate care facility (ICF) An institution that provides less intensive care than skilled nursing facilities. Patients are generally more mobile, and rehabilitation therapies are stressed.

Interns Doctors in their first year of postgraduate training in a hospital. The term is being replaced by "first-year resident."

Intravenous lines Tubes placed within, or connecting to a needle placed within, a vein to administer fluids and drugs.

Licensed practical nurse (L.P.N.) or licensed vocational nurse (L.V.N.) A person who has undergone training and been granted a license to provide general care to the sick. Considered less well trained than a registered nurse (R.N.), but functions may overlap considerably, depending on state law.

Living Will A document executed prior or early in the course of an illness, expressing one's wishes in regard to medical treatment if one becomes unable to direct the course of it personally. May or may not be explicitly permitted by the laws of the individual states.

Maximum allowable actual charge (MAAC) An amount, set by Medicare, that is the highest amount a doctor may charge a Medicare beneficiary for a service. The maximum allowable actual charge applies only to doctors who do not take assignment, since the Medicare approved charge is all that the doctor may charge for assigned claims.

Medicaid A federal/state program, established by Title XIX of the Social Security Act, which provides medical care to the poor.

Medically needy Eligible for Medicaid not because of absolute lack of income, but because income, less accumulated medical bills, is below state income limits for the Medicaid program.

Medical necessity The state of being thought to be required by the prevailing medical consensus. What is medically necessary in one period, or one area, may not be so in another.

Medical necessity determination A formal judgment, usually made for purposes of insurance payment, that a treatment was or was not medically necessary.

Medical technician An individual with training that allows him or her to carry out some of the functions of holders of the M.D. or D.O. degrees, especially in emergency situations outside of hospitals and during transport to hospitals, when limited but intense life support services must be provided. Medical technicians may be more highly trained in their limited areas of expertise than nurse practitioners or physicians' assistants.

Medicare insured group (MIG) An experimental approach to providing care to Medicare beneficiaries in which a traditional provider of retiree benefits, such as a corporation or union welfare plan, takes over responsibility for all care to those 65 or over in return for a set payment from Medicare.

Medicare-participating physician A doctor who has agreed to accept assignment on all claims from all Medicare beneficiaries in return for certain incentives.

Medigap policy An insurance policy sold as a supplement to Medicare, usually but not always having coverage of copayments and deductibles as its main features.

Metastasis A secondary growth, in a location of the body apart from the original site, of a cancer.

Nasogastric tube A tube placed through the nose and into the stomach to drain secretions or deliver food and medications.

Nonprofit voluntary hospitals Entities organized to provide hospital services on a nonprofit and nongovernmental basis, generally with alleged oversight from the community they serve via self-perpetuating boards of trustees. The classic American hospital.

Notarized affidavit A document, signed in the presence of a notary public, in which an individual asserts, under penalty of perjury, that an assertion is true. An informal, written form of testimony.

Nuclear medicine The branch of medicine concerned with the use of radioactive chemicals, as opposed to electromagnetic radiation, for therapy and diagnosis. Overlaps with radiology and radiation therapy.

Nurse practitioner A registered nurse (R.N.) who has taken additional training and is certified to handle some of the functions of a holder of the M.D. or D.O. degree.

Office of Management and Budget (OMB) The agency of the executive branch of government which prepares the budget the President submits to Congress each year and supervises spending by government agencies during the year.

Operating room A portion of a hospital, or other facility, specially equipped for surgery.

Ophthalmologist A holder of the M.D. or D.O. degree who specializes in treatment of diseases of the eye with drugs and surgery. May or may not prescribe corrective lenses.

Optometrist A holder of the degree of Doctor of Optometry, who specializes in prescribing corrective lenses and diagnosing, but not treating, conditions of the eye that require surgery or medication.

Outliers Cases that fall outside the statistical norms of the DRG system, either in total cost or in days of hospitalization required. Medicare makes additional payments for outliers if the peer review organization approves.

Out-of-area care Care that is given to a member of a health maintenance organization when the member is outside the service area of the HMO. This is an issue largely because federal laws for HMO certification require the definition of a service area. Depending on the HMO, arranging for out-of-area care can be a problem.

Out-of-pocket limit An amount no more than which an insured individual is required to pay, after which his or her insurance policy pays all costs for the services it covers, regardless of other provisions.

Outpatient Having to do with a person, or treatment given to that person, when he or she is not admitted to the hospital; e.g., "outpatient surgery."

Outpatient prescription drugs Drugs that can be given outside a hospital in some or all cases, usually written on the orders of a physician.

Outpatient surgery Surgery performed without admission to a hospital, even though the surgery may be performed in the hospital.

Outpatient treatment Treatment at a hospital, or in a setting outside a hospital, that does not require admission or temporarily residing at the hospital.

Over-the-counter drugs Drugs that may be sold without prescription. Examples:

aspirin, some decongestants and antihistamines, antibiotic ointments, low-dose cortisone creams, soothing eyedrops.

Pacemaker   A medical device, implanted in the body, which sends the heart electrical signals to beat when the normal mechanism for generating such signals is defective.

Packed red cells   Blood cells that have been separated from the plasma and are administered separately.

Participating physician agreement   An agreement a doctor signs with HCFA to accept assignment on all Medicare claims and to follow certain procedures; renewed annually.

Pathologist   A doctor specializing in examining tissues removed from the body and in performing autopsies.

Peer Review Organizations (PRO)   Groups of doctors who have contracts with the Health Care Financing Administration to evaluate the medical necessity of care rendered to Medicare beneficiaries under the Medicare program and to investigate the quality of care in providers serving Medicare beneficiaries.

People's Medical Society (PMS)   A large health care consumer organization.

Permanently and totally disabled   A term of art under the Social Security Act, applying to those persons who meet the definition of disability in the act and qualify for Social Security payments and Medicare on that basis.

Permanent vegetative state   A condition in which higher brain functions are permanently suppressed.

Perverse incentive   A motivation provided by a system that defeats the system's purpose. In fee-for-service systems, there is a perverse incentive to overtreat; in prepaid systems, there is a perverse incentive to undertreat.

Physiatrist   A doctor who specializes in giving and prescribing physical therapy, primarily for rehabilitation.

Physicians' assistant   An individual trained to carry out some of the functions of holders of the M.D. or D.O. degree, usually with more training than a nurse practitioner or a medical technician.

Physician extenders   Individuals who are trained to do a part of what a holder of the M.D. or D.O. degree can do. They include nurse practitioners, physicians' assistants, and medical technicians. They are used heavily in health maintenance organizations.

Podiatrist   A holder of the degree of Doctor of Podiatric Medicine (D.P.M.), concerned with treatment of diseases of the feet.

Power of attorney   A legal document giving a person the power to act as the representative of the other in certain situations, which can be defined in the power-of-attorney document.

Practice patterns   Statistically detectable tendencies for individual doctors, or groups of them, to treat certain conditions in a certain way.

Preferred provider organization (PPO)   An arrangement in which patients are "locked in" to a group of providers, usually by restrictions on payment for services provided by those not in the group of providers, in return for discounts or expanded services. A wide variety exists, some resemble traditional insurance plans, some resemble health maintenance organizations.

Primary care physicians   Physicians who, by training, preference, or necessity, practice a very broad range of medical services for persons not in need of highly specialized medical services. Usually cited as including general practitioners, family practitioners, general internists, pediatricians, and gynecologists who take care of both their patients' gynecological and general medical needs.

Primary diagnosis The chief medical reason for an encounter with a health care provider or admission to a hospital.

Private room In a hospital or nursing home, a room occupied by only one person, as opposed to the standard two-person room or a ward.

Private duty nursing Care given by a nurse who is hired to care for one individual exclusively in a hospital or nursing home and is paid directly by the individual or his or her family.

Procedure A manipulation of the body to give a treatment or perform a test; more broadly, any distinct service a doctor renders to a patient; all distinct physician services have "procedure codes" in various payment schemes.

Prognosis A medical prediction of the course or probable outcome of an illness or condition.

Prospective payment Payment made before a service is rendered, and accepted as payment in full by the provider. The opposite of fee-for-service payment.

Protocol A written plan for caring for a particular condition, intended as a guideline to physicians, and usually adopted by a medical institution such as a clinic, hospital, or health maintenance organization.

Provider A generic term for any person (a doctor) or entity (a home health agency, a hospital) approved to give care to Medicare beneficiaries and to receive payment from Medicare.

Pulmonary specialist or pulmonologist A doctor specializing in lung diseases.

Quarter of coverage One-fourth of a calendar year during which a person earns enough, in employment covered by Social Security, to have the quarter counted toward the number needed (usually forty) to ensure entitlement to Social Security and Medicare.

Radiologist A physician specializing in taking diagnostic X rays and administering radiotherapy.

Radiotherapy Treatment for cancer and some other conditions using electromagnetic radiation of several varieties.

Recovery room A place in a hospital where patients are brought after surgery for close observation until they are ready to be taken to their floors or special care units.

Registered nurse (R.N.) Generally, the highest trained of nurses, one licensed by a state to provide general nursing services after passing a qualifying examination. May or may not hold collegiate degrees.

Resident A doctor taking postgraduate training in a hospital, often working towards certification in a specialty area. Much of the training involves the care of patients under the supervision of more experienced physicians, both those based in the hospital and those who admit patients there.

Respirator A medical device that takes over breathing functions for patients who are permanently or temporarily unable to breathe on their own (e.g., after open heart surgery).

Retrospective payments Payment to a provider after care is given, fee-for-service payment.

Rider An attachment to a standard form of insurance policy, obtained for an additional premium, that provides benefits not covered by the standard policy.

Risk pooling The fundamental idea behind insurance. A large number of people with a low probability of high-cost events share the cost, reducing their individual risks to the amount of their insurance premium, rather than the full cost of the event, such as an accident or illness. The fundamental concept of insurance.

Secondary diagnosis   A condition that exists in addition to the one that is the chief reason for an encounter with a health care provider or admission to a hospital.

Sensitivity   The ability of a medical test to detect something wrong, even if it cannot distinguish among various diagnoses. Contrast with *Specificity*.

Serum   Biological material remaining after an animal or plant fluid is coagulated or centrifuged.

Service area   The geographical region in which a health maintenance organization or other prepaid health care plan has agreed to provide services.

Sheltered, or custodial, care   Care that is primarily nonmedical. Residents of sheltered or custodial care facilities do not require constant attention from nurses and aides, but need assistance with one or more daily activities or no longer want to be bothered with keeping up a house. The social needs of residents are met in a safe, secure environment free of as many anxieties as possible.

Skilled nursing facility (SNF)   An institution that offers nursing services similar to those given in a hospital, to aid recuperation of those who are seriously ill. Distinguished from intermediate care and custodial care, which may meet some minor medical needs but are intended primarily to support elderly and disabled individuals in the tasks of daily living.

Social health maintenance organizations (SHMO)   Experimental programs that try to provide for the medical and social needs of the elderly and disabled in one, prepaid package. These have, so far, not been too successful because they were more expensive than was hoped.

Social Security Administration (SSA)   The part of the Department of Health and Human Services that operates the various programs funded under the Social Security Act and determines eligibility for Medicare.

Social Security office   Local offices of the Social Security Administration, found throughout the country, which take applications for Social Security and Medicare and handle processing of Medicare requests for reconsideration and appeals.

Social Security number (SSN)   A unique number assigned to each individual by the Social Security Administration for tax and benefits purposes. Also used as a unique personal identifier by many other government programs and private enterprises.

Somatize   To involuntarily express emotional concerns as physical symptoms.

Special care units   Portions of a hospital organized and staffed to take care of one kind of (usually serious) problem, such as a cardiac care unit, an intensive care unit, a burn unit, and so on.

Specialist   A physician who has elected to practice, and usually has special training in, some branch of medicine other than primary care, such as surgery, or an exclusive focus in one area of primary care, such as allergy, gastroenterology, ear-nose-and-throat care, and so on. Especially in urban areas, specialists are expected to have certification from specialty societies or boards that they have had adequate training in the specialty.

Specificity   The ability of a medical test to identify a specific diagnosis or condition. Contrast with *Sensitivity*.

Staff model health maintenance organization   A health maintenance organization staffed by doctors who are its employees and are not in individual or group practice.

Stop-loss provision   See out-of-pocket limit.

Streptokinase   A drug, produced by bacteria of the beta-hemolytic streptococcal strains, used to abort heart attacks by dissolving clots that block the arteries of the heart.

Subluxation of the spine   A partial dislocation of one of the bones of the spinal column.

Supplemental Security Income (SSI)   A program that provides small stipends to the elderly, blind, and disabled who for one reason or another are not eligible for other, more generous welfare programs.

Swing beds   Hospital beds approved by Medicare for use as hospital or skilled nursing facility beds, depending on demand.

Terminally ill   Having an illness that is expected to end in death.

Thrombophlebitis   Irritation of a vein caused by a blood clot.

Tissue plasminogen activator   A drug, naturally occurring in small amounts in the human body and produced in quantity by genetically engineered bacteria, used to abort heart attacks by dissolving clots that block the arteries of the heart.

Tumor   An abnormal growth of a component of the body that is not inflammatory and possesses no physiological function.

Urgent   A situation, less grave than an emergency, in which care is required in the near future to prevent death, serious injury, or deformity. Contrast with emergency.

Usual, customary, and reasonable reimbursement system   A means of determining payments to doctors based on statistical profiles of their, and their colleagues', history of charges.

Utilization review committee (URC)   A group of doctors in a hospital who review lengths of hospital stays and treatments to make sure that they are medically necessary.

Vaccines   Biologically produced drugs designed to provide or enhance immunity to specific diseases or disease families.

Waiver of liability   A legal removal of an individual's responsibility to pay for a treatment in an instance where Medicare or Medicaid does not pay for it.

X rays   Electromagnetic radiation capable of penetrating soft tissue and producing pictures of the inside of the body; also, pictures taken with such radiation.

Index

Join the *People's Medical Society* now. Only $15 a year. (That's less than the cost of just one office visit with your doctor.) And your contribution is 100% tax deductible.

People's Medical Society
MEMBERSHIP FORM

☐ **Yes,** I want to join. Start my subscription to the PMS Newsletter. My $15 annual membership dues are enclosed.

☐ Send me more information about membership in the People's Medical Society.

Name _____

Address _____

City/State/Zip _____

Please make your check payable to *People's Medical Society*.

People's Medical Society
462 Walnut Street
Allentown, PA 18102
(215) 770-1670

MME

The *PEOPLE'S MEDICAL SOCIETY* is a nonprofit citizens' action group committed to the principles of better, more responsive and less expensive medical care, and dedicated to the belief that people, as individuals or in groups, can make a difference. To this end, the *PEOPLE'S MEDICAL SOCIETY* is involved in the organizing of community efforts around local health-care issues, and in the national debate over the future of the medical care system.